SACKRED Birth

SACKRED Birth

Mobilizing a New Quality Paradigm in Obstetric Care

Karen Antoinette Scott

LEXINGTON BOOKS
Lanham • Boulder • New York • London

Published by Lexington Books
An imprint of The Rowman & Littlefield Publishing Group, Inc.
4501 Forbes Boulevard, Suite 200, Lanham, Maryland 20706
www.rowman.com

86-90 Paul Street, London EC2A 4NE

British Library Cataloguing in Publication Information Available

Library of Congress Cataloging-in-Publication Data

Names: Scott, Karen Antoinette, author.
Title: SACKRED birth: mobilizing a new quality paradigm in obstetric care / Karen Antoinette Scott.
Description: Lanham: Lexington Books, [2024] | Includes bibliographical references and index.
Summary: "This book offers a new obstetric quality paradigm to address violations of physical and emotional safety during childbirth hospitalization. It's a vital call for prioritizing Black mothers' expressions, expectations, and experiences in clinical practice, decision-making, and care delivery"—Provided by publisher.
Identifiers: LCCN 2024042768 | ISBN 9781666938395 (cloth ; alk. paper) | ISBN 9781666938401 (ebook)
Subjects: MESH: Maternal Health—ethnology | Black or African American | Systemic Racism | Pregnant Women—ethnology | Delivery, Obstetric—standards | Obstetrics—standards | Pregnancy Outcome—ethnology | United States
Classification: LCC RG950 | NLM WA 310 AA1 | DDC 362.19820089/696073 —dc23/eng/20241118
LC record available at https://lccn.loc.gov/2024042768

Contents

Acknowledgments

I am deeply honored for the privilege and responsibility to share the ideas birthed through, with, and within this book. I felt I had abandoned the little Black girl in me when I chose medicine twenty-eight years ago. Writing this book represents a second chance for the little Black girl in me to reclaim her voice and power to freely become and be HER. Her is me. The stories of thirty-six Black mothers planted themselves in the soil of my heart, mind, body, and spirit over five years ago. Like seeds, the stories waited patiently in great anticipation for the optimal conditions, opportunities, and options to germinate within me, facilitating a rooting down and shooting up, bridging my past and future selves to my present.

I am grateful for God, my ancestors, and given and chosen family for being with me on this journey. Birthing this book now in 2024 reminds me that I no longer fear or grieve my past choices. I will always choose the red pill, no matter the costs. I am also grateful for the founding mother of Black women's health, THE Byllye Avery, and prolific scholar activist in anthropology, the late Leith Mullings. Both Avery and Mullings remain my North Star for how I can continue to actualize my dreams of curating a Black feminist movement in the professionalization and provision of obstetric care and the evaluation of obstetric quality and patient safety.

Thank you, Ryn Edwards, for teaching me, for believing in me, and for introducing me to Byllye Avery in your course, Biology of Female Sexuality. Your course taught me about the healing and transformative power of women building community and organizing themselves and others to activate and actualize their full autonomy and agency over their bodies and their minds to speak truth to power in all aspects of their lives.

Along this journey, a number of individuals and organizations stood up for me publicly and privately while I navigated violent systems and structures, and the people leading and funding them. From the depths of my heart, I thank you for taking time to respond to a text, email, phone call, audio message, or a request to feed and drink with me. Jann-Murray García, Shakti Butler, Melanie Tervalon, Monica McLemore, Laura Jelliffe-Pawlowski, Shari Dworkin, Mama Linda Jones, Wenonah "Elder Coach V" Valentine, LeConté Dill, Stephanie and Larnie Bray, and Joia Crear-Perry. Many of you participated in my 2019 and 2020 research studies at two different yet similarly harmful academic institutions as patient, community, and content experts. I appreciate Dana-Ain Davis, Emily White VanGompel, Jin-Shei Lai, Francesca Carlock, Tamentanefer Camara, Brianne Taylor, Chakiya Clary, Ashlee McCorkle-Jamieson, Safyer McKenzie-Sampson, Caryl Gay, Amanda Armijo, Lillie Lapeyrolerie, Lavisha Singh, Jessica Roach, Susan Perez, Audrey Lyndon, Brittany Chambers Butcher, iDREAM for Racial Health Equity, Diversity Uplifts, SisterWeb, Beloved Birth Black Centering, Black Women Birthing for Justice, Growth Mindset, CinnaMoms, California Black Women's Health Project (CBWHP), CHOICES Center for Reproductive Health, Expecting Justice, Growth Mindset, and UCSF Preterm Birth Initiative, Public Health Foundation Enterprise WIC, Kindred Space LA, Black Women for Wellness (BWW), African American Breastfeeding Cultural Outreach Taskforce (BCOT).

My understanding of the warfare and fear as well as the sanctity and power of a hospital birth would be myopic and meaningless without the brilliance, leadership, and humanity of Tanefer, Brandi Gates-Burgess, and Allana Samuel from BCOT and BWW's Janette Robinson Flint and Raena Granberry (now with CBWHP). Many thanks to Ifeyinwa Asiodu for introducing me to BCOT.

Without you, the soil of my spirit would lack optimal water, oxygen, light, and temperature. Thank you for nurturing and nourishing me, transporting me to and from the emergency department, or acting as my virtual Long COVID doula: Ana Delgado, Janice Tinsley, April Bell, Aimée Tom, Timika Simpson, Grace Howard, Jessica, and Brittany.

Dána, Lynn, and Audrey, thank you for seeing me, hearing me, holding space for, believing me, believing in me, and for reading and editing my work from the original memos to the final book. Terry J. West, Jr., you are the best Big Bro ! PERIODT!

My gratitude to Lexington Books, my editor Courtney Morales, your assistant Breasia Boyd, and my production team, Kayla Cunningham and Sanjana Premkumar, for your support and guidance.

I also want to express my gratitude to Black and Indigenous women activists, artists, advocates, scientists, and scholars whose curiosity, courage, creativity, and work continue to inspire me, such as Sweet Honey in the Rock, the Combahee River Collective, Marteja Bailey, Jernicya Onyekwelu, bell hooks, Audre Lorde, Leith Mullings, Irma McCLaurin, Linda Tuhiwai Smith, Camara Phyllis Jones, and more.

I dedicate this book to the SACKRED 36, the remaining 98 percent who birth in hospitals by choice, force, and coercion, and all the little Black girls waiting in great expectation for the manifestation of your highest self.

Welcome to the future of obstetric quality where peace, love, safety, liberty, justice, laughter, pleasure, light, legacies, and the Divine abide in the wombs of Black reproducing bodies.

Chapter 1

When Existing Paradigms Never Served Us

In December 2018, Dana-Ain Davis first introduced obstetric racism into the lexicon of childbirth experiences among Black women in the United States (U.S.) (Davis 2018). Specifically, her ethnographic analysis of U.S. Black women's reproductive care before and after childbirth carefully described mechanisms of reproductive control and domination that manifest as a coordinated set of beliefs, practices, and behaviors imposed upon the Black reproducing body by any health care professional. According to Davis, obstetric racism poses a threat to positive birth outcomes, transcending the boundaries of violence captured by the obstetric violence and medical racism (Davis 2018). Within the global context, Latin American childbirth activists and legal scholars first described obstetric violence in 1993 as consequences of structural violence manifesting as excessive rates of medical interventions, non-consented care, disrespect, and other abusive practices enacted against women during childbirth (Sadler et al. 2016). Within the U.S., medical racism described how the health profession or professional responds to the race of a patient thereby, influencing the diagnostic decision-making process and treatment modalities in the broader context of medical provision, and requires the racialization of every aspect of every organ of every Black body, thereby placing the patient at risk for inadequate or inappropriate care (Hoberman 2012). While obstetric violence optimally described a form of gender-based violence enacted against any obstetric patient resulting in their subordination because of their positionality as an obstetric patient within the medical industrial complex, obstetric violence fails to take into consideration racial stratification of life and reproduction that track along histories of anti-Black racism and eugenics that uniquely impact Black women and girls in the U.S. Therefore, Davis selected the term obstetric racism to describe both as analytic and phenomenon that embodied an extension of racial stratification and revealed gendered dimensions of medical racism emerging from histories of stigma, stigmatization, and other forms of reproductive abuses, experimentation, exploitation, and extraction of Black women in reproductive, gynecological, and obstetric care (Berry 2017; Owens 2017), from the near eradication of Black Grand midwives in favor of white public health nurses and white male obstetricians (Wilkie 2003; Goode 2014), and from Black women's memories of encounters and interactions with physicians, nurses, and other health care professionals during and after pregnancy and childbirth (Davis 2018).

In this book, I explain how and why I chose to define obstetric quality and patient safety during childbirth hospitalization in the U.S. among Black women through the expectations, expressions, and experiences of Black women. By defining obstetric patient safety in hospital settings as a manifestation of Black women's anticipated and actual experiences, then Black women's imaginations become the standard by which hospitals and insurance companies measure, monitor, and maintain a certain threshold, or quality, of care. Essentially, I argue for normalizing Black women's patient-reported experiences of hospital-based obstetrics care as the standard quality metric for evaluating the overall value, performance, safety, and quality of the U.S. maternal health system. By August 2018, I successfully defended my master's thesis in the pursuit of my MPH in Applied Epidemiology. My thesis research study involved the first-ever application of public health critical race (PHCR) methodology (Ford and Airhihenbuwa 2010) in a quantitative population health research study, for the purposes of interrogating the racialized social and clinical phenomenon of preterm birth among Black women with gestational diabetes in California and elucidating patterns and predictors of preterm birth based on nativity. My study established a precedent for my current scholarship in terms of ethical, theoretical, and methodological approaches. First, the utilization of PHCR established two fundamental assumptions that remain true and consistent throughout the scholarship: (1) structural racism creates a hierarchy of human value, knowing, knowledge, power, domination, and privilege based on skin color, genitalia, gender, partner preferences, body ability, and body size in society that impacts the distribution and manifestation of diseases, discomforts, disabilities, health, deaths, and near-deaths as well as differential access to and utilization of resources to meet and maintain basic social needs (i.e., food, housing, water, family/community stability, employment, and safety); and (2) the structural context and conditions of living as a Black woman in the U.S. impact perinatal and reproductive health (PRH) and health care outcomes and experiences in a manner not reported nor described in white women or foreign-born Black women (Scott et al. 2020). Second, the intentional decision to exclude white women or any other non-Black women as the referent group acknowledges and affirms the complex, nuanced, and rich heterogeneity of Black femininity, Black womanhood, and Black girlhood (Scott et al. 2020). Disrupting the practice of prioritizing white women as the referent group in public health and maternal child health research serves as an act of epistemic refusal of race as a biological construct and epistemic resistance against Blackness and Black womanhood as biologically inferior and socially inadequate. Choosing inclusion and exclusion criteria and sampling techniques that resulted in a study sample of Black women representatives of the African Diaspora facilitates within-group analysis and subsequent detection of differences to better support customization of care and disease prevention, mitigation, and treatment modalities that consider individual variability in genes, environment, and lifestyle, also known as precision medicine.

In 2018, no one in the field of obstetrics and gynecology or obstetric patient safety publicly named racism as the driver of the disproportionate yet predictable, preventable, and unfair rates of deaths and near deaths among Black women in the U.S. Standard reporting and dissemination practices in public health, epidemiology, maternal child health, medicine, and nursing led to superficial oral and written discussions of mortality and morbidity that emphasized white: Black comparisons. Prior to Davis' introduction of obstetric racism, the existing obstetric quality and patient safety paradigm lacked both scientifically and culturally appropriate frameworks and corresponding topologies, meanings, manifestations, measurements, and metrics by which to register and report harm as defined for, by, and with Black women and girls. Despite quality improvement initiatives, clinical safety bundles, technological advances, and social protections such as higher education, higher income, and marriage between men and pregnant women, current hospital safety programs failed to protect Black mothers and birthing people from harm during and after childbirth. In 2018, the call to action in obstetric patient safety was to simultaneously improve the quality of care and advance health equity during the provision of obstetrics care in U.S. hospitals. However, the blueprint for advancing care quality and equity centered primarily on improving care outcomes selected by health care, health equity, quality, or patient safety professionals, scientists, data analysts, evaluators, or economists. The blueprint, formally called a patient safety bundle, is an organized series of evidence-informed actions and best practices for improving care processes and patient outcomes in pregnant and postpartum women and people, developed by a group of experts from different clinical disciplines. Examples of patient safety bundles include obstetric hemorrhage, severe hypertension in pregnancy, safe reduction of primary cesarean birth, cardiac conditions in obstetric care, and sepsis in obstetric care (AIM n.d.). A second gap was the absence of a theoretical framework that substantiated assumptions about Black women and the power relations, differentials, and dynamics that shaped how Black women show up, speak up, speak out, shut down, move, and make decisions in society and in the health systems. The third gap was the lack of historical context and conditions that explained the origins of anti-Black racism and anti-Black misogyny in the U.S. that manifested in the provisions and processes of contemporary hospital-based obstetric care.

When thinking about the multiplicity of my positionality as a Black queer feminist southern woman, a dissident community-trained and practicing OBGYN, an OB Hospitalist, an applied epidemiologist, a mixed methodologist, a survey developer, a paradigm leader, an infopreneur, and an improvement and implementation scientist, practitioner, and researcher, I made a conscientious decision to disrupt the obstetric patient safety paradigm by asking the question, "What if the experience is the outcome?" Instead of prioritizing and measuring change in clinical pathology as the outcome of interest, I sought out to design the most accurate and precise measure of care experience that best aligned with the feelings, thoughts, words, expectations, experiences, and expressions of Black women seeking help or health care during labor, birth, and immediate postpartum in hospital settings. This book demonstrates the application of a Black feminist praxis and precision medicine in obstetric quality measure development and validation. The six fundamental steps included in the making of a measure consist of: (1) determine the theoretical framework; (2) develop a preliminary conceptual model; (3) review existing measures to start developing an item bank; (4) design new items if needed; (5) revise your item bank with patient, community, and content experts; and (6) pilot test and perform psychometric analysis. Maintaining fidelity to precision medicine in instrument validation means that before one can improve care outcomes, by advancing quality, equity, and safety, one must first practice courageous curiosity to name, define, and describe particular harms experienced by Black mothers and birthing people and enacted by hospital clinicians, staff, and administrators against Black mothers and birthing people. Davis' online publication in December 2018 gave me permission to speak truth to power about the egregious violations of obstetric quality and patient safety with a great sense of Black feminist pride, purpose, passion, and power. In this chapter, I describe the methodology for designing and conducting a Black feminist hermeneutic phenomenology of childbirth hospitalization based on the pregnancy, labor, birth, and postpartum expectations, expressions, and experiences of Black mothers in Los Angeles and Oakland, California. First, I situate the discussion of quality of care within the larger context of the U.S.-based patient safety literature and lexicon by first introducing the reader to the Agency for Healthcare Research and Quality (AHRQ). Second, I offer a high-yield overview of the importance of establishing a just culture and patient safety paradigm. Third, I discuss the limitations and hypocrisy of the existing patient safety paradigm, including the lack of transparency, rigor, relevance, responsiveness, and accountability. Fourth, I discuss three phenomena, the near eradication of Black Grand midwives, the establishment of the Maternal Mortality Collaborative and subsequent Pregnancy Mortality Surveillance System, and the March of Dimes 2023 report, to illuminate the existence and exacerbation of a chronic and pervasive manufactured Black maternal and infant health crisis in the U.S. Fifth, I explain the challenges and limitations in prioritizing outcome-only measures as hospital performance indicators. Sixth, I describe the methodological approach to my research. Finally, I close the chapter with the guiding principles of the SACKRED Birth Framework.

Hospitals, health plans, and quality organizations define safety as the absence of preventable harm in health care delivery. Existing patient safety literature from the AHRQ Patient Safety Network (PSNet), a national web-based resource on patient safety, describes three concepts and definitions that inform the operationalization of reporting systems: adverse event, near miss, or error (AHRQ PSNet n.d., a). An *adverse event* is defined as any unintended injury resulting from or contributed to by medical care or management, rather than the underlying disease, that requires additional monitoring or treatment, prolongs the hospitalization, produces a death or disability at the time of discharge, or all three. Identifying something as an adverse event does not imply "error," "negligence," or poor quality care. Labeling a care outcome as an adverse event simply indicates that an undesirable clinical outcome resulted from some aspect of diagnosis or therapy, not an underlying disease process. Subcategories of adverse events include preventable (those that occurred due to error or failure to apply an accepted strategy for prevention); ameliorable (events that, while not preventable, could have been less harmful if care had been different); and neglectful/negligence (events that occurred due to care that falls below the standards expected of clinicians in the community) (AHRQ PSNet n.d., a). Two additional terms define violations of patient safety that do not result in harm (where harm is traditionally and repeatedly defined by systems and structures of power within the patient safety field: *near miss*, an unsafe situation that is indistinguishable from a preventable adverse event except for the outcome whereby a patient is exposed to a hazardous situation but does not experience harm either through luck or early detection; and error, a broader term referring to any act of commission (doing something wrong) or omission (failing to do the right thing) that exposes patients to a potentially hazardous situation (AHRQ PSNet n.d., a).

Within the context of maternal and pregnancy-related health, the World Health Organization (WHO) defines a near miss maternal morbidity as a pregnant woman or person who nearly died because of a complication that occurred during pregnancy, childbirth or postpartum up to 42 days after the end of a pregnancy (WHO 2011, 12). In decreasing order of severity from a near miss maternal morbidity, severe maternal morbidity (SMM), as defined by the WHO, represents "any health condition attributed to and/or aggravated by pregnancy and childbirth that has a negative impact on the woman's wellbeing" (Firoz et al. 2013). In comparison, the Centers for Disease Control and Prevention (CDC) define SMM as "unexpected outcomes of labor and delivery that result in significant short- or long-term consequences to a woman's health" (CDC 2017). In decreasing order from SMM, the CDC defines maternal morbidity as an unexpected health condition attributed to or complicating pregnancy and childbirth that has a negative impact on wellbeing or functioning (Say et al. 2009). In general, getting pregnant in the U.S. results in 60,000 women or gender-expansive individuals experiencing SMM and 700 pregnancy-related deaths (DeClercq and Zephyrin 2021). Thus, for every pregnancy-related death in the U.S., approximately eighty-five women or gender-expansive individuals will experience a near miss.

Multiple studies demonstrate inequities in the rate of SMM based on race as a proxy to racism, age, region, community-level income, and hospital type. The highest rates of SMM occurred among Black women and individuals, and women and individuals under the age of twenty or over the age of forty, residing in the northeast and southern states, living in the poorest communities, and experiencing childbirth in public hospitals. Additional data revealed worsening inequities in SMM based on race as a proxy for racism, among Black women utilizing both public and commercial insurance (DeClercq and Zephyrin 2021). The Commonwealth Fund analysis further revealed a pattern whereby women and individuals who experienced an SMM are much more likely to be readmitted to the hospital during the postpartum period compared to women and individuals who did not experience SMM. Regarding costs, the Commonwealth Fund presented data showing that births affected by SMM cost about 40 percent more than births without SMM, independent of public or commercial insurance, during the prenatal and postpartum periods of care provision (DeClercq and Zephyrin 2021). Similarly, the CDC asserts that the consequences of increasing SMM prevalence and health implications vary and include factors such as increased medical costs and duration of hospitalization. Thus, the CDC offers two strategies to reduce SMM prevalence: monitoring SMM trends and implementing interventions to improve the quality of maternal care (CDC 2017). However, a host of challenges pose as barriers and burdens to reducing the rate of SMM, such as the absence of mandated reporting of SMM across birthing hospitals and community settings (e.g., birthing centers, home births), and a consensus on SMM definitions, measurements, monitoring strategies, and prevention and mitigation actions. The most egregious examples of structural and institutional barriers to addressing SMM include the absence of curious, courageous, and disruptive leadership, ethics, knowledge, and science to name and address obstetric racism as a singular threat to curating, sustaining, and advancing a culture of obstetric quality and patient safety within and across U.S. birthing hospitals.

Existing literature describes key components to establishing a culture of patient safety, such as operationalizing consistent safe practices, curating a blame-free environment where reporting occurs without fear of retaliation, and promoting collaboration across disciplines and levels of power and positionality. Current evidence also describes ongoing threats to advancing patient safety, such as variations in perceptions of safety within and across health systems, poor teamwork and communication, a culture of low expectations, and power relations and dynamics. Despite safety culture definitions, safety measures, teamwork training, executive walk rounds or clinical debriefing, unit-based safety teams, rapid response teams, and standardized communication methods during patient-hand offs, provision of high-quality, safe, and equitable care remains a major challenge for U.S. hospitals and health systems. The "no blame" spirit in the early patient safety movement may no longer best serve organizations, especially when certain errors are deemed blameworthy and demand accountability. For example, the CDC 2022 report found 84 percent of all pregnancy-related deaths (a total of 1,018) from 2017 to 2019 among residents of thirty-six states to be preventable (Trost et al. 2022). Thus, current efforts must focus on establishing a just culture that reconciles the dual needs for a no-blame culture and appropriate personal accountability. According to Dr. Dekker, a just culture within patient safety requires identifying and addressing systemic and structural factors that permit individuals within health systems to participate in unsafe language and behaviors while maintaining individual accountability by establishing zero tolerance for reckless behavior (Dekker 2017). Dr. Dekker also offers three distinctions as an alternative to the dominant "no-blame" approach: human error (e.g., slips), at-risk behavior (e.g., taking shortcuts), and reckless behavior (e.g., ignoring required safety steps). In a just culture, the unit, departmental, and organizational response to an adverse event, error, or near miss is determined by the type of behavior, regardless of intent, associated with the patient safety violation, and not the severity of the event. For example, reckless behavior, such as a physician or nurse refusing to obtain informed consent prior to a vaginal/cervical exam, would warrant disciplinary action, even if the patient experienced a normal labor course and birth outcome (absence of harm as defined by authoritative figures in patient safety).

The implementation, spread, and scale of a just culture and patient safety paradigm in health care, particularly in hospital-based obstetrics, without the historical and contemporary contextualization of racism as a well-defined and measurable adverse event is irresponsible, unethical, inhumane, and unjust. The willful ignorance and exclusion of medical racism, obstetric violence, or obstetric racism, regardless of intention, as a single threat or a series of ongoing threats to patient safety for Black women and reproducing capable people seeking help or health care for any pregnancy-related reason reifies the hierarchy of human value based on skin color, genitalia, and gender. More importantly, the systemic and structural exclusion and/or erasure of Black patient experiences and community wisdom in shaping terminology, meanings, and measurement selection further silences the voices and undermines the agency and self-efficacy of Black mothers and birthing people in advancing quality and equity in patient safety. Consequently, the perpetrators of harm are then protected and even incentivized by the very system that's supposed to protect patients and hold individuals within the organization accountable for the provision of care in a just and safe culture of care.

Standardized perinatal safety and quality measures primarily focus on physical outcomes, effectively excluding experiential, spiritual, and ancestral knowledge of patients and community wisdom (Jolivétte 2015). The structural and systemic exclusion of patient and community knowledge and experts limits the capacity of existing outcome measures to provide sound information about the safety of care provided to Black mothers and birthing people as defined for, by, and with Black mothers and birthing people (Scott 2021, 2019a, 2019b; Scott et al. 2021; Scott and Davis 2021). Thus, naming obstetric racism as a patient safety indicator is an essential first step in the measurement, monitoring, evaluation, and reporting of harm as defined by patient and community knowledge in hospital performance. Yet the ahistorical and atheoretical evaluation of quality in hospital-based obstetrics serves to procure and protect the interests, power, and spaces of predominantly white, male, physicians, or quantitative data analysts. The security and sustainability of white, male, physician or white male physician positionality as epistemic gatekeepers require committed multi-level actions that facilitate the structural exclusion, erasure, and eradication of the intellectual thoughts and activism of Black women and people as patient, community, and content experts. The fathers of obstetric quality improvement and implementation science, practice, and research follow in the steps of their brethren, the fathers of obstetrics and gynecology (Scott 2021).

The inception and proliferation of the professionalization and commodification of childbirth with the advent of obstetrics and gynecology required forced exploration of, experimentation on, and extraction from enslaved Black women's bodies (Owens 2017; Washington 2006). In the eighteenth century, reports of the European man midwife explained his perception of obstetrics as rewarding but unprofitable. Many complained of both exhaustion and low compensation when attending births and preferred to spend their time serving the diseased and discomforted and dispensing prescriptions. Yet, many realized the unintended negative consequence of abandoning midwifery was the loss of their families to their competitors. Thus, "deliver the babies and you will have the family for life" became the strategic motivation for the tethering of general practice and the management of childbirth (Loudon 2008). From the nineteenth century to mid-nineteenth century, Black Grand midwives attended the majority of births in the U.S. and provided holistic care to entire communities. In 1900, 5 percent of births occurred in hospital settings (Thomason and Treber 2008). Medical advances such as the development and utilization of forceps to "extract breech babies" and cesarean "abdominal" or "surgical" births and changes in the medical training of physicians made working and organizing in hospitals more attractive and lucrative to general practitioners and obstetricians. By the mid-twentieth century, the near eradication of Black Grand midwives by white male physicians, white female public health nurses, and white nurse midwives facilitated the design, implementation, spread, and scaling of models of prenatal care and birth that prioritized the privatization of health care and medicalization of birth (Goode 2014; Goode and Rothman 2017; Oparah and Bonaparte 2015). The near eradication of Black Grand midwives occurred despite the equal rates of maternal and infant mortality among births attended by midwives or physicians. One study in the 1930s revealed lower rates of maternal and infant mortality in Alabama among Black women whose births were attended by midwives compared to the rates reported among white women whose births were attended by physicians (Vollers 2023). In 1912, the U.S. established the Children's Bureau to investigate and report on concerns for child welfare throughout the country, specifically the "problems of infant and maternal mortality and child labor." By 1921, the U.S. passed federal legislation drafted by Julia Lathrop, the first Chief of the U.S. Children's Bureau, titled the Sheppard-Towner Maternity and Infancy Protection Act. The federal legislation awarded grants to states and Washington D.C to build up and utilize public health nurses in the provision of health services and instruction, nursing education in schools and universities, and through other educational pathways. The curricular content focused on hygiene for mothers and children, well-child conference centers, adequate confinement care, and hospital facilities for mothers and children (Madgett 2017; Gathercole 2024). Depending on positionality, power, and privilege, an analysis of Lathrop's influence would credit her leadership at the federal level in reducing maternal and infant mortality and supporting advancements in prenatal care services at the state level among recipients of federal grants. However, the passing of the Sheppard-Towner Maternity and Infancy Protection Act reproduced and reinforced hierarchies of knowing, knowledge, and professionalism grounded in class exploitation and racism, resulting in the near eradication of Black Grand midwives and midwifery in the United States (Madgett 2017; Gathercole 2024). By 1929, Congress allowed the law to expire. However, within an eight-year period, the U.S. federal government disbursed grants to forty-five states (Madgett 2017; Gathercole 2024). Consequently, white male obstetricians and white public health nurses conspired to undermine the value, work, reach, and impact of Black Grand midwives. The near eradication of Black Grand midwives disrupted traditional care relationships, methods, and settings in favor of physician-attended births in hospital settings (Vollers 2023; Goode 2014; Goode and Rothman 2017; Suarez 2020; ACNM Admin 2021). From 1900 to 1950, the proportion of births in hospital settings increased remarkably from 5 percent to 80 percent, with midwives, in general, attending less than 10 percent of U.S. births, despite the unfavorable rates of infant and maternal mortality associated with physician-attended births (Vollers 2023; Goode 2014; Goode and Rothman 2017).

The paradigm shift, from birthing at home in the company of women, assisted by a midwife, to birthing in hospitals in the company of mostly white male physicians, began by 1940, when the proportion of out-of-hospital births (also known as community births or birthing in the community at home or at a midwifery-led birthing center) fell to 44 percent. By 1969, the prevalence of community births dramatically decreased to 1 percent, where it remained throughout the 1980s (Wertz and Wertz 1989; MacDorman, Menacker, and Declercq 2010; Grove and Hetzel 1968). By the 1950s, birthing in hospitals meant erosion of autonomy, agency, self-efficacy, and memory with the administration of drugs during labor such as barbiturates (e.g., morphine) to mitigate the pain of childbirth and an amnesic agent (e.g., scopolamine) to nearly eradicate the memories of birth (Alves 2018; Dekker 2013; Oregon Health & Science University n.d.).. The inappropriately widespread use of twilight sleep, in combination with the unnecessary application of forceps and performance of episiotomies upon crowning (emergence of the newborn's head from the vagina), "just in case something might go wrong," demonstrated the dominant culture of obstetric violence and the complicity of obstetricians in silencing women's voices and stealing women's power in childbirth (Dekker 2013). Birthing in the U.S. during the 1950s and 1960s meant birthing in hospitals with mostly white male obstetricians who initiated another paradigm shift that reimagined birth as potentially dangerous, establishing and spreading new norms and narratives leading to the professionalization, medicalization, pathologization, and commodification of childbirth (Rothman 2007; Dekker 2013; Bonaparte 2014; Suarez 2020).

Additional drivers in the near eradication of Black Grand midwives and the increased rates of childbirth hospitalization among Black women demonstrated the heterogeneity of intention and expectation about birth attendants and settings within the Black community. Black social and political organizations such as the National Association for the Advancement of Colored People (NAACP) failed to support midwifery and community births. The movement to desegregate society within and across systems and structures within the workforce, education, law, and health care aligned with the right to seek help or health care in desegregated hospitals. For example, public leader and sociologist, W. E. B. DuBois, supported hospital birth for Black mothers (Goode and Rothman 2017; Suarez 2020). At the same time, more and more affluent Black women within higher socioeconomic strata deliberately pursued childbirth in hospital settings with physicians as a symbol of their Black class privilege and pride (Goode and Rothman 2017). The passage of the Hill-Burton Act in 1946 presented another facilitator in the paradigm shift from midwifery-led community births to physician-led hospital births.

The Hill-Burton Act provided funds to build hospitals and health clinics for underserved communities while simultaneously maintaining "separate but equal medical facilities" (Hill 2016). One outcome of the Hill-Burton Act was the disproportionate amount of funds distributed within the South, establishing more segregated health care facilities and hospitals, particularly in rural communities. Consequently, increasing numbers of Black women in the South experienced childbirth in hospitals with physicians, contributing to the erasure and exclusion of Black Grand midwives in birth work and overall reproductive health care.

While Black women continued birthing in hospitals, some white women began mobilizing around their right to bodily autonomy during childbirth and raising their voices in resistance to twilight sleep, forceps, and episiotomies and in favor of natural childbirth (Wertz and Wertz 1989; Rothman 2007; Suarez 2020). Specifically, middle-class white women felt drawn to the natural childbirth movement as part of the larger women's rights movement in the 1960s and 1970s. The movement sparked the return of midwifery in the 1970s and 1980s, notably white midwives for affluent white women, who organized to reclaim birth as a physiological and communal experience, with minimal to no interventions and in the company of midwives and family members at home or within midwifery-led birth centers (Oregon Health & Science University n.d.).

Throughout the prior thirty years, from the 1950s to the 1980s, no authorized medical or government entity mandated any birthing hospitals or maternal health care facilities to collect, monitor, and report data on pregnancy and birth outcomes or obstetric quality and patient safety (Koonin et al. 1988). By the end of the twentieth century, the CDC started to record the number and causes of maternal deaths in 1985, dating back to 1980. In a collective effort to better define the incidence, causes, and risk factors associated with maternal deaths, the CDC's Division of Reproductive Health and Center for Chronic Disease Prevention and Health Promotion coordinated a study by the Maternal Mortality Collaborative (MMC), a Special Interest Group of the American College of Obstetricians and Gynecologists (ACOG). In 1983, ACOG's MMC established a voluntary surveillance of maternal deaths for the years 1980–5. The MMC ultimately reported on 601 maternal deaths from nineteen reporting areas for 1980–5, representing a maternal mortality ratio of 14.1 maternal deaths per 100,000 live births (Koonin et al. 1988). One benefit of coordinating the MMC study was an increase in the number of overall reported maternal deaths by 39 percent, when reported by the ACOG's MMC compared to the reporting of the same areas by the National Center for Health Statistics. In summary, the MMC report on 601 maternal deaths from 1980 to 1985 identified risk factors at the intersection of race and age. Women over thirty years of age had a higher risk of dying than younger women. Across each age group, Black women and non-Black women of color had a greater risk of dying than white women, with Black and non-Black women of color who were thirty years and older having the highest risk. The first MMC report identified the following medical conditions as the leading causes of maternal deaths: embolism (deadly blood clot formation), hypertension in pregnancy, conditions or complications associated with ectopic pregnancy—a pregnancy located outside of the uterus (e.g., hemorrhage, tubal rupture, death) hemorrhage, cerebrovascular accidents (stroke), and anesthesia complications. Of the 111 nonmaternal deaths, 90 (82 percent) were attributed to unintentional (e.g. motor vehicle accidents) or intentional injuries (e.g., homicide or suicide). When examining the distribution and determinants of deaths by race, the lives of Black women and other non-Black women of color were more likely than white women to die from each cause, especially from complications related to ectopic pregnancy, anesthesia, and abortion (Koonin et al. 1988).

In 1986, the CDC initiated a national surveillance of pregnancy-related deaths to better address knowledge gaps in the identification and understanding of the multifactorial causes of death (National Center for Chronic Disease Prevention and Health Promotion (U.S.). Division of Reproductive Health 2023). From 1987 to 2019, the CDC implemented the Pregnancy Mortality Surveillance System (PMSS) to describe the distribution, determinants, and trends of pregnancy-related deaths. During this thirty-year period, the number of reported pregnancy-related deaths increased from 7.2 deaths per 100,000 live births in 1987 to 17.6 deaths per 100,000 live births in 2019. According to the PMSS data, the reasons for the overall increase remain unclear, despite improvements in the identification of pregnancy-related causes using computerized data linkages between death records and birth and fetal death records by states, changes in the coding of causes of death, and the addition of a pregnancy checkbox to death records. Yet, errors in the reporting of pregnancy on death records occur, which may potentially lead to an overestimation of the number of pregnancy-related deaths. Based on the PMSS data from 2017 to 2019, three non-Hispanic groups in the U.S. suffered the greatest losses of lives and legacies to pregnancy (National Center for Chronic Disease Prevention and Health Promotion (U.S.), Division of Reproductive Health 2023). For every 100,000 live births in their communities, Native Hawaiian or Other Pacifici Islander communities lost approximately sixty-two lives; Black communities lost forty lives, and American Indian or Alaska

Native communities lost thirty-two lives. During this same time periods, three groups in the U.S. experience the greatest preservation and proliferation of lives and legacies through pregnancy with the least losses. For every 100,000 live births in their communities, non-Hispanic white communities lost fourteen lives, non-Hispanic Asian communities lost thirteen lives, and Hispanic communities lost twelve lives (National Center for Chronic Disease Prevention and Health Promotion (U.S.), Division of Reproductive Health 2023). What is the common shared history for Native Hawaiian or Other Pacific Islander communities, Black communities, and American Indian or Alaska Native communities? Each community was forced to survive and thrive despite centuries of navigating colonialism, including imperial power, planter, settler, and transport colonialism (Shoemaker 2015). To date, pregnancy in the afterlife of colonialism is not one of the CDC-approved causes of pregnancy-related deaths.

The 2023 March of Dimes Report (March of Dimes Peristats n.d.) revealed indicators of maternal and infant health and evaluated state efforts based on reporting the rate of preterm birth (prior to thirty-seven weeks pregnancy age) and assigning a letter grade for performance. According to the 2023 report, over 380,000 babies were born preterm in 2022, representing 10.4 percent of all births, the highest rate in ten years, despite a 1 percent decline in 2021. Based on data from 2018 to 2022, the maternal mortality rate has nearly doubled since 2018, increasing from 17.4 deaths per 100,000 to 32.9 in 2021, disproportionately and unjustly impacting Black women persistently for nearly forty years, based on data from the initial 1980–5 report from ACOG's MMC. Although the infant mortality rate declined 10 percent over the last ten years (6.0 infant deaths per 1,000 live births in 2012 to 5.4 infant deaths in 2021), the rate among babies born to Black birthing people from 2019 to 2021 was nearly two times the national rate (10.5 and 5.4, respectively). Just like the racial inequities and injustices captured by the reporting of the rates of maternal and infant mortality in the U.S., the preterm birth rate among babies born to Black mothers and birthing people was one and a half times higher than the rate among all other non-Black babies (14.6 percent compared to 9.0–12.2 percent among Asian, white, Hispanic, American Indian/Alaska Native, and Pacific Islander mothers and birthing people). Upon evaluation of efforts to prevent preterm births at the city level, the 2023 report showed that one third of the one-hundred U.S. cities with the greatest number of live births earned a preterm birth grade of F in 2022. Sixteen states earned a grade of D while eight states and one U.S. territory earned a grade of F. Rightfully so, the U.S. earned an overall preterm birth grade of D+ for two consecutive years (March of Dimes Peristats n.d.).

For decades, studies of anti-Black racism, nativity, intersectionality, or Black feminism challenged norms and narratives that reinforce Blackness as biologically inferior to whiteness, justifying the disparate death rates among Black people (David and Collins 1997; Rich-Edwards et al. 2001; Mullings 2005; Dominguez et al. 2009; Dominguez 2011; Davis 2018; Hardeman et al.

2018; Davis 2019; Black Women Scholars and Research Working Group for the Black Mamas Matter Alliance 2020; Bridges 2020; Ekeke et al. 2020; Hardeman and Karbeah 2020; Hardeman et al. 2020; Scott 2018, 2019a, 2019b, 2021; Scott et al. 2020; White VanGompel et al. 2022). Lest we forget that sociologist W. E. B. DuBois reported on the infant mortality rate for the year 1900, among Black babies in Philadelphia in 1906 during the eleventh conference for the study of the Negro problems, held on May 29th, 1906 in Atlanta, GA at Atlanta University Press (DuBois 2003; DuBois 1906). Nearly 118 years ago, DuBois shared that 25 percent of the 1,467 Black babies born in Philadelphia in 1900 died prior to celebrating their milestone first solar return. Evaluating disparate deaths, disabilities, and near deaths that persistently impact Black people, particularly Black women and gender-expansive individuals during pregnancy and postpartum, one must name and explain racism in health services provision and research as the primary driver for yielding disparate outcomes, biased interpretations, and the spread of inaccurate and imprecise information (Davis 2018; Hardeman et al. 2018; Davis 2019; Black Women Scholars and Research Working Group for the Black Mamas Matter Alliance 2020; Bridges 2020; Ekeke et al. 2020; Hardeman and Karbeah 2020; Hardeman et al. 2020; Scott 2018, 2019a, 2019b, 2021; Scott et al. 2020; Scott and Davis 2021; White VanGompel et al. 2022). A more precise and accurate approach to interpreting Black women's medical encounters within the U.S. health system is to situate both race and gender as forms of knowledge production by which we make meaning of Black women's expectations, experiences, and expressions (Davis 2018; Davis 2019; Davis 2020). The CDC 2022 report on the distribution and determinants of pregnancy-related deaths from 2011 to 2017 revealed that 84 percent of pregnancy-related deaths are preventable, and that Black women disproportionately represented 33 percent of lives lost due obstetric quality and patient safety violations, despite only representing 12 percent of the U.S. women's population (Trost et al. 2022).

From 1980 to 2024, the staggering inequities and injustices in pregnancy and postpartum persist and worsen in certain geographies, disproportionately, predictably, and unfairly impacting Black women and the families and communities left behind to grieve a past, present, and unexpected future (Bridges 2020; Harper et al. 2004; Somer, Sinkey, and Bryant 2017; Howland et al. 2019). Racial capitalism and racialized medical procedures without voluntary consent (e.g., labor inductions, cesarean births, sterilization, long-acting reversible contraceptives) continue to force and constrain Black women's reproduction and control and stratify both fecundity and fertility (Scott and Davis 2021). Twelve years after the MMC report of maternal deaths, Dorothy Roberts illuminated the intricate ways that state and institutional policies, actors, and agents conspire to obliterate and/or obstruct Black lives and legacies through the criminalization of addiction, particularly Black women navigating pregnancy or parenting among (Roberts 1997), parent—child separation, and family and community destabilization and devastations, across and with generations. Thus, the synergistic policies, practices, procedures, processes, and programs within these oppressive systems and structures function to achieve one shared perpetual goal: "killing the Black [reproducing] body." At the same, one must consider the parallel near eradications of knowledge and practices from three groups of Black women: Black Grand midwives, Black women, and Black women scholars.

The genocide of Black life, Black people, Black thought, and Black activism is real. On December 17, 1951, William Patterson and Paul Robeson simultaneously delivered a petition from the Civil Rights Congress (CRC) to the United Nations (U.N.) titled, "We Charge Genocide: The Crime of Government Against the Negro People." Signed by nearly one-hundred U.S. intellectuals and activists, the document accused the U.S. of genocide against Black people. Mr. Robeson, known for his exceptional talent as an athlete, lawyer, actor, singer, cultural scholar, author, and political activist, delivered the petition to the U.N. headquarters in New York, while CRC Secretary Patterson delivered the petition to the U.N. headquarters in Paris (Civil Rights Congress 1951; Zinn Education Project n.d.). From the preface, written by Ossie Davis: "This is not the first time the Black people of the U.S. have issued a warning. W. E. B. Du Bois himself said it plain in 1900: "The problem of the 20th century is the problem of the color line." We say it again, we will submit no further to the brutal indignities being practiced against us; we will not be intimidated, and most certainly not eliminated. We claim the ancient right of all peoples, not only to survive unhindered, but also to participate as equals in man's inheritance here on earth. We fight to preserve ourselves, to see that the treasured ways of our life-in-common are not destroyed by brutal men or heartless institutions. We Charge Genocide! Indeed we do, for we would save ourselves and our children. History has taught us prudence—we do not need to wait until the Dachaus and Belsens and the Buchenwalds are built to know that we are dying. We live with death and it is ours; death not so obvious as Hitler's ovens—not yet. But who can tell?" (Civil Rights Congress 1951, v). The opening paragraph of the Introduction states: "Out of the inhuman black ghetto of American cities, out of the common plantations of the South, comes this record of mass slayings on the basis of race, of lives deliberately warped and distorted by the willful creation of conditions making for premature death, poverty, and disease. It is a record that calls aloud for condemnation, for an end to these terrible injustices that constitute a daily and ever-increasing violation of the United Nations Convention on the Prevention and Punishment of the Crime of Genocide. It is sometimes incorrectly thought that genocide means the complete and definitive destruction of a race or people. The Genocide Convention, however, adopted by the General Assembly of the United Nations on December 9, 1948, defines genocide as any killings on the basis of race, or, in its specific words, as "killing members of the group." An intent to destroy, *in whole or in part*, a national, racial, ethnic, or religious group is genocide, according to the Convention. Thus, the Convention states, "causing serious bodily or mental harm to members of the group" is genocide, as well as "killing members of the group." We maintain, therefore, that the oppressed Negro citizens of the U.S., segregated, discriminated against and long the target of violence, suffer from genocide as the result of the consistent, conscious, unified policies of every branch of government (Civil Rights Congress 1951, xiv).

When examining data from 1900 to 2023, one thing remains true: the absence of declaring racism as the driver for lost lives and legacies disproportionately, persistently, and unfairly stolen by the inactions of health care providers, administrators, educators, financiers, researchers, and policymakers before, during, and after human pregnancy and childbearing among Native Hawaiian or Other Pacific Islander communities, Black communities, and American Indian or Alaska Native communities. Inaction in the face of need is institutionalized racism (Jones 2000). Inaction is the catalyst and accelerant for genocide.

On September 23, 2022, the CDC released findings from a new analysis that included data on 1,018 pregnancy-related deaths from Maternal Mortality Review Committees (MMRCs) across thirty-six states from 2017 to 2019 (Trost et al. 2022). As described by the CDC, MMRCs are multidisciplinary groups of experts who meet regularly in a structured manner at the state or local level to comprehensively review maternal or pregnancy-related deaths that occur during or within 1 year of the end of pregnancy. The CDC works with MMRCs to improve review processes, procedures, and practices that inform recommendations for preventing future pregnancy-related deaths. Although MMRCs may differ from state to state, the CDC offers a logic model, or roadmap, to guide the work. The logic model was developed to demonstrate the general inputs, activities, and outcomes of an optimal, fully functional MMRC. The CDC encourages MMRCs to view the logic model as a foundation by which to organize, customize, and/or adapt to the context, conditions, and resources available to the local or state-based MMRC (CDC 2021).

The most egregious finding from the 2022 CDC report on pregnancy-related deaths was that 84 percent of pregnancy-related deaths in 2020 were preventable. Among pregnancy-related deaths with information on timing, 26 percent of deaths occurred during pregnancy, 27 percent occurred on the day of childbirth or within 7 days after, and 47 percent occurred between 7 days and 1 year after childbirth (Trost et al. 2022). Although Black women make up 12.9 percent of the total representation of women in the U.S.

based on 2019 data (U.S. Census Bureau 2020), nearly one in three (31.4 percent) mothers and birthing people who died during or after pregnancy and childbirth identified as non-Hispanic Black persons, based on 2019 population estimates by age, sex, race, and Hispanic origin. The leading underlying cause of pregnancy-related deaths included mental health conditions (including deaths due to suicide and overdose/poisoning related to substance use disorder). When the data was disaggregated by race and ethnicity, the leading causes of pregnancy-related deaths manifested differently: Cardiac and coronary conditions (non-Hispanic Black people), mental health conditions (Hispanic and non-Hispanic White people), and hemorrhage (non-Hispanic Asian people). Among pregnancy-related deaths with information on the place of last residence, 82 percent of mothers and birthing people who died lived in urban counties. The following fourteen states do not currently have MMRCs: Idaho, Kentucky, Maine, Maryland, Montana, Michigan, North Dakota, Nevada, Rhode Island, South Carolina, South Dakota, Utah, and Vermont. According to Wanda Barfield, MD, MPH, director of CDC's Division of Reproductive Health at the National Center for Chronic Disease Prevention and Health Promotion, "The majority of pregnancy-related deaths were preventable, highlighting the need for quality improvement initiatives in states, hospitals, and communities that ensure all people who are pregnant or postpartum get the right care at the right time" (CDC 2022).

The CDC 2022 report demonstrates the ongoing failures of U.S. health systems to protect mothers and birthing people, particularly structurally marginalized and minoritized birthing communities in urban settings. Despite the emphasis on individual-level interventions (e.g., weight loss, avoiding late childbearing) and social protections (e.g., marriage, higher education, higher income), the 2022 CDC report reinforces a widely unaccepted truth: the primary drivers of preventable deaths and harms are variations in quality and safety within and across U.S. hospitals and the absence of meaningful accountability measures and reporting systems. Despite a focused emphasis on safety meanings and measures, patient safety culture, teamwork training, executive walk rounds, rapid response teams, and standardized communication methods, current evidence describes ongoing threats to advancing patient safety (e.g., variations in safety perceptions, poor teamwork/communication, culture of low expectations, power, and "no blame" approach). Current perinatal QI and patient safety efforts must focus on establishing a just and equitable culture that demands appropriate individual, departmental, institutional, and structural accountability and oversight (Dekker 2017).

INTRODUCING A NEW OBSTETRIC QUALITY AND PATIENT SAFETY FRAMEWORK

The *SACRKED Birth* framework argues that the existing ethics and epistemology of quality and patient safety in hospital-based obstetrics contribute to the worsening death and dying gap between Black and non-Black mothers and birthing people. The dominant measurement selection and monitoring strategies prioritize outcome measures as the standard measures of quality and safety. Yet, outcome measures continuously fail to capture hospital performance based on how well or how poorly hospitals see, hear, believe, support, want, and celebrate Black birthing families during care provision. By 2022, I decided to begin all my presentations with the following declaration: outcome-only measures cannot, do *not,* and will likely *never* capture the patient and community experiences of care, specifically the hidden narratives of disproportionate, preventable, predictable, and unfair hurt and harm of reproducing, birthing, lactating, parenting, and partnering for pleasure and/or family building while Black in *any* U.S. societal system or structure.

Consider the image and messaging of a Black mother and child who "achieve positive birth outcomes" based on traditional standards of high quality and safety: full-term pregnancy, absence of medical conditions or comorbidities, optimal prenatal care utilization, vaginal birth with a small laceration that required an uncomplicated repair, normal weight infant at term (normative range between 2.5 and 4.0 kilograms, or 5.5 and 8.8 pounds), healthy infant with no need for high-resource care or admission into the neonatal intensive care unit (NICU), and optimal breast-, chest-, body-feeding with effective latching, suckling, and swallowing. Under the existing obstetric quality and safety paradigm, one would likely label this Black birth and the birthing hospital as "high performing, high quality, and safer."

However, when asked about the alignment between her expectation and experience of hospital care, a Black mother in Los Angeles reflected on her experience and shared the following memory of holding her baby during the repair of a birth laceration, "We're human. Treat the human. We know you're going to sew me back up. But I feel like a rag doll. Just because you stitched me back up don't mean I'm whole again." The Black mother's experience and how she made sense of her experience, in contrast to the existing quality and patient safety paradigm, highlight the limitations in quality improvement ethics, leadership, knowledge, science, measurement selection and monitoring, and data quality that prioritize outcome measures over patient experience measures. In the above Black mother's reflection on her birth, we see the stark contrast between the meaning and measurement of a physical outcome and a patient's expectation, expression, or experience of the physical outcome. The difference between an outcome identified by the health system and an experience defined by patients reveals the limitations and dangers in evaluating hospital quality and safety through outcomes-only data. The prioritization of clinical outcome measures as performance indicators facilitates the development and sustainability of an unjust culture of care provision during entire hospital shifts regardless of the hospital worker's race, gender, positionality, specialty, or discipline. Upholding an unjust culture of care during childbirth hospitalization reproduces acts of epistemic injustice and corresponding violations of patient safety, agency, and self-efficacy in interactions, communication, counseling, decision-making, and documentation and dissemination of health care information in electronic health records.

The critical questions we need to consider in conflating a positive birth outcome with a positive birth experience: Is this a *safe* or *unsafe* Black Birth? Who gets to define, measure, monitor, and report on safety? Who gets to determine accountability and oversight mechanisms of actions for evaluating hospital performance? Who determines approval or denial of reimbursement based on quality and safety? What is the proximity between these structures and systems of power AND Black mothers and birthing people in terms of equity, inclusion, belonging, and justice?

Health plans, hospitals, quality leaders, data scientists, public health practitioners, and maternal and child health leaders continue to miss opportunities to bridge the gap between hospital intention and community impact. The ongoing structural and systemic denial of community harm in prioritizing outcome measures reveals epistemic ignorance, arrogance, or both, in understanding nuanced differences across system intention, community impact, and opportunities for innovation, disruption, and transformation in obstetric quality and patient safety paradigms. The system intention is to evaluate hospital performance in quality and safety using outcome measures usually based on a patient's physical or clinical characteristics. In reality, outcome measures evaluate the physical performance of the Black birthing body in response to the quality of care provided by hospital workers and to centuries of structural and systematic violence, control, and dominance within and across multiple generations. Likewise, outcome measures can create a false narrative of quality, value, and safety. Thus, disaggregating outcomes-only data by race alone is not going to save Black mothers and birthing people from harmful and hurtful acts of obstetric racism. When hospitals, health plans, and state perinatal quality collaboratives disaggregate the data by race and the data teams don't see racialized differences in outcomes, then hospitals make false assumptions that they provide color-blind or anti-racist care. For example, several hospitals in the U.S. northeast, southeast, and west report being actively engaged in providing anti-racist health care and/or implementing anti-racism initiatives as noted on their websites or in online news articles, such as Duke Health, University of California San Francisco (UCSF) Benioff

Children's Hospitals (BCH), Mount Sinai, and Mass General Brigham (Duke Health n.d.; UCSF BCH n.d.; Mount Sinai n.d.; McFarling 2022).

Examining the quality of care and patient safety through clinical outcomes establishes two lies as truths: (1) Blackness is biologically inferior, particularly the Black reproducing body, Black women, and Black babies are broken, deficient, and more vulnerable or susceptible to disparate birth outcomes; and (2) The absence of clinical pathology signifies the presence of perinatal equity. A high Black vaginal birth rate does not mean hospital workers are routinely present, engaged, and responsive to the expressed care needs of Black mothers and birthing people. Systems can't change what systems fail to recognize, name, measure, monitor, and mitigate. However, a validated patient-reported experience measure (PREM) of the quality during childbirth hospitalization designed for, by, and with Black mothers and birthing people can enhance our understanding of the experience of care as the patient, beyond the boundaries of outcome, process, balancing, and satisfaction measures. According to the Center for Medicare & Medicaid Services (CMS), "quality is defined by the National Academy of Medicine as the degree to which health services for individuals and populations increase the likelihood of desired health outcomes and are consistent with current professional knowledge" (CMS n.d.) In comparison, CMS defines quality improvement (QI) as "the framework used to systematically improve care." The CMS website explains that the purpose of QI is to "standardize processes and structures to reduce variation, achieve predictable results, and improve outcomes for patients, healthcare systems, and organizations." CMS also provides examples of structural (e.g., technology, culture, leadership, and physical capital) and process (e.g., knowledge capital such as standard operating procedures or human capital such as education and training) factors or measures. By affirming, amplifying, and analyzing real-life hospital birthing narratives from Black mothers in California, the SACKRED Birth framework identifies and characterizes limitations in the existing structural and process factors in existing obstetric quality measurements and QI frameworks. The current QI ethics, knowledge, leadership, science, measurement selection and monitoring strategies, data quality and accessibility, and community participation and partnership no longer serve Black mother and birthing people, and perhaps never served Black birthing families and communities. A PREM of quality during childbirth hospitalization would highlight the many different forms of violence and abuse that any hospital personnel—regardless of race, gender, class, specialty, or intent—perpetuate against all mothers and birthing people, particularly Black mothers and birthing people. Regarding accuracy and precision, a PREM of quality during childbirth hospitalization offers a more wholistic and humanistic examination of the impact of care processes on patient experiences.

My recommendation is for structures and systems to supplement outcome measures with a validated PREM of quality during childbirth hospitalization to more accurately and precisely evaluate hospital performance based on hospital treatment or mistreatment of Black mothers and birthing people. In a 2022 article written by Akilah Johnson and published in the *Washington Post*, I publicly spoke on record naming the existing measurement selection and monitoring strategies as a primary driver of the manufactured Black maternal health crisis. The scientific, medical, and cultural obsession with examining diseased and dead Black pregnant and birthing bodies deters us from exploring the biological etiologies that protect white mothers and birthing people from experiencing significantly higher rates of adverse pregnancy and birth outcomes and experiences. "Just because you don't see the pathology that you define doesn't mean someone's not being hurt or harmed," said Scott, who created an instrument to measure Black patients' experiences of obstetric racism, capturing what she describes as the misalignment between hospital intentions of providing safe and high-quality care and patients' actual experiences. (Johnson 2022).

In 2023, my co-authors and I published "Emotional safety is patient safety" in *BMJ Quality and Safety* (Lyndon et al. 2022). We justify the need for a new patient safety paradigm using obstetric racism as the exemplar. Obstetric racism, as defined by Dána-Ain Davis, PhD, MPH, is both an event and a framework that sits at the intersection of obstetric violence and medical racism (Davis 2018; Davis 2019). With the introduction and explanation of the six dimensions of obstetric racism by Davis in 2018, we can more accurately and precisely explain how the U.S. maternal health system devalues, dehumanizes, controls, and abuses Black women and their babies in ways that track along histories of anti-Black racism and eugenics or population control. We must interrogate and reconcile "being safe" as defined by systems and "feeling safe" as defined by patient experiences and community wisdom. If we don't, then we create and perpetuate epistemic and testimonial injustice, thereby covering up the realities of harm and hurt. First, prioritizing safety as defined only for, by, and with systems and structures dismisses patient feelings and testimonies of safety and harm as real outcomes. Second, prioritizing structural and systematic paradigms of safety diminishes the value of patient testimonies and positions patient testimonies as subjective truths, which hospital systems, teams, and individual clinicians and staff judge as lacking credibility. Third, prioritizing being safe displaces the onus of responsibility, recognition, reporting, repair, and reconciliation *from* the system to the patient, patient-provider dyad, and health care or hospital teams. Fourth, standardizing safety meanings, manifestations, and measures defined by systems and structures denies the possibility, imagination, innovation, disruption, and transformation of patient safety beyond the absence of physical injury or reduction in adverse outcomes (Lyndon et al. 2023).

Approximately one year after our commentary on the limitations of the current patient safety paradigm, US News and World Report announced a list of twenty-six hospitals across thirteen states achieving excellent outcomes for cesarean section and unexpected newborn complications among Black patients (US News and World Report 2024). Prioritizing patient outcomes at the exclusion and/or erasure of patient experiences means the U.S. holds a myopic view of quality and safety in maternity care. Hospitals can reduce the rate of cesarean births and unexpected newborn complications among Black women and gender-expansive individuals and *still* provide harmful care that reinforces inequity, anti-Black racism, misogynoir (Bailey 2016; Bailey and Trudy 2018; Bailey 2021), and obstetric racism (Davis 2018; Davis 2019). The intersection of the racial empathy gap, white racial frame, and anti-Black feminism facilitates the devaluation of the lives of Black mothers and birthing people, as evidenced by the absence of empathy as a manifestation of obstetric racism during service provision (Hardeman 2020; Bernhardt and Singer 2012; Forgiarini et al. 2011; Hardeman et al. 2016; Davis 2018; Scott 2021; Scott and Davis 2021; White VanGompel et al. 2022; Lyndon et al. 2023). The prioritization of individual behaviors, without a structural analysis of power and obstetric racism, as the basis for perinatal inequities, perpetuates positivism and reproduces a culture of "mother blame" care. Consequently, the stigmatization, scapegoating, increased surveillance, and criminalization of Black bodies and Black motherhood fester in the absence of empathy and erode the autonomy of Black mothers and birthing people (Davis 2018; Scott et al. 2019; Scott 2021; Scott and Davis 2021; White VanGompel et al. 2022; Lyndon et al. 2023). Thus, the conflation of reducing pathology-centered outcomes with advancing equity and dismantling anti-Black racism and misogynoir is very concerning.

The SACKRED Birth framework and quality domains that emerged from the 2019 Black feminist phenomenology of the quality and culture of childbirth hospitalization birthed the first and only patient-reported experience measure of obstetric racism©, also known as the PREM-OB Scale® (White VanGompel et al. 2022). Study findings from the first publication of the PREM-OB Scale® showed that 806 Black mothers and birthing people across 348 hospitals and 34 states, including DC, experienced obstetric racism independent of their pregnancy age, BMI, and birth modality (vaginal birth vs. cesarean birth) (White VanGompel et al. 2022). Therefore, the ongoing system denial of the limitations in outcome measures to monitor and evaluate the quality of childbirth hospitalization must be continuously interrogated in public and ultimately addressed through legal, legislative, political, social, or financial recourse.

Nearly six years after Davis' first online publication detailing the different dimensions of obstetric racism (Davis 2018), the current quality and patient safety paradigm in the U.S. continues to deny the historical contextualization and contemporary implications of obstetric racism as a well-defined, measurable, reportable, predictable, and preventable adverse event. *The SACKRED Birth: Mobilizing a New Quality Paradigm in Obstetric Care* offers a Black feminist hermeneutic phenomenology of the process and culture of childbirth hospitalization for Black women through meaning-making of text describing the lived experiences of thirty-six cis-gender Black mothers in Oakland and Los Angeles, California. A Black feminist hermeneutic phenomenology of obstetric quality during childbirth hospitalization means I believe that race and gender serve as modes of knowledge production in bridging the subjectivity and objectivity of birthing while Black in hospital settings (Collins 1990; Davis 2018; Crowther and Thomson 2023). A Black feminist hermeneutic phenomenology gives me permission, as a dissident and recovering OBGYN physician, public health scholar, applied epidemiologist, and quality improvement and implementation scientist, to ground myself, my scholarship, my activism, and these written narratives in our world through a profound understanding of experience, consciousness, and awareness. In choosing a Black feminist hermeneutic phenomenology as the methodological examination of the quality of childbirth hospitalization as a Black woman, I feel I can more authentically and reflexively integrate my evolving engagement, attachment, and relationship with the written Black hospital birth narratives and my memory of the sounds, thoughts, and feelings of co-designing and co-facilitating the two different focus groups with Black community and content experts and non-Black allied content experts (Crowther and Thomson 2023). A Black feminist hermeneutic phenomenology gives me permission to be courageous, honest, and transparent (Crowther and Thomson 2023), which aligns with my 4T model of inquiry, ingenuity, and innovation: truth-telling, transparency, trust, and transformation (Birthing Cultural Rigor 2024). *SACKRED Birth* is a book that provides a more nuanced, accurate, and precise description of how Black mothers navigate systems of control and dominance during the pursuit of a SACKRED birth in hospital settings through the words, feelings, and thoughts about Black women and hospital personnel as described exclusively by Black women themselves.

In Fall 2018, as the token co-founding director of the California Birth Equity Collaborative, I engaged two California-based Black women-led and serving community-based organizations (BWCBOs): the African American Breastfeeding Cultural Outreach Taskforce (BCOT) in Oakland and Black Women for Wellness (BWW) in Los Angeles. I invited them to co-design and co-implement an approach to curating space for community dialogue that acknowledged and affirmed the lives of Black mothers, birthing people, their children, and their community as worthy during hospital births and hospital-based perinatal quality improvement and implementation science.

The BWCBOs represented organizations with prior experience in providing services, supports, and advocacy to Black women, mothers, and people with the capacity for pregnancy, miscarriage, abortion, labor, birth, postpartum, and lactation. Together we formulated a structure for research activities that included a racially and culturally concordant and affirming space, plentiful food, adult and youth community caretakers onsite to assist with children, and encouragement of participants to speak up and speak out, or to step out and step back as indicated to meet participants' respective needs. Spaces considered for study events had to support breast-, chest-, and body-feeding and inclusion of infants, small children, and adolescents. Based on our mutually expressed needs, verbal and nonverbal communication, attitudes, and interactions in the spaces reproduced and reinforced messages and images of the power, potential, passion, and promise, not pathology, of Blackness, Black bodies, Black births, Black womanhood, and Black motherhood/parenthood.

Racial and cultural concordance between researchers and the researched was vital in illuminating the power relations, differentials, and dynamics that Black mothers and birthing people navigate to achieve and sustain self-determination in both research and service provision through the intellectual thoughts and political activism of Black mothers and birthing people, Black women community leaders, Black women birth workers, and Black women scholars. Study participants engaged in two 90-minute research activities: a focus group and temporal-spatial mapping dialogue. Question design was guided by a Black feminist critical ethnographic and phenomenological approach, inspired by Leith Mullings' Harle Birth Right Project (Mullings et al. 2001). The study was conducted with the state perinatal quality collaborative in California and received ethical review and approval from Stanford University Human Subjects Review Board.

Current strategies to address the death and dying gap between Black and non-Black birthing communities continue to perpetuate mother blame and biological determinism through investments in and implementation of individual-level interventions designed by white-led research teams guided by anti-Black ethics, epistemologies, leadership, methodologies, and messaging. The overreliance and misuse of clinical outcome measures and claims data as key performance indicators perpetuate Black testimonial and hermeneutical injustice by creating a false narrative of quality and safety (Scott 2021). Structural extraction of Black talent, knowledge, and social capital without equitable compensation or representation as principal investigators or program directors leads to ongoing epistemic redlining and epistemic injustice. Structural erasure and exclusion of Black scholarship, specifically the intellectual thoughts and activism of Black women and gender-expansive people, becomes the norm to which the dominant leadership in quality and patient safety aspire to establish and maintain. Consequently, Black women-led interventions to advance quality and equity in patient safety programs are labeled by the dominant leadership as inferior, fraudulent, and non-feasible (Scott et al. 2020; Scott 2021).

Thus, my role as a recovering board-certified OBGYN, applied epidemiologist, public health scholar, improvement and implementation scientist, and activist-scholar, whose intellectual genealogy is grounded in anthropology, is to facilitate knowledge uptake and understanding of the limitations in prioritizing outcomes data during the evaluation of maternal, infant, or perinatal quality and safety, using childbirth hospitalization as an exemplar. As the granddaughter of the Black domestic help employed by two white wealthy families who wore white girls' hand-me-down Sunday's best dresses, and as the maternal and paternal sister of Black women who survived and thrived after recurrent pregnancy losses, shortened cervix, premature birth, teen pregnancy and parenting, and postpartum stroke, I offer a Black feminist critique and analysis of epistemic redlining in the field of perinatal quality improvement and patient safety in the afterlife of slavery. *SACKRED Birth* argues that outcome-only measures cannot, do not, and will likely never capture the patient and community experiences of care, specifically the hidden narratives of preventable and unfair hurt and harm of birthing while Black in U.S. hospitals.

The application of a Black feminist praxis throughout this hermeneutic phenomenology of the quality of care during childbirth hospitalization as a Black woman in the U.S. emancipates the stifled expressions of daily harm enacted against Black mothers, their babies, their partners, and their given and chosen kin by hospital systems, teams, and individual administrators, clinicians, and staff. *SACKRED Birth* is organized into eight chapters that provide the reader with a Black feminist critique and analysis of the ethics and epistemologies of quality and patient safety in hospital-based obstetrics and perinatal care through the exploration of birthing while Black in California hospitals (chapter 1). Each subsequent chapter (chapters 2 through 7) offers a Black feminist reimagining of labor, birth, and immediate postpartum during childbirth hospitalization through seven patient-identified quality care domains named and defined by the words, feelings, thoughts, and lived experiences of Black mothers. The arc of the book transports the reader from characterizing the drivers of the manufactured epidemic of the Black death and dying gap through Black feminist scholarship, such as Mullings' Sojourner syndrome, Davis' obstetric racism, and Scott's reproductive and perinatal apartheid (an adaptation of Harriet Washington's *Medical Apartheid*), to conceptualizing the solutions to advancing quality and patient safety through operationalizing a novel Black feminist quality framework, SACKRED Birth, and a novel validated instrument, the patient-reported experience measure of obstetric racism©, also known as the PREM-OB Scale® suite. Cultural rigor, which I defined in 2020, sits at the intersection of cultural humility (Murray-García and Tervalon 2014) and scientific rigor (National Institutes of Health n.d.; Lauer 2016), and simultaneously operationalizes Black feminist praxis, reproductive justice, and research justice across four modalities: analytic, praxis, vision, and movement (Scott et al. 2020). Cultural rigor then informs the direction, breadth, and depth of the book's arc.

This book is written to transform the knowledge, abilities, skills, and language of professionals and learners in health care, public health, quality improvement, and data science, working in academia, government, and industry. By mobilizing a movement to decolonize, destigmatize, and democratize childbirth hospitalization, the book compels its audience to reimagine hospital quality through the lived experiences and perspectives of Black mothers. In naming obstetric racism as an adverse event that creates preventable and unfair harm and violates patient safety, the author uncovers the hidden legacy of epistemic injustice in the field of quality improvement and offers novel and nuanced ethical, theoretical, and methodological approaches in measurement selection and strategies, data quality and accessibility, and community participation and partnership.

In 2020, I obtained permission to elaborate on the concept of cultural humility from the two California-based Black women physicians and public health scholars, Melanie Tervalon, MD, MPH, and Jann Murray-García, MD, MPH, who first defined the tenets of cultural humility in 1998. Cultural rigor sits at the intersection of scientific rigor, as defined by the National Institutes of Health, and cultural humility, as defined by Dr. Tervalon and Dr. Murray-García. Cultural rigor simultaneously operationalizes reproductive justice, Black feminism, and research justice across four modalities: analytic framework, social movement, vision, and praxis. In the application of cultural rigor, patient, community, and content experts and expertise are equally and equitably prioritized, as explained through research justice. Likewise, cultural rigor situates gender and race at the center of knowledge production, as defined in Black feminism. The hierarchy of knowledge and knowing in the traditional quality and patient safety paradigm deprioritizes patient experiential, cultural, and spiritual knowledge, relegating the title (and corresponding compensation) of experts to individuals with formal education and researcher to individuals who acquired formal skills and training. Thus, research justice requires a reimagining of the researched as the researcher and the experts with cultural and spiritual knowledge, experiential knowledge, and mainstream (or institutional) knowledge. Research justice offers a strategic vision with principles and practices to acknowledge, affirm, activate, and amplify the political power and legitimacy of structurally marginalized and minoritized communities as valid knowledge incubators and producers. Consequently, research justice situates patient and community experts in the position to leverage all three types of knowledge to drive policy-making decisions in rectifying historical and contemporary power inequities and advancing social justice (Jolivétte 2015). Weaving cultural rigor throughout the obstetric quality and patient safety paradigm also supports women and gender-expansive individuals in their right to have children, the right not to have children, and the right to nourish and nurture their existing children in safe and healthy environments as outlined in the tenets of reproductive justice (Ross and Solinger 2017; Ross et al. 2017).

As a social movement, cultural rigor catalyzes a new obstetric quality and patient safety paradigm that is continuously dismantling the hierarchy of knowing and knowledge production and its consequences, including structural arrogance and absence of empathy. According to a commentary published by Elizabeth Snively in 2022 (Snively 2022), the six domains of healthcare quality emerged as recommendations for systemic changes in response to a book, *To Err is Human: Building a Safer Health System*, published in 2000 by the Institute of Medicine, now the National Academy of Medicine (Donaldson et al. 2000). The book established a national agenda to improve patient safety at the systems level in response to medical errors made by "good people working in bad systems that need to be made safer," resulting in approximately 98,000 patient deaths occurring in hospitals in any given year. The high annual patient mortality from medical errors exceeded losses of human life from motor vehicle accidents, breast cancer, AIDS, or workplace injuries, four causes of death that had received much higher public attention. The book humanizes making mistakes in the provision of healthcare and places the onus of preventing and mitigating medical errors, not on individuals, but on the health system. By adopting a systemic approach that focuses on operationalizing a framework made of six domains, the expectation was for healthcare organizations to increase the likelihood of simultaneously reducing errors and improving the overall quality of healthcare they provided to patients and communities. Snively explained that each of the original six domains of healthcare quality corresponded to specific components of practice. Initially established by the Institute of Medicine (IOM), now known as the National Academy of Medicine (NAM) (IOM 2001), the AHRQ defined each of the six quality domains in the following manner (AHRQ 2015):

- *Safe*: avoiding harm to patients from the care that is intended to help them;
- *Effective*: Providing services based on scientific knowledge to all who could benefit and refraining from providing services to those not likely to benefit (avoiding underuse and misuse, respectively);
- *Patient-centered*: Providing care that is respectful of and responsive to individual patient preferences, needs, and values, and ensuring that patient values guide all clinical decisions;

- *Timely*: Reducing waits and sometimes harmful delays for both those who receive and those who give care;
- *Efficient*: avoiding waste, including waste of equipment, supplies, ideas, and energy;
- *Equitable:* Providing care that does not vary in quality because of personal characteristics such as gender, ethnicity, geographic location, and socio-economic status.

From a patient's perspective, the six-domain framework of quality could serve as a communication tool for patients to evaluate care quality and their satisfaction with the care they received. However, I am unable to identify utilization of the six-domain framework of quality in any of the participatory studies examining the drivers of suboptimal quality and safety during the provision of hospital-based obstetric care to Black mothers and birthing people. The literature rarely discusses the relationship between poor perinatal health outcomes, philanthropy, and traditional quality improvement ethics, epistemology, and methodology. In 2020, Scott *et al.* provided a critical interrogation of the role of philanthropy in shaping the research agenda, questions, and leadership (Scott et al. 2020a). The authors interrogated the inability of the philanthropic sector to prioritize the examination of birthing while Black in the U.S. through the expertise, experience, and filter of Black women scholars. The authors interpreted philanthropy's resistance or refusal as either an unintended oversight or an explicit denial of the value and relevance of navigating oppressive and exploitative structures and systems within society and across public health, legislative advocacy, health services research, and improvement and implementation science. Consequently, the authors offered different pathways and strategies forward through the conceptualization and operationalization of cultural rigor across four modalities (social movement, analytic framework, praxis, and vision). The authors concluded with a call to action for funders to embody cultural rigor as a mechanism to advance structural equity and racial justice and to sustain community engagement in research (Scott et al. 2020a).

Despite a proliferation of anti-racist statements by academic institutions in 2020, the establishment of state perinatal quality care collaboratives (PQCs), advances in reproductive technologies, and social protections such as higher education and optimal prenatal care utilization, U.S. hospitals do not keep Black mothers and birthing people safe. The problem with perinatal QI innovation and transformation is the hypervisibility of Black women as victims and the structural exclusion and erasure of Black women as patient, community, and content experts (Scott 2021). Despite the widespread media attention and rapid release of funding proposals to examine the relationship between structural racism and perinatal health care experiences, outcomes, and policies, very few, if any, perinatal QI safety bundles or standards of best practices have acknowledged, adopted, or amplified Black women's leadership, intellectual thoughts, and political activism (Scott 2021). At the time of writing this paper, only three state PQCs among fifty states and five territories inhabited by people in the U.S. are led by a Black woman (Mississippi, Louisiana, and Massachusetts) based on an informal Twitter inquiry. The ongoing unwillingness to recognize and accept obstetric racism as a primary driver of inequitable perinatal care experiences and outcomes should raise concerns about the ethics and epistemology of QI science. Obstetric racism explains the forms of violence and abuse that hospital personnel routinely perpetuate against Black women and people seeking help or health care for any pregnancy-related concern (Davis 2018; Davis 2019; Davis 2020; Scott and Davis 2021).

For decades, QI leaders and health services researchers assigned greater value to outcomes data from big administrative databases and medical-record review as the preferred method to evaluate and improve quality and safety. The hidden ranking system in perinatal epistemology created fertile ground for a harvest of two byproducts of epistemic redlining: epistemic injustice and hermeneutical injustice (Fricker 2007; Scott 2021; Lyndon et al. 2023). Epistemic injustice discounts the credibility of Black women's voices and narratives of their lived experiences, resulting in testimonial injustice, while hermeneutical injustice renders Black women as incapable of making sense of their own experiences and of having their expressed experiences be understood by others (Fricker 2007; Scott 2021; Lyndon et al. 2023). A deeper analysis of perinatal QI reveals an abusive overreliance on outcome measures from "diseased or dead Black female bodies." Consequently, the overreliance and prioritization of outcome measures weaponizes race as a biological construct, reinforces race as a risk factor, and undermines the critical role of patient-reported experience measures in QI innovation and systems transformation. Thus, traditional QI ethics, theories, methods, and outcome measures reproduce epistemic injustices that continuously and violently undermine Black women and people as knowledge incubators, generators, accelerators, and disseminators (Scott 2021).

Despite state and national quality improvement initiatives, clinical safety bundles, technological advance, safe motherhood initiatives, and social protections such as marriage, higher education or higher income, hospitals in the U.S. do not keep Black women and people safe throughout pregnancy, childbirth, and postpartum including up to one year after childbirth. Throughout the field of patient safety, the literature describes various concepts and definitions. As of August 7, 2024, the website for the AHRQ Patient Safety Network (PSNet) defines "patient safety as avoiding harm to patients from care that is intended to help them" (AHRQ PSNet n.d.(b); Committee on

Quality of Health Care in America, Institute of Medicine 2001). The website for AHRQ PSNet also defines patient safety as "the prevention and mitigation of harm caused by errors of omission or commission in healthcare, and the establishment of operational systems and processes that minimize the likelihood of errors and maximize the likelihood of intercepting them when they occur" (AHRQ PSNet n.d.(b); National Quality Forum 2006). Existing ethics, leadership, science, measurement selection, monitoring strategies, data quality, and community partnership and participation in quality and safety paradigms fail to highlight the many different forms of violence and abuse enacted against Black mothers and birthing people by hospital systems, teams, and individual clinicians and staff, regardless of race, gender, class, specialty or positionality. To address quality and safety variations during the provision of hospital-based obstetrics and perinatal care specifically to pregnant and postpartum Black women and gender-expansive individuals, we need a Black woman—person focused theoretical framework of obstetric quality and patient safety.

The methodologies for this study were informed by Black feminist, participatory research praxis and the theoretical frameworks of obstetric racism (Davis 2018), reproductive and perinatal apartheid (Scott 2019b; Davis and Scott 2020; White VanGompel et al. 2022), and Sojourner syndrome (Mullings 2005). Drawing on Mullings' use of Community Dialogue Groups (Mullings et al. 2001), I co-developed a study with community partners using a strategy that included both community-based focus groups and community-based consensus dialogue to develop the patient-driven domains of SACKRED Birth (Scott 2018; Scott 2019a; Scott 2019b). First, I engaged two California-based Black women-led and serving community-based organizations (BWCBOs) in Oakland, BCOT, and in Los Angeles, BWW, to co-design and implement an approach to curating space for community dialogue that acknowledged and affirmed the lives of Black birthing people, their children, and their community as worthy during hospital births and hospital-based perinatal quality improvement and implementation science.

In 2018, prior to BWCBO participation and partnership, I led a paradigm shift in perinatal quality and patient safety to use more inclusive language such as Black mothers and birthing people. My intention was to facilitate psychological safety and connectedness, or belonging, awareness, acknowledgment, and acceptance of the various identities, roles, and responsibilities held by individuals, couples, families, and communities. A singular focus on cisgender heterosexual women as the only pathway to pregnancy, motherhood, and family planning perpetuated harm and hurt, independent of intention. I called for a culture shift in obstetric quality and patient safety language to dismantle heteronormativity, avoid homo-, queer-, or transphobia, and expand our messaging and imaging to curate diversity (representation), inclusion (participation), belonging (psychological safety), and equity (decision-making on opportunities, options, and optimal conditions to achieve the patient's and community's best as defined for, by, and with patients and community). Although we used the term Black mothers and birthing people, all participants identified as females.

Study participants engaged in two in-person 90-minute research activities in Oakland, during a two-day session on February 12, 2019, and February 19, 2019, and in Los Angeles, in a full one-day morning and afternoon session on March 10, 2019: a focus group and temporal-spatial mapping dialogue. The question design was guided by the ethnographic approach of the Harlem Birth Right Project (Mullings et al. 2001). The plan for both activities was informed by the BWCBOs, who provided feedback on the focus group guides and the temporal-spatial mapping dialogue guides in January 2019. Study activities were conducted in Oakland and Los Angeles in February and March 2019, respectively, and were structured similar to community events with music, food, non-alcoholic beverages, childcare, and moments of silence, gratitude, and meditation to honor new ancestors, a BCOT member, and Black mothers who transitioned beyond life on Earth.

BWCBOs led the recruitment of community participants, also known as patient experts. Black women leaders from the BWCBOs made outreach to their respective communities to identify and invite eligible individuals to participate. In Oakland, the same participants took part in the focus group and temporal-spatial mapping dialogue that occurred on different days, except for one person who did not attend the second date. In Los Angeles, both data collection events occurred on the same day, with a break between activities. Written informed consent and a media release was provided by participants for all activities. Participants received a $125 gift card in consideration of their time and travel to and from the events.

The focus group activity was led by me and comprised of 8–10 Black-identified women discussing their prior planning, preparation, expectations, and experiences around birthing while Black in hospital settings in California within two years of study recruitment and enrollment in January 2019. The interview guide consisted of thirteen questions organized into the following four areas of interest: readiness and responsiveness to birth; birth expectations and experiences; birth supports and resources; and birth priorities and autonomy. Focus groups were audio-recorded and professionally transcribed for analysis. The focus groups and temporal-spatial mapping groups occurred simultaneously. Black mothers consented to participate in both groups.

Temporal-spatial mapping groups were each facilitated and led by two Black women leaders of the BWCBOs who were trained by me as the lead principal investigator on focus group moderation and the study research methods. The BWCBOs and I obtained permission from study participants for a non-Black Asian woman member of the research team, recruited by California's state perinatal quality collaborative, to be present and available during the temporal-spatial mapping group to provide technical support to ensure mapping and discussion were effectively captured. BWCBO recruitment efforts resulted in 17 and 19 Black mothers and birthing people participating in the data collection activities in Oakland and Los Angeles, respectively.

BWCBO community outreach and recruitment efforts resulted in the screening, consent, and enrollment of thirty-six study participants in Oakland (seventeen participants, 47.2 percent) and Los Angeles (nineteen participants, 52.8 percent). For the purpose of sharing thirty-six Black birthing narratives, I used pseudonyms to protect the identities of participants. These pseudonyms were chosen to reflect cultural and contextual relevance, ensuring confidentiality while maintaining the authenticity and integrity of the participants' expressions, expectations, and lived experiences in the study. Table 1.1 lists the study participant demographic information. The average participant age was 30.6 years (Oakland = 29.8 years; LA = 31.3 years). All study participants identified as being racialized as a Black person, with one participant who also identified as a multi-racialized Black and white person. Black women participants in the study were also identified collectively as patient experts and represented communities from thirty-six different zip codes in California. Twenty of thirty-five (57.1 percent) study participants who reported their insurance type for childbirth hospitalization relied on public insurance such as Medicaid, also referred to as Medi-Cal, California's Medicaid health care program. The highest reported income before taxes was $25,000 to $49,999, representing thirteen of thirty-five (37.1 percent) patient experts. The second highest reported income before taxes was less than $25,000, representing ten of thirty-five (28.6 percent) patient experts. The highest reported educational attainment was some college, representing sixteen of thirty-six (44.4 percent) patient experts. The second highest reported educational attainment was a college degree or higher, representing thirteen of thirty-six (36.1 percent) patient experts. Half (50.0 percent) of the patient experts reported having one child, while seven (19.4 percent) and six (16.7 percent) reported having two and three children, respectively. Four (11.1 percent) of the thirty-six patient experts were born outside of the U.S. in one of the following four countries: Eritrea, Nigeria, Guinea, and Jamaica. Three (75.0 percent) of the four patient experts born outside of the U.S. also reported speaking a language other than English at home (e.g., Tigrinya, French, and Twii). All thirty-two (89.9 percent) patient experts born in the U.S. reported that the parents or adults who cared for them as a child were also born in the U.S. All but one patient expert reported an experience with a hospital birth. A different patient expert reported having prior birthing experiences in a hospital setting and community setting (e.g., Midwifery-led

Table 1.1 Characteristics for Patient Experts (Focus Group Participants) in Los Angeles and Oakland, California, 2019, N = 36

Item	*N* *(not all values add up to 36 due to nonresponse)*
Location	
Oakland	17
LA	19
Insurance for hospital birth care, n = 35	
Public	20
Private	14
No insurance	1
Income before Taxes, n = 35	
< $25,000	10
$25,000–$49,999	13
$50,000–$74,999	6
$75,000–$99,999	5
> $100,000	1
Highest level of education completed, n = 36	
College degree or higher	13
Some college	16
Trade school	3
High school / GED	4
Number of children, n = 36	
1	18
2	7
3	6
4	3
5	1
6	1

birth center). One patient expert reported a prior childbirth experience in a community setting, specifically in her home.

The purpose of the temporal-spatial mapping, first developed by me in 2019, was to find shared language, meaning, manifestations, and measures to better describe the embodied experiences and emotions of participants across time and space from their perceived onset of labor through discharge from the hospital following birth. In response to the lack of scientific rigor and cultural humility, or cultural rigor, and patient involvement in survey development from design to dissemination, I felt compelled to design and implement a novel method to illuminate the words and wisdom of Black mothers and birthing people navigating power inequities in knowledge about, access to, and utilization of various types of birth services and supports along the pathway of seeking help or health care for a hospital birth. Phases of experience—for example, onset of labor, reaching out for help, getting to the hospital—were identified and placed on large sheets of paper on the walls.

Led by me, the research team identified eight terms from a literature review, Black women scholars with expertise in maternal and perinatal care, Black women community and academic experts in reproductive justice and birthing justice, non-Black women allied health services researchers and a focus group comprised of leaders from local BWCBOs that serve Black mothers and birthing individuals in Oakland and Los Angeles. The final terms identified were *Safety, Loved, Empathy, Trust, Listened to, Respect, Dignity,* and *Equity*. Participants were asked to identify and write words describing their feelings, thoughts, and experiences from the discernment of recurring abdominal pain as uterine contractions (e.g., labor) to hospital discharge, across the eight phases of experience on sticky notes, and to place these words in the corresponding phase of the temporal-spatial map created on the wall using large poster paper. The words most frequently used in each temporal-spatial phase were then identified and discussed by the group. The group defined their general meaning and understanding of the words or how they would define and recognize each word. On the large poster paper, a scribe, an Asian non-Black woman academic scholar, captured participants' definitions for each of the words (meaning). Next, the two Black women community experts (representatives of the BWCBOs with credentials as International Board Certified Lactation Consultants (IBCLCs)) guided the group to share how these words "showed-up" or how they would expect these words to "show-up" during care provision in action, behavior, language, and the different ways the hospital cared for participants during interactions, communication, counseling, and decision-making during their birth experience (manifestation and measurement). These definitions and responses were recorded on multi-colored sticky notes and placed on the walls. The research team also took photographs of the completed activity for documentation. Participants also had the opportunity to share through writing of their meanings and measurements as another way to capture their experiences from the onset of labor to hospital discharge.

During data analysis, the two BCOT members with a prior history of conducting qualitative research, coding, and data analysis; a total of three Black women scholars in academia, including myself; and one allied academic Asian woman scholar read and re-read focus group transcripts, co-developed the codebook, and then identified and coded units of meaning by assigning labels and definitions to concepts related to the hospital birth planning, preparation, expectations, and experiences of thirty-six Black mothers and birthing people in Oakland and Los Angeles, California. BCOT was the only BWCBO that participated in the coding of focus group transcripts from June 2019 to August 2019 and the in-person PREM convening in August 2019 in Oakland. The second BWBCO, BWW, withdrew and disengaged from the study during the coding and PREM convening due to inappropriately delayed compensation from Stanford University for work completed from January 2019 to March 2019. After many conversations around economic injustice, structural racism, tokenism, exploitation, and extraction with the 2019 senior leadership of California's state PQC and the funder, a state-based healthcare-focused philanthropic foundation, Stanford University and California's PQC compensated both BCOT and BWW in late August 2019.

The original theoretical concepts identified during the pilot planning grant based on literature review and stakeholder interviews in 2018 included the DREEMS framework: **D**ignity, **R**espect, **E**quity, **EM**pathy, and **S**afety. The revised theoretical concepts, based on data from the 2019 focus groups, 2019 temporal-spatial mapping, and the 2018 World Health Organization (WHO) network strategic objectives to improve quality of care for maternal, newborn, and child through quality, equity, and dignity the following conceptual framework called MASQUERADE: **M**easuring **A**utonomy, **S**afety, **QU**ality, **E**quity, **R**esponsiveness, **A**ccountability, **D**ignity, and **E**mpathy. Initially, thirty-four codes or themes were developed, organized into two overarching themes: Birth planning, preparation, and expectation (11 codes) and birth experience (23 codes). Two additional themes were added by community researchers from the Oakland BWBCO, BCOT, that represented strategies to mitigate obstetric racism during hospital birth expectation or birth experience. These thirty-six codes were then organized into eight categories summarized as MASQUERADE, which represented the dual performance engaged by Black birthing people and the hospitals where they sought care: Black birthing people engaged in masquerade performance to survive their hospital treatment, and hospitals engaged in a masquerade thinking they are doing the right thing by providing care to ensure the fallacy "safe motherhood" when they are often actively engaged in harming Black birthing people.

Temporal-spatial mapping data were analyzed by reviewing the photographs of the wall spaces and sticky notes placed on the large posters on the wall spaces for the two groups in Oakland and the two groups in LA. The words, meanings, manifestation, and measurements for the existing eight terms selected by the research team and the new twenty-four terms identified by the study participants in Oakland (8) and LA (16) were extracted from the photos and sticky notes and stored and organized in an Excel file by the following eight temporal-spatial domains/phases of experience:

- Where Did Labor Begin?
- Getting to the Hospital
- Getting to the Labor and Delivery Floor
- Getting Registered/Checked In
- Going to Your Assigned Room and Giving Birth
- Getting Care and Support After Childbirth
- Going to the Postpartum Floor/Room
- Going Home/Hospital Discharge

The words, meanings, manifestations, and measurements for the eight existing terms and the new twenty-four terms across the above phases of experience were then compared to the MASQUERADE categories from the focus groups and considered in relationship to the seven dimensions of obstetric racism (Daviss 2018; Davis 2019; Davis 2020; and Davis 2021). Then, in an effort to maintain fidelity to an asset-based approach to uplifting the power, potential, and promise, not pathology, of Black bodies, Black births, and Black motherhood/parenthood, I made the decision to develop a conceptual framework that reflected the complex and dynamic acts of resistance and resilience in response to various types of anticipated and actual acts of oppression imposed on the lives and bodies of Black women, mothers, and birthing people during labor, birth, and postpartum in hospital settings. The deliberate selection and utilization of Leith Mullings' Sojourner syndrome as a quality improvement ethical standard and explanatory framework strategically counters the hypervisibility of Black women and people as voiceless and choiceless victims predicated to birthing death and dying. Second, Mullings' scholarship curates nuanced knowledge and insight into the various types of privilege, positionalities, pathways, and strategies that Black women and people utilize to exert or benefit from power when seeking to activate their autonomy and honor their truths (Scott 2021). As the lead researcher, I further organized the thirty-six codes into the conceptual framework of SACKRED birth; each letter represents one of six theorized domains of healthcare quality during childbirth hospitalization: **S**afety, **A**utonomy, **C**ommunication and Information exchange, **R**acism, **E**mpathy and Humanity, and **D**ignity in Blackness. Three additional domains were identified by community as pathways, strategies, and solutions to mitigate the onset, frequent, duration, and magnitude of obstetric racism during perinatal service provision in hospital settings: Accountability, Social Capital/Network & Kinship, and Holistic Care with the restoration of Black Midwifery Models of Care and Black Doula Support.

Based on focus group and temporal-spatial mapping data, the domain name, meaning, and measurements of six theorized domains of healthcare quality emerged as the SACKRED Birth model of hospital-based perinatal service evaluation in the following configuration:

- **S**afety and Accountability
- **A**utonomy and Social Capital/Network and Kinship
- **C**ommunication and Information Exchange
- **R**acism—anti-Black racism, gendered racism, and misogynoir
- **E**mpathy and Humanity
- **D**ignity in Blackness & Holistic Care

Strategies for maintaining rigor and reflexivity throughout analysis included ongoing re-reading of narratives, journaling, writing memos on individual excerpts, focus group dialogue, and six theorized quality domains, re-reading of Black feminist scholarship in anthropology, and frequent discussions with mentors in nursing, patient safety, and anthropology such as Audrey Lyndon, RN, PhD, FAAN, and Dána-Ain Davis, MPH, PhD (Charmaz 2006; Altman et al. 2019). Over the five years between data collection and group analysis, I spent the last four years focusing on how we do things in quality improvement and implementation science, how we desperately need to do things differently, how to adopt the spirit and praxis of Black feminist hermeneutic phenomenology, and how to be fully open and receptive to the hurts, harms, and hopes of Black mothers as they experience being, knowing, and living as a Black woman during childbirth hospitalization in a U.S. hospital given the historicity of their background (Crowther and Thomson 2023; Heidegger 2010). My primary goal was to better understand the lived experience of childbirth hospitalization as a Black woman and the invisible meanings of childbirth hospitalization that matter most to Black women and their given and chosen kin. Only then could I, as a dissident and recovering Black woman OBGYN and improvement and implementation scientist, better understand how to both interrogate the obstetric quality and safety of childbirth hospitalization and offer a new paradigm for measurement selection, evaluation, and monitoring strategies, and data analysis, interpretation, synthesis, triangulation, sovereignty, and dissemination. As a result of being transformed by staying open and attuned to the way of a Black feminist hermeneutic phenomenology, I noticed the role of kinship showing up across all six theorized domains as Black mothers leverage both given and chosen kin as sources and tools of protection and comfort. Thus, I dissociated kinship from autonomy and named kinship as a seventh theorized quality of care domain. Hence, SACRKED Birth includes the letter K.

To create initial working definitions of the hypothesized seven patient-identified quality domains in the SACKRED Birth model of care and identify existing scales pertinent to these domains, we undertook a systematic review of the existing literature using search terms related to the theoretical concepts and names of Black women authors across diverse disciplines. The list of theoretical concepts included: Black feminism, Black womanism, reproductive justice, obstetric racism, cultural humility, Sojourner syndrome, levels of racism (e.g., structural, institutional, interpersonal), gendered racism, and reproductive oppression and injustice. We reviewed close to 3700 articles. In developing the item pool, we identified thirty-five articles with metrics that had face validity for potential relevance to the PREM, which contained 1036 items and their source, domain, subdomain, and question text. During a two-day working group meeting held in Oakland in August 2019, the

PREM Team and BWCBOs came together to map these existing items onto the theoretical domains defined through the formative qualitative work. For each theoretical domain, group members reviewed existing items and offered suggestions for exclusion or inclusion. The item pool encompassed over 400 items represented by the surveys listed in the Databank.

By September 2019, California's PQC notified its Birth Equity team that there were no additional funds to support the compensation of BWCBOs and Black mothers and birthing people to participate in future cognitive pretesting (n = 25) and validation (n = 600) of a draft PREM. Likewise, the current approval by Stanford University's Human Subjects Review Board did not support subsequent and vital research to develop and implement the tools needed to elicit expert feedback and conduct cognitive interviewing and validation. Thus, California's PQC terminated all contracts and ended the PREM development with the above academic and community research collaborative of patient, community, and content experts.

Chapter 8 contains additional details about the subsequent PREM development and validation study, titled SACKRED Birth During COVID-19 study, and designed and led by me as the principal investigator. In chapter 8, I describe the specific methodology of the **P**atient-**R**eported **E**xperience **M**easure of **OB**stetric racism©, also known as the PREM-OB Scale® suite. Likewise, I also share key points from two publications about the novel validated instrument. As explained in chapter 8, six of the seven theorized domains in the SACKRED Birth quality framework were retained after evaluation of the survey items within each theorized domain using factor analysis and item response theory. The validated PREM-OB Scale® suite is organized into three independent yet related scales:

- Humanity, which consisted of thirty-one retained items from four subdomains: safety and accountability, autonomy, communication and information exchange, and empathy and humanity
- Kinship, twelve items
- Racism, nine items

Prior to chapter 8, I periodically describe the predictive utility of the PREM-OB Scale® suite in the absence of quantitative data generated from the completion of the online instrument by an eligible English-speaking Black-identifying mother or parent recently discharged from the hospital after childbirth. Study findings demonstrated that all three measures were significantly associated with separate non-retained items with strong face validity as measures of safety, mistreatment, or inequity. Higher agreement on items representing patient dissatisfaction with care (table 1.2, items S10, E66, D74, and R56) showed direct association with each IRT scaled score. In calculating the important difference in IRT scaled score for each scale in the suite, we chose four non-retained items consistent with national perinatal quality improvement goals as anchors to estimate important differences. Higher agreement on items representing optimum care and minimally acceptable care showed an inverse association with all three IRT scaled scores. For example, when a Black mother reports alignment between her care expectations and care experience across any phase of care (e.g., "I feel the hospital supported the experience I wanted [during labor] [during birth] [during postpartum]"), then the Black mother is 72 percent–78 percent less likely to experience racism (anti-Black racism or misogynoir); 83 percent–87 percent less likely to experience disrupted kinship, and 84 percent–89 percent less likely to experience dehumanizing care throughout labor, birth, and immediate postpartum (table 1.3).

For non-retained items that measure minimally acceptable care (e.g., "I felt the hospital staff were available and paid attention to me when I needed help"), a Black mother who agreed with the statement was 87 percent less likely to experience anti-Black racism and misogynoir, 90 percent less likely to experience disrupted kinship, and 97 percent less likely to experience dehumanizing care. All items displayed medium to large effect sizes when moving from strongly disagree/disagree to neutral or from neutral to agree/strongly agree. Higher agreement on items representing patient dissatisfaction with care (table 1.2, E66, D74, and R56) showed direct association with each IRT scaled score. For example, dissatisfaction non-retained items represented three categories of Black hospital birth experiences: (1) Black mothers who would seek out any Black birth worker to be part of their hospital if they could "re-do" their hospital birth; (2) Black mothers made to feel grateful for surviving birth despite having a poor quality experience; and (3) Black mothers who desired to have more Black mother-Black birthing person focused information and support about lactation and breast/chest/body-feeding. Any Black mother who strongly agreed or agreed with any of the dissatisfying care items was 2x to more than 8x more likely to experience harm across any of the three subtypes of obstetric racism, with the most egregious harm associated with the survival narrative, more than 8x more likely to experience dehumanizing care. Thus, the PREM-OB Scale® can be used as a predictive tool to estimate the overall experience of harm and quality of care based on subtype of obstetric racism, based on higher agreement with non-retained items that measure optimum care, minimally acceptable care, safety, mistreatment, care alignment, and cultural concordant care and support in the form of a person or information.

Table 1.2 Cumulative Proportional Odds Logistic Regression of Scale Scores on Representative Perinatal Quality improvement items, S10, E66, D74, and R56.

IRT scaled score	*I felt the hospital staff were available and paid attention to me when I needed help (S10) OR (95% CI)*[a,b]	*I would seek out a Black physician, midwife, doula, lactation educator, or nurse to be part of my hospital birth team, if I could re-do my 2020 hospital birth. (E66) OR (95% CI)a,b*	*The hospital made me feel that because my baby and I survived birth, my experiences in labor, birth, and postpartum did not matter. (D74) OR (95% CI)a,b*	*I wished I had more information and support about lactation, breastfeeding, or chest feeding that was specific to Black mothers and birthing people. (R56) OR (95% CI)a,*
Racism	0.13 (0.10–0.17)	2.84 (2.36–3.42)	6.43 (5.02–8.24)[c]	2.07 (1.73–2.47)
Kinship	0.10 (0.08–0.13)	3.03 (2.51–3.66)	5.60 (4.38–7.15)	2.59 (2.15–3.12)[c]
Humanity	0.03 (0.02–0.04)	2.89 (2.42–3.46)	8.36 (6.24–11.21)	2.33 (1.96–2.77)

[a] All P-values were statistically significant (<.0001).
[b] Probabilities modeled are accumulated over the lower Ordered Values (3-Strongly agree/Agree, 2-Neutral, 1-Disagree/Strongly disagree).
[c] Proportional Odds Assumption does not hold. For the four variables violating the proportionality assumption, if the ORs from the nonproportional odds model were within the 95 percent confidence interval of the proportional odds model, the OR (95 percent CI) from the proportional odds model were used.

Table 1.3 Cumulative Proportional Odds Logistic Regression of Scale Scores on Representative Perinatal Quality Improvement Items, Alignment between Expectation and Experience

Alignment between Expectation and Experience			
IRT SCALED SCORE	During labor OR (95% ci)[a,b]	**At birth** OR (95% ci)[a,b]	**Postpartum care** OR (95% ci)[a,b]
Racism	0.22 (0.18–0.27)	0.28 (0.23–0.34)	0.27 (0.22–0.33)[c]
Kinship	0.13 (0.10–0.17)	0.16 (0.12–0.21)	0.17 (0.13–0.22)
Humanity	0.11 (0.08–0.14)	0.16 (0.13–0.21)	0.16 (0.13–0.21)[c]

[a] All P-values were statistically significant (<.0001).
[b] Probabilities modeled are accumulated over the lower Ordered Values (3-Strongly agree/Agree, 2-Neutral, 1-Disagree/Strongly disagree).
[c] Proportional Odds Assumption does not hold. For the four variables violating the proportionality assumption, if the ORs from the nonproportional odds model were within the 95 percent confidence interval of the proportional odds model, the OR (95 percent CI) from the proportional odds model were used.

SACKRED Birth is a theoretical framework of guiding principles, as defined by me that shapes attitudes, values, intentions, skills, conditions, practices, and behaviors around Black Mamas and Black birth, birth care, birth spaces, birth work, and birth partners. SACRKED birth celebrates sexuality, sexual pleasure, and birth as affirming aspects of human life and development. SACRKED birth is a radical attitude toward human births, specifically Blackness, Black bodies, and Black births that regards all birth activities as fundamentally normal, healthy, spiritual, familial, magical, transformative, erotic, communal, emancipatory, and power activating. SACKRED birth encourages diverse and inclusive birth pleasure, practices, care, spaces, options, partners, communities, and experiences. The SACKRED birth movement advocates for safer, respectful, dignified, high-quality "participatory" birth care, conditions, experiences, and outcomes, and improved workforce diversification, development, sustainability, and restoration of Black Midwifery care and Black Doula support models as part of its campaign," (Scott 2018; Scott 2019a; Scott 2019b).

Chapter 2

Racism

Manifestations of Anti-Black Racism and Misogynoir

The daily denial of the role of racism, specifically anti-Black medical racism and anti-Black misogyny, or misogynoir, in the examination of Black women's perinatal deaths, reinforces the lie that race is a biological construct (Scott 2021; Scott and Davis 2021; Hardeman et al. 2020; Metzl and Roberts 2014; Roberts 2011). More importantly, racism denial in society (Jones 2000), in public health literature (Hardeman et al. 2018), and in obstetric quality and patient safety literature (Scott 2021) facilitates the creation and spread of mother blame narratives (McLemore 2018; Scott, Britton, and McLemore 2019). Essentially, mother blame permits professionals and their corresponding organizations in public health, medicine, nursing, epigenetics, medical risk and liability, quality, and patient safety to place the onus of disparate deaths, near deaths, and disabilities on the individual behaviors and individual choices of Black mothers (McLemore 2018; Scott, Britton, and McLemore 2019). Consequently, fundable research, improvement, implementation, and policy initiates focus exclusively on screening, surveillance, and control of "aberrant Black behavior" as solutions to save and protect Black children. By blaming individual choices and behaviors, instead of addressing the oppressive and inhumane structural, socioeconomic, and political conditions that shape Black mothers' options and opportunities to experience life, liberty, and the pursuit of happiness, then these very systems and structures never have to do better. According to Dr. Camara Jones, in her very compelling explanation of the levels of racism using the allegory of the gardener's tale in the 2000 peer-reviewed publication in the *American Journal of Public Health*, institutionalized racism is often evident as inaction in the face of need (Jones 2000). Based on the evidence as reported from 1900 to 2023, inaction to name racism (e.g., structural racism, institutional racism, interpersonal racism, internalized racism, gendered racism, obstetric racism) in the face of needing to explain persistently worsening racial inequalities, inequities, and injustices in experiencing life, liberty, and the pursuit of happiness through pregnancy and childbirth is, in fact, institutionalized racism.

Like the fathers of gynecology, the fathers of perinatal and maternal quality improvement assigned a higher value and visibility to the expressions and experiences of white male physicians or any person adjacent to and protective of whiteness, a practice called epistemic redlining. By establishing a hierarchy of knowing and knowledge that relegated Black women silent or silenced through diseases, disabilities, and deaths, systems and structures excluded or erased Black women's voices, intellectual thoughts, and activism through the support of philanthropy and funders (Lyndon et al. 2023; Lett et al. 2023; White VanGompel et al. 2022; Scott 2021; Scott and Davis 2021; Scott, Bray, and McLemore 2020). In resistance to and refusal of the silence and silencing of Black women as patients, community, and content experts, we invited Black mothers to reclaim the sound and movement of their mouths. We curated sacred spaces of connectedness and psychological safety, honoring Black women's innate worth as human beings. In holding sacred spaces for Black women to speak and the sound to be heard, received, recorded, transcribed, interpreted through a Black feminist hermeneutic phenomenology, remembered, and shared with informed consent feels like doing the work of God. The privilege and responsibility of translating stories into strategies to transform the obstetric quality and patient safety paradigm is spiritual work. Listening to and learning from and with thirty-seven Black women changed me in immeasurable ways. What these brilliant, bold, and beautiful Black women created stands as the first and only shared language and understanding of the meanings and measures of racism, specifically anti-Black medical racism and anti-Black misogyny, or misogynoir, during pregnancy, childbirth, and postpartum. The four most common meanings of racism during pregnancy, labor, birth, and postpartum included: (1) Perpetuation of an anti-Black racist stereotype about Black people that adversely impacts service, support, and care provision and utilization (anti-Black medical racism); (2) Perpetuation of an anti-Black misogynistic stereotype about Black women or Black motherhood that adversely impacts the provision of affirming care or utilization of care, services, and supports (anti-Black gender racism, or misogynoir); and (3) differential birth care, outcomes, and experiences based on differential access to and utilization of services and supports, including certified nurse midwives (in relation to hospital births) and doulas (particularly the Black and Brown birth workforce), and life-affirming versus life-negating state resources (e.g., Black Infant Health, Child Protective Services (CPS)).

Three specific scenarios or narratives of anti-Black medical racism and misogynoir dominated the individual responses and focus group dialogue. First, Black mothers and birthing people feared conforming to historical and contemporary stereotypes such as the "angry Black woman" or being labeled in patient sign-offs or the health record as "too demanding or difficult patient" if they persistently asked for help or clinical attention after initial and/or prolonged periods of clinical neglect, indifference, denial, dismissal, and/or delay. Subsequently, Black mothers and birthing people modified their behavior, attitude, language, or appearance to avoid any type of negative interaction or experience or other forms of retaliation (i.e., worsening care, involvement of hospital administration as a form of censorship or silencing, and punitive actions such as involvement of security, CPS, psychiatry/mental health, or police/law enforcement to facilitate the separation of the Black mother from her child, her partner, her mother, her community doula or midwife, or any other community support person without hospital affiliation or alignment). Second, Black mothers also discussed ways in which Black men or masculine presenting partners and loved ones modified their behavior, attitude, language, and/or appearance when wanting to appear more accepting to the white gaze, white authority, or any dominating figure on the hospital team in proximity to whiteness, particularly during periods of advocating for self, partner, and/or baby. The self-imposed transformations as well as code switching occurred as protective strategies to avoid conforming to the historical and contemporary stereotype of "Black brute" or "animal-like savage." Third, Black mothers expressed the fear of conforming to the narrative of "being a drug-seeker" reminiscent of the "historical crack epidemic" if they dared to ask for or eventually demand the initial, subsequent, or prolonged administration of general analgesic or opioid medications. The majority of the quality violations during pain (mis)management occur in the setting of Black suffering and inadequate pain control associated with labor contractions, rough handling of the Black body during a cesarean birth, and postoperative pain control after a cesarean birth during hospitalization. The details of the language, attitude, and behavior of hospital physicians and nurses represent a stark contrast to the contemporary opioid epidemic response, in the afterlife of slavery, crack crisis, and the War on Drugs campaign (Shachar et al. 2020; Associated Press, 2017). The contemporary response to the opioid epidemic includes an abundance of empathy, grace, humanity, dignity, and resources, including forgiveness and restoration, extended to a different group of mothers racialized as non-Black. Thus, Black mothers in pain for medically related and valid reasons avoid seeking help or clinical attention even after major abdominal surgery, such as a cesarean birth.

Black mothers in Oakland and Los Angeles feel that anti-Black medical racism and misogynoir show up in clinical & social interactions, communications, consent, decision-making, and documentation and dissemination of healthcare information in patient signoffs, patient handoffs, and electronic or paper health records. Anti-Black medical racism and misogynoir manifest in the following two ways: (1) Differential access to and utilization of birth resources, pain management options, visitation policies, senior staff for procedures, consent, refusal, and the four Ts: time, trust, truth, and transparency to make decisions (Birthing Cultural Rigor n.d.); and (2) Presence and proliferation of language, actions, and behaviors by hospital administrators, clinicians, and staff rooted in myths and misconceptions that Black people don't feel pain, have a higher threshold of pain, or exaggerate their pain, creating barriers and burdens to optimal clinical recognition, responsiveness, and resolution, and overall birth experience around pain (mis)management.

One of the dominant experiences of harm enacted through isolated or repeated violations of safety and accountability, autonomy (e.g., decisional, bodily, informational, care), communication and information exchange, empathy and humanity, and dignity in Blackness and holistic care was, is, and remains the (mis)management of Black pain and discomfort. Repeatedly, the evidence shows that failure to end Black "emotional, mental, cultural, or physical" suffering in the provision of obstetrics care is one of the most insidious and impactful tools to break the human spirit, individually and collectively. "Institutionalized racism is often evident as inaction in the face of need," Dr. Camara Jones, PhD, MH, MPH (Jones 2000). In my own attempts to understand how the lack of oversight, accountability, and justice toward the inhumane conditions of experiencing and navigating pregnancy, labor, childbirth, and postpartum while Black, I had to consider the motivations for ignoring Black suffering while creating Black suffering. And I was not the only one thinking about the motivations and justifications of inaction. When asking Black mothers why they believe hospital clinicians and staff treat them differently as Black women compared to the treatment of white women and act without any remorse, oversight, or accountability, one particular response from a Black mother in Los Angeles comes to mind. "You push out the baby, and then you go back on the fields, and you keep picking the cotton. I am in pain. But you are looking at me like I don't feel pain. I'm just being ignored. I'm talking, but nothing's coming out of my mouth." Her critical reflections of her own hospital experiences affirm and justify ethical, epistemological, and methodological approaches to examining atrocities of the U.S. maternal health systems and structures through histories that track along anti-Black racism and eugenics in the afterlife of slavery at the intersection of medical racism and obstetric violence, which is Davis' analytic and phenomenon that she first defined in an online publication in December 2018, obstetric racism (Davis 2018).

In the context of Black mothers exploring the motivations for the rise in forced inductions and forced cesarean births among Black mothers, and the widespread unmitigated dismissiveness and denials of Black suffering combined with the lack of motivation to end Black suffering involved in a spontaneous or forced birth by way of forced pregnancy in the afterlife of slavery and in a post-Dobbs world—this is obstetric racism—and capitalism is the driver. In describing one meaning of anti-Black racism in obstetrics care, Black mothers stated that racism is the perpetuation of a racist stereotype about Black people in general and Black mothers and birthing communities in particular, held by hospital clinicians, administrators, and staff, in public or private, that adversely impacts the provision of hospital-based perinatal services, care, and support in three key areas. The corresponding belief and behavior show up as hospital administrators, clinicians, and staff hold myths or misconceptions that Black people don't feel pain or have a higher threshold of pain, creating barriers and burdens to optimal clinical recognition, responsiveness, and resolution, and the overall birth experience. The dominant exemplars for demonstrating the presence and permeation of anti-Black medical racism in obstetrics focused on the (mis)management of pain during and after childbirth, particularly among Black mothers who utilized the epidural during a vaginal or abdominal (cesarean) birth.

> *Keisha:* Oh, yeah, my C-section was planned. But I had a really bad experience because they were expecting me to be okay with the pain because I had a couple [prior surgeries]. So, they read my history and were thinking that oh, let me just brush her off. Because I could feel it. Like my husband was there. I could feel it going so hard. And then after that I asked her a question. I said why were you going so hard on me. Because I could feel it like, you know. Oh, you had a lot of muscle. I said that's not an excuse. And also, with the pain killer, she was like oh—one of the nurses was like I don't think you need this. I said I'm in pain. Yeah, like now you thinking for me? Because they read that, you know, that I had surgery before that I'm used to the pain. I'm like I'm really in pain. Like I need something right now. So, yeah.
>
> *Jada:* You had a lot of muscle, come on.
>
> *Keisha:* Yes. I said there's no muscle there. It was all weight so. And then I asked her a question, but they always had an answer for something. (Two Black mothers in a focus group dialogue, March 2019, Oakland)

Through the speaker's story of a planned cesarean birth, in the context of a history of prior abdominal surgeries, one learns of the audacity of the obstetrician as the primary surgeon to dismiss their patient's explicit and expressed discomfort during a major abdominal surgery. To boldly ignore the patient in the presence of the husband in the operation room shows an even greater level of arrogance combined with a lack of fear of harming a Black mother. The primary surgeon's confidence and comfort in knowing the nurses and support staff would remain complicit in the violation of a patient's ethical and legal right to optimal pain management during a major abdominal surgery speaks volumes. When reflecting on the "white gaze of white" physicians and nurses "upon Black bodies, one wonders what is that thing that white" health professionals "force themselves to see or not see when they gaze upon the dark bodies" (Yancy 2016a; 2016b) of reproducing, birthing, or lactating Black people, particularly the same Black bodies within the context of pain and suffering. Again, Dr. Camara Jones asserted in her 2000 publication that inaction in the face of need is institutionalized racism (Jones 2000).

When Keisha persisted in her inquiries to the primary surgeon about the rough nature of the surgery, the primary surgeon identified characteristics of the Black mother's body (i.e., a lot of muscle or dense adhesion, scar tissue from prior surgeries) as the reason for suboptimal intraoperative pain management. In this situation, the racism escalated as the primary surgeon participated in the medical mob mentality of displacing blame and accountability for suboptimal pain control onto Black bodies. In this series of harmful clinical interactions, we see the manifestation of Davis' obstetric racism as a tool of anti-Black medical racism through the reproduction of neglect, intentional causing of pain, and medical abuse. The lack of recognition and response to persistent pain during and after a major abdominal surgery by the primary OB surgeon, anesthesiologist, and the entire OB surgical team of nurses and support staff represented neglect, dismissiveness, and disrespect when medical professionals ignore or dismiss a person's expressed need for reproductive help or care and/or treat them with disdain. Keisha shared additional details about the unsolicited banter and judgments imposed onto her condition that only further dismissed her suffering and diminished her valuation of being worthy of white benevolence during Black suffering. "Oh, you had a lot of muscle. I said that's not an excuse. And also, with the pain killer, she was like oh—one of the nurses was like I don't think you need this. I said I'm in pain."

When the primary OB surgeon and the postoperative or postpartum nurse fail to appropriately manage her pain, we must not ignore that the reason for a medical mob mentality in denying, dismissing, or diminishing patient-reported experiences of pain among Black people is grounded in racialized beliefs about pain immunity. Nearly twenty-four years ago, researchers conducted a study in an urban emergency department (ED) in Atlanta, Georgia that examined the independent effect of a patient's race (or the ED clinician's response to a patient's race in the provision of medical care) on utilization of pain medications while controlling for the effect of other factors (Todd et al. 2000). The researchers measured the proportion of Black patients versus white patients receiving ED pain medications. To reframe, the primary outcome was the extent to which ED physicians and nurses reproduce anti-Black medical racism in the recognition and response to Black and white patients presenting to the ED with new, isolated long-bone fractures over a 40-month period at an urban ED in a Black mecca such as Atlanta, Georgia. Data collection required blinding the physician and nurse reviewers from knowing the patient demographic information, including racialized identity and ethnicity. The physician recorded characteristics of the patients' injury and treatment, while the nurse recorded the administration of the analgesic, pain medication. Study findings revealed the urban city ED in Atlanta practiced anti-Black medical racism in pain management to Black patients experiencing long-bone fractures. The study sample consisted of 217 patients; 41.4 percent identified as individuals racialized as white and 58.5 percent identified as individuals racialized as Black. Yet, in a Black majority study sample, the ED physicians and nurses were significantly more likely to administer ED analgesics to white patients compared to Black patients (74 percent versus 57 percent, $p = 0.01$), despite similar or equal records of pain complaints in the medical record. The risk of the ED clinician's response for denying analgesic administration was 66 percent greater when the ED clinician responded to (or cared for) a Black patient compared to a white patient. The effect persisted even after controlling for other factors (Todd et al. 2000).

Immediately, "equal pain, separate care" comes to mind as the simplest meaning, measure, manifestation, and mechanism of anti-Black medical racism in facilitating unmitigated Black suffering in medical spaces. The lack of oversight and accountability in addressing the U.S. standard of "equal pain, separate care" based on these data is yet another example of institutionalized racism and inaction in the face of need. Ironically, at the time of writing this paragraph, U.S. Congressman and physician, Dr. Greg Murphy, MD, introduced the Embracing anti-Discrimination, Unbiased Curricula, and Advancing Truth in Education (EDUCATE) Act to ban race-based mandates at medical school and accrediting institutions on Mar 19, 2024. "American medical schools are the best in the world and no place for discrimination," stated Congressman, Dr. Murphy (Offices of U.S. Congressman Gregory F. Murphy, MD 2024). As a dissident and recovering OBGYN physician for 22 years and counting, who is firmly grounded in Black feminist ethics, ethos, and praxis, I agree with the last part: U.S. medical schools are no place for discrimination, especially if they are beneficiaries of any type or form of federal funds.

The discriminatory, specifically anti-Black medical racism, in the provision of care for patient expressions of pain extends beyond adult Black bodies. Fifteen years after the demonstration of equal pain, separate care by physicians and nurses in the ED in Atlanta (Todd et al. 2000), a different set of clinician scientists sought to address the longstanding history of equal pain, separate care in the ED by first considering the possibility of biases, including spectrum bias (Goyal et al. 2015). Given the disproportionate use of the ED as a primary source of health care for nonurgent care, among other reasons, the researchers justified the past evidence as racial and ethnic differences in ED use rather ED management, as minorities may be more likely to present to the ED for nonsurgical or less intense causes of abdominal pain. The assumptions and rationale for justifying equal pain, separate continue to displace the onus of suboptimal pain management, specifically the lack of motivation to end Black suffering, on individual "unfit" Black bodies and behaviors. To eliminate biases, the researchers decided to evaluate pain management of appendicitis. The motivation for this type of evaluation was based on two assumptions. First, appendicitis is the most common surgical cause of pain in the ED. Second, the provision of analgesic medication in the ED for appendicitis is accepted and supported as the standard of care. Thus, the researchers decided to examine racial differences (really, these are racial inequities and racial injustices in pain management, carryon) in the overall administration of general analgesia and opioid analgesic, after controlling for factors such as demographics, ethnicity, visits, and pain score among children aged twenty-one years or younger in the ED. The study sample consisted of nearly one million children diagnosed as having appendicitis. To reframe the meaning and significance of study findings, I use active voice, instead of passive voice, in data interpretation and dissemination. The use of active voice shifts the focus to examining the behaviors of ED teams in response to children's accounts of pain within the context of manifesting medical racism in the diagnosis of appendicitis and administration of analgesic medications (both general and opioid) (Goya et al. 2015)

The ED teams administrated any type of analgesic to about 60 percent of all children, with the ED teams administering more opioid analgesics to white children compared to Black children (43.1 percent versus 41.3 percent). When examining ED pain management based on children's pain scores and controlled for race and ethnicity, the ED teams were less likely to administer any analgesic to Black children with moderate pain from appendicitis compared to white children reporting equal pain. Similarly, the ED teams were less likely to administer opioid analgesics to Black children in severe pain compared to white children with equally severe pain. After controlling the effect of many factors, the researchers found no statistically significant differences in the overall rate of analgesic administration by race. On the contrary, the odds of administering opioid analgesic medication by the ED team to children in pain due to appendicitis is 80 percent lower if the ED teams care for a Black child in pain (Goyal et al. 2015).

Independent of ED "over or inappropriate" utilization by structurally marginalized and minoritized individuals and communities or ED management of pain for conditions deemed acceptable, the abundance of evidence is clear. Equal pain, separate care is pervasive throughout the U.S. health system, including the maternal health system. A Black mother from Oakland, Rhonda, shared her thoughts on the ubiquitous denial of Black women's testimonies of their pain particularly during childbirth:

> I think they automatically think like women of color—like not just women of color, but Black women, like oh, you're just trying to use the drug situation, and stuff like that. I think that's what it is; they automatically think we're just trying to get the drugs, you know what I mean, and this child birthing a joke. And they're like we're lying about our pain or something like that.

The ease with which any person indoctrinated into medicine or nursing, independent of race or gender, can willfully, boldly, and repeatedly ignore Black pain is a manifestation of Davis' obstetric racism (Davis 2018; Davis 2019; Davis 2020; Davis, Varner, and Dill 2021). When one or more individual health care professionals with state-issued licenses to practice nursing or medicine fail to appropriately manage pain, then three things can be true. One, the motivation is grounded in racist antebellum popular culture disseminated in many literature realms, including natural and social sciences for the promotion of domination through subordination and chattel slavery. Two, the acceptance of, and possibly, pleasure in the onset, duration, continuation, and exacerbation of Black suffering demonstrates an act of bodily terrorism, fueled by the absence of empathy for Black people's suffering, including emotional, cultural, and physical suffering. Three, the lack of internal motivation to alleviate or reduce Black suffering likely stems from implicit biases passed on since the antebellum period and from a lack of systemic or structural oversight and accountability within the hospital or state licensure agency. The brutality and inhumanity of public beatings to death and lynchings facilitated subjugation. The white gaze upon the Black reproducing body in pain within the context of power dynamics between a hospital physician or nurse and a Black female patient "replicates the history of whiteness as terror. The scene is one of spectacle. Gazing upon the despised and violated Black body is also a site of white racist pleasure, masochism, and dominance" (Yancy 2016a, 13). Therefore, widespread denials of Black discomfort and suffering maintain control and domination in the hierarchy of humanity. The perpetual denial of Black suffering is also a manifestation of medical abuse, as defined by Davis (Davis 2018; Davis 2019; Davis 2020). Medical abuse can occur when health care professionals engage in experimentation and/or repetitive behavior that serves to validate the clinician's self-worth and upholds their domination over the patient, with no regard for the patient's desires, experiences, or concerns.

In December 2019, months after the completion of the Oakland and Los Angeles focus groups in February and March 2019, respectively, researchers published a study evaluating racial and ethnic differences in postpartum pain scores, inpatient opioid administration, and discharge opioid prescriptions among women (Badreldin et al. 2019). To reframe, the researchers examined the pain management behavior of physicians and nurses at a single, high-volume tertiary care center from December 2015 to November 2019, in response to women's race. The three primary outcomes of interest included: (1) patient-reported postpartum pain scores at discharge (on a scale from 0 to 10); (2) inpatient opioid dosing during postpartum hospitalization; and (3) receipt of an opioid prescription at discharge. Researchers examined the association between race-ethnicity and the three primary outcomes among 9,900 eligible postpartum women using statistical methods beyond the scope of this chapter and book. Again, to reframe, the researchers used race-ethnicity as a proxy for exposure to medical racism, where the source of exposure is postpartum pain management by hospital physicians and nurses. The impact of exposure to postpartum pain management includes postpartum pain experiences of Hispanic, non-Hispanic Black, and non-Hispanic white women (Badreldin et al. 2019). By identifying non-Hispanic white women as the referent group for a phenomenon by which they benefit as patients in pain, independent of their knowledge, consent, or participation, the exposure is not medical racism. The correct exposure, when placing white women's pain as the standard expectation, experience, or expression of postpartum pain in comparison to Hispanic and Black women, is more accurately and precisely identified as white women's privilege in postpartum pain prevention, treatment, and mitigation. With an anti-bias, anti-racist, anti-oppression, anti-privilege, equity-focused, and humanistic reframing, one better appreciates how hospital management of pain in response to whiteness and white women's suffering protects, values, affirms, and reassures white women's privilege and comfort, at the cost of inaction toward Black suffering in the face of need, which is institutionalized racism (Jones 2000).

Compared to white women's experiences of postpartum pain, Hispanic (1.6x) and Black women (2.2x) were more likely to report pain scores of 5 or greater on a pain scale from 0 to 10 (Badreldin et al. 2019). Despite higher patient-reported experiences of pain among Hispanic and Black women, with both statistical and clinical significance, hospitals acted as a system to respond to evidence of pain by administering significantly fewer doses of morphine each day during postpartum hospitalization to Hispanic and Black women. Within the context of higher patient-reported pain scores and lower doses of opioid administration during hospitalization, the hospital system responded by distributing significantly lower numbers of opioid prescriptions to Hispanic and Black women upon discharge compared to white women. Joan is a Black mother who participated in the online meaningful community checking for alignment and/or revisions of the patient-identified quality domains for SACKRED Birth, under the Racism domain. She shared her knowledge of white denial of Black suffering in the action of need and subsequent bodily terrorism against a collective of Black reproducing bodies, including her cousin.

> Yeah, it really just pisses me off. Like I have watched a lot of videos and then, like I said I've heard a lot of feedback from different moms as far as them acting out because of pain and literally been labeled as crazy and more like when you're alone. For instance, I have a cousin who actually had a baby in Alexandria and she didn't have any medicine and they were just yelling, you know, she was screaming and they assumed that she was crazy and she was just giving this feedback because she was alone out there. She felt like nobody had her back and just because you're letting them know that you're in pain and they're telling you that, "Oh, it's not that bad," you're supposed to just agree with them. Even with me, I had a good experience but I believe this type of stuff happens a lot because doctors have even admitted to the same that they believe that we exaggerate our pain and for you to say that just because of race or what we've been through, because they automatically look at the chart. They're looking at our charts when we come in so they're going based off of what—they've already stereotyped us, so this type of stuff just upsets me.

What motivates an entire hospital system to conspire, independent of intention or collective planning, to protect, save, and soothe white women and prioritize white women's discomfort, even in the face of statistically and clinically greater need among Black women? According to Accapadi in their essay titled "When White Women Cry: How White Women's Tears Oppress Women of Color," they assert that white women navigate male privilege at the intersection of their race and gender, where one socially constructed identity is privileged, as a white person, and the other identity is oppressed, as a woman (Accapadi 2007). Accapadi also cites the work of Palmer, who explains that one challenge for white women is that acceptance of their privilege is based on accepting the norms and narratives of goodness. And that white women's goodness is articulated as powerlessness that informs the nature of white womanhood. Within these constructs that support operating systems and structures of power and control, "male privilege positions the meanings, manifestations and mechanisms of womanhood while whiteness or white privilege situates a white woman's existence as the universal standard of womanhood through histories of various forms racial, sexual, reproductive and perinatal injustices" (Accapadi 2007).

Additionally, as Palmer states, "the problem for white women is that their privilege is based on accepting the image of goodness, which is powerlessness" (Palmer 1994, 170). This powerlessness informs the nature of white womanhood. Put in simple terms, male privilege positions the nature of womanhood, while white privilege through history positions a white woman's reality as the universal norm of womanhood, leaving a woman of color defined by two layers of oppression (Palmer 1994; Accadia 2007; Collins 1996; Crenshaw 1991). According to Accapadi's essay, white women and individuals with a one up/one down identity must recognize when their privileged identity is the operating norm. For white women, we invite them to consider power, privilege, protection, and promotion tethered to their whiteness. Similarly, Black men are invited to consider when and how power, privilege, protection, and promotion come with their maleness (Accapadi 2007; Crenshaw 1991). What sets white women apart from marginalized and minoritized groups is that these operating systems and structures of power and control permit white women to freely move between being a white person or a woman. At the intersection of both, society permits white women to exhibit *helplessness* without taking on the helplessness of the entire racialized group of all white people and *powerful* by taking on the positionality of power as any white individual (Accapadi 2007).

In the provision of obstetric care in the U.S., the standard of humanity protects, privileges, and prioritizes white women. In 1826, a physician named Dr. Philip Tidyman wrote about the peculiar physical characteristics of enslaved Black people or Africans in the South, compared to Europeans, in "A Sketch of the Most Remarkable Diseases of the Negroes of Southern States." Tidyman, like other white antebellum physicians, conducted inhumane experiments and concluded that Africans were stronger than whites when it came to surgeries. White physician scientists and surgeons concluded that Africans had a greater tolerance for pain. Another Louisiana physician peer of Tidyman, Samuel Cartwright, shaped racist ideology and medical understanding on the differences between Africans and whites, including his self-proclaimed calling to justify slavery as the only appropriate condition for the Negro race (Bankole 1998). In the focus group dialogue between myself and LaToya, a Black mother in Oakland, she shares an account of severe physical pain during the intravenous (IV) administration of an antibiotic, penicillin, as a form of prophylaxis against infection by Group B Streptococci (GBS) in a newborn during birth, if GBS is found in the urine or vulvovaginal-rectal culture of the pregnant individual. This critique in the quality of care focuses less on the indication for IV antibiotics and more on the (mis)management of her pain.

> *LaToya:* I agree 100 percent. I had a shift change. When my water broke on the 2nd. I didn't have her until the 3rd. And I actually had her two weeks early. So, on the 31st I had an appointment for the infection check where they just make sure you don't have that infection or whatever. Yeah, so since I ended up having her on the 2nd, they didn't get my results back. So, they had to give me antibiotics just in case, you know, they handled her. Because I didn't have it, they didn't

have to give her but they gave me antibiotics. So, the [antibiotic] medicine they gave me. But it was the most excruciating—I had a bad reaction. It was the worse pain ever. It was worse than my contractions. It made me want to cut my arm off. I would just start crying. I couldn't even take it. And I explained that to them and they cut the medicine down to where they were giving me smaller doses. Now when the shift changed, the lady told me before she left [she] let them know do not up your dose because you're having a bad reaction to this antibiotic. As soon as the lady came in, I told her immediately because that pain was just unbearable. And she still upped the dose. It made me want to choke her. I just couldn't believe that you're making me go through this pain. It was the worse pain. It was worse than labor. I'd rather take the contractions for another 24 hours than go through that pain. And she still upped the medicine.

Dr. Scott: Were you able to tell anyone other than her that she wasn't following what the prior nurse did?

LaToya: No.

Dr. Scott: Okay. Got it. Along those lines, and I know, but I want you to say it for our person who's listening [the transcriber]. Do you feel that your voice was heard?

LaToya: No. I told her and she still did it.

Because penicillin is thicker in consistency than normal saline, the patient may experience an injection site rejection (not to be confused or conflated with an allergic reaction), which may include any one of the following symptoms or signs: pain, swelling, bruising, skin changes, or a hard lump where the medicine was injected. From the patient's perspective, the patient may report increasing pain. Possible responses to mitigate the pain for the nurse include slowing down the infusion rate (while keeping the dose the same), applying a compress, or possibly stopping the infusion to take a break, depending on extenuating clinical circumstances, such as proximity to birth of the newborn. In the current scenario, LaToya explains in detail the agony and severity of her pain and the mitigation steps taken by her first nurse to reduce her suffering. Shift changes represent deal breakers in the pursuit of high-quality, safe, equitable, and culturally affirming care. Within the confines of her assigned quarters during childbirth hospitalization, LaToya initiated a series of steps to shield herself from future harm and to maintain her suffering at a minimum. Racial reconnaissance describes the Herculean efforts made by Black women to avoid or mitigate racist encounters, including being hypervigilant about procedures (Davis 2019; Davis 2020). Prior to change of shift, LaToya obtained confirmation from the departing nurse that the patient handoff to the new nurse would include both awareness and acceptance of the problem (e.g.,

Black suffering via injection site reaction) and solution (e.g., lower infusion rate). Upon the new nurse's immediate arrival, LaToya spoke up about the problem and agreed to a successful solution that involved lowering the infusion, as mutually agreed upon by LaToya and the former nurse. Instead, the new nurse brazenly dismissed LaToya's suffering and proceeded to increase the infusion, knowing her action would result in greater Black pain and suffering in a Black reproducing body.

One must then consider the origins of sadist tendencies and practices in the health care industry and in individual health care professionals, particularly physicians and nurses in obstetrics and perinatology. Further examination of antebellum popular culture created by pro-slavery intellectuals, who simultaneously adorned themselves in white coats in the role of physicians and surgeons, revealed subordination and dehumanization of enslaved Black women. In 2001, Black feminist scholar Ruppe Simms argued that slave owners shaped the construction of three key controlling images across several literary realms for the purpose of mobilizing their domination of plantation society (Simms 2001). For the purposes of this chapter, I will focus on one controlling image that slave owners applied to enslaved African women, the mule. Re-imagining African women as "insensible brutes and subhuman beasts, only to be valued for her labor," authenticates the extraction, exploitation, and experimentation of enslaved Black women by slave masters, overseers, speculators, auctioneers, breeders, and any men who profited from chattel slavery and plantation colonialism (Simms 2001, 883). In 1866, a pro-slavery and anti-abolitionist scientist, known as Reade, wrote, "The women of Africa are very inferior. Their very virtues, with their affections and their industry, are those of well-trained domestic animals" (Simms 2001, 886). The reconstruction of enslaved Black women's being and existence as subhuman and beastlike justified the horrific beatings, forced labor, and every imaginable inhumane and atrocious action enacted on, with, in, and through Black reproducing bodies.

With the topology of obstetric racism introduced first by Davis in 2018, we now possess a living bridge between the histories of anti-Black racism and eugenics and the contemporary ideologies, images, and practices of U.S. obstetrics and gynecology (Davis 2018). The postpartum and postoperative pain management studies offer such meaningfully overt evidence of the manifestations of obstetric racism, as neglect, dismissiveness, and disrespect, intentionally causing pain, and medical abuse, and evidence of the manifestations of institutionalized racism, as inaction to ameliorate Black suffering in the face of need. A second study published in 2022 examined racial/ethnic differences in postoperative pain experiences and opioid medication use within the first twenty-four hours after a cesarean birth at a single center from January 2016 to December 2017 (Poehlmann et al. 2022). The sample included 2, 228 patients whose pregnancies culminated in a cesarean birth. To reframe, the study examined postoperative pain management within the first twenty hours after a cesarean birth based on the hospital clinician's response to a patient's race. Similar to Badreldin et al. in 2019, the outcomes included the average pain score of all documented patient-reported experiences of pain (from 0 to 10) during the first twenty-four hours post-cesarean birth and oral morphine equivalents used in the first 24 hours post-delivery. When contextualizing the study design, results, conclusions, and implications within the context of antebellum pro-slavery and anti-abolitionist physician and scientist-centric ideologies, researchers used race-ethnicity as a proxy for exposure to systemic and structural power to protect, privilege, and prioritize white women's whiteness (power), helplessness (gender), and humanity (permission to be both). By identifying non-Hispanic white women as the referent group, the more accurate and precise exposure is white women's privilege in postoperative pain prevention, treatment, and mitigation. Study findings from Badreldin et al. 2019 and Poehlmann et al. 2022 provide evidence of inaction as institutionalized racism (Jones 2020) during postoperative pain management in obstetrics. Study findings demonstrated hospital practices that maintained fidelity to antebellum ideologies that relegated Black lives to subhuman and brute beasts, particularly Black women to the status of a mule. Maintaining fidelity to antebellum pro-slavery ideologies looks like non-Hispanic Black mothers and gender-expansive individuals reporting significantly higher pain scores than white women after a cesarean birth, while the hospital team administered equal amounts of morphine. The equal pain, separate care ideology and practices dominate obstetrics culture, care, communications, and documentation and dissemination of information in patient handoffs, patient sign-outs, and electronic or paper health records. When controlling for patient-reported pain scores, hospital teams administrated significantly lower doses of morphine to non-Hispanic Black patients (who reported significantly higher levels of pain) and Non-Hispanic Asians (who reported similar pain scores), compared to white women (Poehlmann et al. 2022).

Intentionally causing pain, one of six dimensions of obstetric racism, describes actions and decisions made by hospital clinicians and staff to refuse to address and alleviate Black physical suffering (Davis 2018; Davis 2019; Davis 2020). When a Black mother repeatedly expresses any form of pain, discomfort, or dis-ease in her body, and no one on the hospital team affirms her feelings, thoughts, and experiences in her own body, then the hospital chooses violence in the form of neglect, dismissiveness, and disrespect. When a Black mother repeatedly expresses her concerns to multiple members of the hospital team, including the nurses and attending physician, and they dismiss or diminish her account of her own experiences in her own body, then the hospital chooses violence in the form of testimonial injustice

(Fricker 2007; Scott 2021; Lyndon et al. 2023). Increasing evidence in the form of published qualitative and quantitative studies, including Op-eds, blogs, podcasts, and archival data, points to widespread practices throughout the U.S. medical specialty of obstetrics and gynecology that render most, if not all, Black women as incapable of making sense of their own experiences, and of having their own experiences believed and understood by others. Such actions are the very definition of hermeneutical injustice (Fricker 2007; Scott 2021; Lyndon et al. 2023). The experimentation and/or repetitive behaviors that reproduce hospital acts of obstetric racism, such as failing to alleviate Black physical suffering (intentionally causing pain), serve as mechanisms of action that reinforce the hierarchy of value and power in obstetrics, situating the clinician's worth above the Black reproducing body and upholding domination over the patient and her body, which Davis defined as medical abuse.

> *Tasha:* So, I felt like they wasn't hearing me, especially in the operating room. So, I thought why they were doing it and why then—like the room was cold but they were pushing to make—keep pushing to, you know, get the baby out. So, they were pushing me and pushing me. All of that I like really felt sick, light-headed, the room started spinning. I was like throwing up. And I kept telling her I feel sick, I feel sick, I feel sick. He put a vomit had thing up. And then, you know, they were like oh, no one ever feels sick. Like how could you be feeling sick. And I'm telling her like it's, you know, because it's a nurse by here. And whoever you have in the room is over here. And so, I'm telling the nurse who was holding my hand is that I feel sick, I feel sick, I feel sick. Like wake me up or lift me up, give me that thing. She wasn't giving nothing. She said no. She was like no one ever complains about feeling sick. You're the first one ever. I've never heard that in all my years of working. And I'm like but I feel sick. I feel real sick. The room was spinning. And then like I had to tell myself like to just close my eyes and try to breathe. But I just couldn't. And then all of a sudden, the throw up came up. And, of course, that was a whole big old thing. And I'm like I told you. I made sure of it this way. Admit it. She, by the way, was mad but I'm like I told you. And she told me like after it was over—after the baby came out, they put me in a room and I was trying to breast feed her. And they said—and I'm telling her like my whole upper region is numb. Everything—my neck. I just felt numb. And she told me like oh, you're not supposed to be feeling that. Nobody can be feeling that. Your supposed to numb from this, you know, from the abdomen all the way down. And she was like if anything your feet would be numb and this and that. And I'm telling her like my breast feels numb. They was tingling and stuff was going on. And she was just like you can't be numb up there. And I said I am. I don't feel the baby sucking. Like she's sucking, I can hear her.
>
> *Dr. Scott:* You could see her, yeah.

Tasha: But I couldn't feel her because it was just, I felt like all the nerves, I was just tingling. I just remember it was tingling.

Dr. Scott: So, what was her response?

Tasha: Her response was you couldn't be numb. She said you couldn't be numb

Dr Scott: Did anything happen as a follow up or they just basically dismissed what you were saying.

Tasha: No, she dismissed it and it was no like follow up. When the physician came to check on me, I did tell him that I was feeling numb. And it was like okay, well give it about an hour or two and if it doesn't get better then tell your nurse again. And I was like okay. But it did go away the next day. But -

Jada: That's a long time.

Tasha: —still—right. I was just scared because, you know, you have to lactate and I'm like am I having an allergic reaction or. You know, I wasn't feeling no itchiness. It was just constantly tingle, tingle, tingle, tingle. But it was a painful tingle. It was like a hurt tingle.

Dr Scott: And it was all over?

Tasha: Just from the neck down here to my breasts. Like I wasn't feeling nothing down here.

Dr. Scott: So, you had no acknowledgement and no real response to what you're saying. Just dismissing you?

Tasha: Yeah.

Imagine the psychological terror of experiencing a myriad of unexpected, unexplained, and unresolved symptoms in one's body, only to be told by the person licensed, compensated, and assigned to one's care that no other human has ever reported the quality and severity of pain in their entire career as a health care professional. The nurse demonstrates a complete absence of empathy, takes no action to alleviate Tasha's suffering, and even informs Tasha that none of her bodily experiences are real. The only way to dissociate from reality and behave in a cruel manner is to believe that Black women are undeserving of care, tenderness, and compassion because one believes Black women are indeed the mules of the world (Simms 2001). Licensed health care professionals practicing in the field of obstetrics behave in a manner designed to reinforce antebellum ideologies that asserted, with racist science, that Black women, men, boys, girls, and gender-expansive adults and children are subhuman, wild animals, fit only for the role and conditions of chattel slavery.

Tasha continues to share her reflections about the totality of her hospital birth experience in Oakland.

> For me, I think that during my—well, during the stay there was I had a high fever, and there's so many people in there, and [I] just don't think they wanted to hear me. Like I would be lying in bed and I'm sick—high fever. They'll be conversing with their own selves instead of like hey, I'm over here. But I really didn't have the strength to—I was sick probably before that, having a really, really bad sickness. Sick probably before that so, I didn't have the strength to even be yelling at ya'll. You know what I mean. They really, like I said, they wasn't attentive to me. They weren't like trying to see what I wanted, how you wanted. And, like I said, with the C-section it was like okay, you need a C-section. And when I get to ask a question—yes, you definitely need it. It wasn't really—like I found out that the—supposedly the baby's umbilical cord was wrapped around on the way to the room. Like on the way there. Like I don't understand how they get away with that. But, you know, certain stuff like that.

Tasha raises an important issue about the lack of systemic and structural oversight and accountability. Oversight in obstetrics requires acceptance of the responsibility for monitoring the actions of all hospital administrators, clinicians, and support staff involved in the health services design, provision, evaluation, and training. Accountability in obstetrics requires acceptance of the responsibility to uphold hospital administrators, clinicians, and support staff to a standard of actions, behaviors, and language that promote safety for all, not safety for a select few individuals at the top of the hierarchy of human life. Thus, evidence of inaction in the face of obstetric racism is the epitome of institutionalized racism (Jones 2000). One might even argue inaction in the presence of obstetric racism occurs due to a lack of systemic, structural, and disciplinary oversight and accountability, as explained by Angie, a Black mother in Oakland.

> *Angie:* From what I hear from not just you ladies but also my other friends and stuff there's just no accountability. People can just say whatever as an explanation and know that they're not going to get in trouble or reported. And I also heard people say like well Black people don't complain. Like they don't—
>
> *Dominique:* Well that's just a lie.
>
> *Angie:*—report it. There's no consequence to complaining in the moment. You can complain and be loud or whatever but that's ultimately there's no consequence. Like they're not going to lose their job, they're not going to be reprimanded, it's not going to go in their permanent file. And that is the issue, that we are known to not do that. And I only had one issue my entire experience and it was because the girl that was coming in for the new shift had a lot of perfume

> on and it was like a body spray. And that was like a no for my entire pregnancy. And I just knew I wasn't going to be able to get through the next however many hours with her. So, I just politely told the lady before her like that is not going to work for me. And so, she went to just tell her like oh, hey, you know, we're going to have someone else come in instead of you because she can smell your perfume. It's really strong. And the girl like went off, she was like really pissed off and really unprofessional. And when her dad [the father of Lisa's baby] came, he was like, well did you report her. And I was like no, like I'm not going to report. That's a Black girl. You know, like I'm not going to report her. Like she got a good job. I wasn't about to say—and he was like that's the problem, she wouldn't have done that if you were a White patient. Why would she have not done that if you were a White patient? And I'm like, I don't know. And he was like, if you were White, she would have known you would have reported her. And so, I was like oh, never thought of it that way. But that's probably true. She probably went off because she knew that I wasn't going to do nothing.

Angie's reflections on the difference between complaining and reporting inspired me at that moment to include accountability as one of the patient-identified quality care domains of birthing while Black. How can safety be achieved without built-in oversight and accountability in naming, defining, measuring, and monitoring violations committed against Black mothers and birthing people with compensated community participation and partnership? Her initial critique sparked an immediate rejection by a peer in the focus group, Dominique. Then Angie carefully explained the various levers at play that determine whether or not to submit a formal complaint to the hospital, in an effort to report harmful behavior during the provision of care. I began to wonder about the tension in filing a formal grievance against an obstetrician and nurse in labor and delivery, the reconciliation with power relations, dynamics, and differentials between a Black mother and the perpetrator. What happens when the perpetrator of obstetric racism and institutionalized racism is a Black hospital clinician or staff member? Angie's expressed concern for not wanting to threaten the job security of a Black nurse demonstrates an internalization of self-worth beneath that of the Black nurse, where the victim, or person harmed, chooses the comfort and well-being of the violator. When, in fact, both the Black nurse, as a perpetrator of obstetric racism and institutionalized racism, and Angie, as a survivor of harm, behave in ways that reinforce antebellum anti-Black racist and anti-Black misogynistic ideologies that deny Black women's innate worth, or dignity, and therefore Black women's humanity, guaranteeing assurances to unalienable rights including life, liberty, and the pursuit of happiness. At the same, Angie's Black male partner offered a different perspective, shedding more insights into the widespread commitment to protecting, privileging, and prioritizing white women's dignity and humanity, including the active role white women play in maintaining white heteropatriarchal supremacy through the weaponization of white tears (e.g., reporting any form of discomfort, whether valid or not) (Accapadi 2007).

Maintaining fidelity to pro-slavery and anti-abolitionist antebellum norms justifies inaction to obstetric racism from all involved, the survivor, the perpetrator, the bystanders, and the institutional, structural, and political structures and systems operating inside and outside of the hospital. Likewise, Black women and people remain fully aware of the grave consequences for initiating action or mobilizing a series of actions to prevent or mitigate harms against Black women and people, as highlighted in the Oakland focus group dialogue between Destiny, Jada, Tiffany, and Ayana.

Destiny: And so, I think we as Black women get labeled for when we do speak up. When we speak up, they feel like well that attitude and anger or, you know, whatever. And it's also it's like the nurse or whoever could say, oh, she had an attitude, or she could make this up. And, you know, and it may not be what happened, or they can, you know, but they'll make it look like that. Oh, she had an attitude, she was just defiant or, you know, she wouldn't let me do anything. So, even though we speak up it's not going to be taken seriously because we have that stereotype of being like attitude or, you know, angry. That's what I'm looking for, yeah.

Jada: And angry without reason.

Tiffany: Yeah.

Destiny: And that's the stereotype, is that we're just angry. Or we should have done it a different way. But if a White person was to do it the same way we did it, it wouldn't be perceived that way.

Ayana: Yeah, it wouldn't be—yeah.

The breaking point for many Black women is reaching that threshold of one too many dismissive, disrespectful, degrading, and dehumanizing words or actions done for the purpose of rendering Black women incapable of saving or protecting themselves. Health reporter, Margo Snipe, at Capital B News published an online piece in 2022, titled "Clinicians Dismiss Black Women's Pain. The Consequences Are Dire" with the following headline. "Black patients are significantly less likely to receive adequate treatment. Often, they're left in agony."(Snipe 2022). And I would add "and angry." Snipe shares a series of stories of Black women, in their own voices, detailing a "persistent pattern of dismissal" of Black pain (Snipe 2022, 2). One story that resonated with me and affirmed the stories of Black mothers in Oakland was

Linda Shaw's narrative. When asked to rate her pain, she felt the 0 to 10 scale limited the magnitude of her pain. Thus, she reported the number twenty as a more accurate evaluation of her pain. Of course, the physicians and nurses humiliated her with their responses, "they'd smirk" (Snipe 2022, 3) and then disregarded her word. "It is very dehumanizing," Shaw said, before pausing and letting out a heavy sigh. "It makes you feel invisible. It makes you feel less than, and to be quite honest, after a while, you get mad" (Snipe 2022, 3).

Once again, the physicians and nurses failed to believe a Black woman's own account of her bodily experiences, committing yet another act of testimonial injustice at the individual level and hermeneutical injustice at the community level (Fricker 2007; Scott 2021; Lyndon et al. 2023). Naturally, the attempt to erase one's existence and exclude one's testimony as truth sometimes feels worse than the physical suffering. One's mind and spirit now hurt at one and the same time. Thus, the ensuing rage that Black women then feel and express needs a place to softly land, to be embraced and addressed in the most gracious, tender, affirming, empathetic, and humane way. Instead, when Black women respond to hospital acts of obstetric racism or to inaction in the face of obstetric racism, which is institutionalized racism (Jones 2020), with rage first, then various systems and structures of domination organize a series of calculated actions to destroy one's credibility and integrity. The focus shifts from addressing acts of obstetric racism and inaction to obstetric racism to sabotaging, silencing, and subduing the inappropriate, loud, scary, unstable, wild, and angry Black woman, as discussed in an ongoing conversation in Oakland between Black mothers, Ayana and Jada.

> *Ayana:* I think there just needs to be more understanding and not just think of us as like just that we're angry or just overexaggerating like—
>
> *Jada:* Yes.
>
> *Ayana:*—like they need to—
>
> *Jada:* Listen.
>
> *Ayana:* Yeah, and bond with us how they would want somebody to bond with their daughter or with someone in their family because they just come in and they're like, oh, no, you're fine, oh, this is typical, oh, this is normal, like you don't know that, this is my pregnancy, I'm experiencing this, not you.

White heteropatriarchal supremacy only makes room for white women's humanity to occupy the duality of helplessness as women and privilege as white people. White women's tears can catalyze a white mob to search for, subdue, and then beat a Black man or Black boy to death. When Black women garner the courage, confidence, both, or neither to name their perpetrator of obstetric racism within hospital systems and structures, then the fight turns to defending your character and protecting your reputation, instead of gathering evidence to support manifestations of obstetric racism and institutionalized racism. One recalls the boldness, clarity, confidence, wisdom, and guidance of the late Toni Morrison,

> The function, the very serious function of racism is distraction. It keeps you from doing your work. It keeps you explaining, over and over again, your reason for being. Somebody says you have no language and you spend twenty years proving that you do. Somebody says your head isn't shaped properly so you have scientists working on the fact that it is. Somebody says you have no art, so you dredge that up. Somebody says you have no kingdoms, so you dredge that up. None of this is necessary. There will always be one more thing. (Forna 2022, 1)

The function of racism is distraction. Racism causes a Black husband to advise his Black pregnant wife to wear her wedding ring as a mitigation strategy against discriminatory treatment in response to the single Black mother or welfare queen trope. Racism distracts hospital clinicians and staff from asking about the expectations and aspirations for pregnancy, labor, birth, postpartum, infant feeding, and parenting as a Black woman. Instead, hospital clinicians and staff focus on inquiring about the paternity status of each child and the whereabouts of the "baby daddy." Inaction to eliminate racist distractions allows for generations of physicians and nurses to focus on gathering information to reinforce archetypes grounded in misogynoir, such as mammy and Jezebel, and not to practice curiosity, compassion, creativity, and critical thinking to provide opportunities, options, and optimal conditions for a Black mother to obtain the highest level of health and wellness. Consider the experience of Chantelle, a married Black mother in Oakland, whose husband focused on strategies and solutions to combat harmful assumptions and discriminatory behaviors in response to the Black single mother or "baby mama" trope.

> It's just like about the lack of support. Because at first, I was judged that, you know, [like] I'm about to be a single mom. Like constantly my husband had to tell me to wear your ring. You're not a kid. . . you already have that nasty look from your own kind, so I don't know. But it's something like that.

Existing obstetric quality and patient safety leadership and initiatives usually dismiss or ignore historical contextualization of contemporary attitudes, actions, behaviors, and language, including cognitive processes, in the provision of sexual, reproductive, and perinatal health services and supports to U.S. Black women. Four centralizing stereotypes emerged in the early nineteenth century that are specific to Black women, originating from the institutionalization of slavery and sexual & reproductive exploitation, experimentation, extraction, and erasure of the virtue and value of Black women as human beings (Childs 2005; Collins 2004; Wyatt 1997). In the literature exploring the sexuality, sexual agency, and behaviors of Black women and girls, four stereotypical roles are characterized; Mammy, Sapphire, Jezebel, and Superwoman (Abdullah 1998; Greene 1995; Greene 1994; Mitchell and Herring 1998; Thomas, Witherspoon, and Speight 2004; West 2012). Prior evidence demonstrates that these four stereotypes of Black women hold unsubstantiated expectations and assumptions about Black women's and girls' sexual expressions. The four stereotypes also place Black women and girls into social categories that limit their agency, autonomy, and functioning. The types and patterns of quality and patient safety violations occurring during childbirth hospitalization that disproportionately impact Black women require quality and patient safety researchers to explore how these four stereotypes impact the cognitive processes of hospital administrators, clinicians, and support staff. Obstetric quality and patient safety researchers and professionals need to also consider the presence, influence, and impact of the four stereotypes in clinical interactions, communications, consent, decision-making, and documentation and dissemination of health information in patient hand-offs, patient sign-outs, and electronic or paper health records. The brief definitions of the four dominant stereotypes include: (1) Mammy characterizes a self-sacrificing, obese, asexual, dark-skinned Black woman with broad features who worked in the master's house, usually as a nanny, housekeeper, and cook (Greene 1995; Greene 1994; Mitchell and Herring 1998; Thomas, Witherspoon, and Speight 2004; West 2012); (2) Jezebel characterizes a seductive, manipulative, hypersexual, animalistic, and exotic Black woman, unable to control her sex drive (Mitchell and Herring 1998; West 2012); (3) Superwoman characterizes a strong, tough, resilient, self-sufficient Black woman, who views asking for help as weak and vulnerable, with expectations to provide for, serve, and support others (Shorter-Gooden and Jackson 2000; Greene 1994; Green 1995; Mitchell and Herring 1998); and (4) Sapphire, a character from the Amos and Andy radio and television show from the 1940s and 1950s, represents a nagging, emasculating, shrill, loud, argumentative Black woman, known as a master of verbal assaults (Mitchell and Herring 1998; West 2012). Black mothers in the Oakland focus group shared their experiences of feeling judged by hospital clinicians and staff about their pregnancy and parenting choices as Black women based on discriminatory assumptions at the intersection of race, gender, age, marital status, and pregnancy status.

> *Imani:* I feel that way too because they do judge you. I feel that I want it to be a reality that we're not just young, single, Black parents. Because my question from three different nurses was oh, is this child by the same father. I didn't

understand why they kept asking me. My daughter's [paternal] grandmother kept saying to me oh, it's just not common in these days [birthing and building a family one man, the biological father] so you shouldn't be offended. But I was offended. Because even if my daughter did have a different dad it's none of your business.

Tiffany: Hey, right.

Imani: But now I feel that if I would have answered yeah, they have different dads you are going to look at me a totally different way. Even though both of them, you know, they both have the same dad.

Dr. Scott: Right.

Imani: But it's like that was an offensive question.

Dr. Scott: Right.

Imani: Would you have asked someone else that or is it just because I'm a young Black woman. I mean three doctors asked me.

Writing this book as a dissident and disruptive OBGYN who also identifies as a Black feminist serves as a validation and liberation of my rage against hospital acts of obstetric racism and inaction in the face of need. Embarking on this journey to name and apply Davis' obstetric racism as adverse events or series of repeated events during childbirth hospitalization embodies Davis' three responses to obstetric racism. First, Davis explains refusal as an act or series of acts of not consenting (or declining) to participate in the medicalization of birthing whereby one deploys one's own will against a system of control and the demands of consent, with a clear awareness, understanding, and acceptance that one rejects the possibility of coercion, medical intervention, abuse, disrespect, and the power that is used to dominate. Refusal represents an understanding that goes beyond understanding the implications of NOT doing something, but rather a deeper knowing and knowledge with appreciation and concern about the risks, barriers, burdens, and other negative consequences of agreeing to do something (Davis 2021; Davis 2022a; Davis 2022b). Second, Davis explains resistance as a strategy whereby one uses their own knowledge to push back against the mandate to intervene, presenting one or more acts of mobilization against a system that can involve questioning the terms of intervention and negotiating various forms of involvement in decision-making. Resistance is rooted in having a vision of how one wants to be treated based on their own terms (Davis 2021; Davis 2022a; Davis 2022b). Third, Davis defines racial reconnaissance as the Herculean acts or efforts made by Black women to avoid or mitigate racist encounters, including (but not limited to) being hypervigilant about procedures and finding providers. Choosing a Black feminist hermeneutic phenomenology as my methodology to making meaning of the lived experiences of pregnancy, labor, birth, postpartum, and infant feeding while Black in U.S. hospitals and health systems through text based on my positionality, is pure rage (Scott 2021) embodied as refusal, resistance, and racial reconnaissance (Davis 2020; Davis 2021; Davis 2022a; Davis 2022b).

Inaction in the face of need is by design when the face is Black and a woman. According to Maya, a Black mother in Oakland, she sees and feels the barriers and burdens of hospital inaction in the face of Black women's dreams and desires for their birth.

> I feel like they don't give us enough options or like care enough to see what we want to do. Like if we would say if I wanted to have a lotus birth, they wouldn't give me that option. I would have to do too much just to have the birth that I want. Like, you know, and then if I wanted to have a water birth, they would make me pay extra money. But if someone like if a white person wants to do it oh, it would be so beautiful and so great like, you know.

When the face in need does not match the face of America's default human and model mother, then U.S. maternal and perinatal health systems and structures are not obligated by any overt or covert standard or agenda to preserve, protect, and secure one's dignity or humanity. Without grounding dignity or humanity in the provision of health and human services, then empathy is obsolete. Without dignity, humanity, or empathy toward Blackness and Black people, then anti-Black racist antebellum norms and narratives of Black women and Black men as savages, without sensibilities to be autonomous human beings with both agency and self-efficacy to govern themselves, their children, or their communities, dominate the consciousness, clinical practice, decision-making, and care delivery.

One anti-Black racist stereotype weaponized against many Black mothers and their communities in the provision of obstetrics, maternity, and perinatal care is the absent Black father or partner. But when the Black father or partner is present, then Black mothers as patients must then become an advocate for their male partner and/or co-parent in order for the hospital team to recognize the presence of Black fathers in care. At the same time, Black mothers must also repeatedly ask for the hospital team to activate and actualize the continuous participation of Black fathers, co-parents, or partners throughout care interactions, communications, consent, decision-making, and documentation and dissemination of healthcare information throughout patient hand-offs, patient sign-outs, or paper and online health records. One Black mother in Oakland, Simone, reflected on manifestations of anti-Black racism during childbirth hospitalizations as reproductions of the absentee Black father trope in the provision of care, *"It's like they count on he's not going to be here."* The reasons for expecting Black men as fathers and partners to be absent are rooted in anti-Black racist narratives about Black family life dynamics. Six years prior to the first planning meeting (January 2019) for designing and conducting focus groups with two Black women-led community-based organizations based in Los Angeles and Oakland, respectively, the CDC published study findings on December 20, 2013, in the 2013 National Health Statistics. The research focused on the participation of fathers in their children's lives. The Fathers' Involvement With Their Children: United States, 2006–2010, study measured how "often a man participated in a set of activities in the last 4 weeks with children who were living with him and with children who were living apart from him" (Jones and Mosher 2013, 1). The research team also measured involvement separately for children aged 0–4 years and children aged 5–18 years. In comparison to white (60 percent) and Hispanic fathers (45 percent), Black fathers (70 percent) who live with their children were most likely to have bathed, dressed, changed, or helped their child with the toilet every day. In comparison to white (74 percent) and Hispanic fathers (64 percent), Black fathers (78 percent) were also more likely to eat meals with their children every day. In comparison to white (20 percent) fathers, Black (27 percent) fathers were more likely to take their children to or from activities every day. And finally, when examining time spent with children on their homework, Black fathers for the win, again. In comparison to white (28 percent) and Hispanic fathers (29 percent), Black fathers (41 percent) in the home were also more likely to help their children with homework every day (Jones and Mosher 2013).

Chantelle continued to elaborate on manifestations of medical abuse in clinical and social interactions and communication in the form of anti-Black racism, by reproducing degrading and hurtful norms and narratives about Black fatherhood, and anti-Black misogyny, or misogynoir, by perpetuating single mother tropes that conjure up images of a whore, welfare queen, or "baby mama."

> They [Black men as parents, partners, family, and friends] shouldn't have to force themselves into being included. But they [hospital clinicians] should ensure that he—any time they asked a question—something, something, something—he was speaking up. [The father gets] all the credit only because she came out looking like him. So, they didn't even know I was the mom. You know, they're like oh, your baby's so cute. They look at me like who's this dark woman. I think it's because they feel like it's not that common that you see Black women—Black couples because even then you're there they're just like, you know, they believe that I've got more than one baby daddy. Or just that I've

> got to be a single mom, so she needs to put her ring on, you know. And I have to let you know to include him. He was included in making this child.

Thus, the act of asking about Black fathers' involvement, in terms of their presence, participation, and persistence of one paternal lineage, outside of inquiries about genetic disorders, is racist. One can assess the Black mother's expectations and aspirations for the involvement of others in her labor, birth, immediate postpartum, and parenting and postpartum after hospital discharge without ever mentioning the words "Black" or "father." The persistent pattern of inquiring about the presence of one paternal lineage, outside of the context of genetic disorders, is a reproduction of obstetric racism in the form of medical abuse. The justification in naming these types of inquiries as medical abuse is explained by Davis' definition of medical abuse and by the origins of inquiry to dehumanize and subjugate enslaved Black men, women, girls, and boys using the law and other policies. Medical abuse occurs when medical professionals engage in experimentation and/or repetitive behavior that is motivated not by concern for the patient but serves to validate the clinicians' self-worth and upholds their domination over the patient (Davis 2018; Davis 2019; Davis 2020; Davis 2021). Therefore, asking mostly Black mothers questions about Black fathers such as "Where is your baby daddy?," "Do all of your children have the same father?," or "Will the father be attending the birth or involved in the baby's life?" is then clinically, socially, ethically, culturally, and scientifically inappropriate and unfounded based on the CDC 2013 data. The 2013 data highlighted the suboptimal presence and participation of two other father demographics, yet the dominant messages and images about deadbeat or absentee dads consist of Black fathers and/or fathers navigating class exploitation and poverty.

In moving from medical abuse to intentionally causing pain, one begins to more clearly see the depth, breadth, and dimension of violence and violations permeating the lived experience of pregnancy, childbirth, postpartum, parenting, and partnering while Black in the U.S. The component of intentionally causing pain, which includes the absence of empathy for Black people's physical suffering and a lack of internal motivation to alleviate or reduce Black suffering, manifests in the clinical attitudes, behaviors, and language of obstetric nurses as well as their cognitive reasoning in the labor and deliver (L&D) triage. The initial dismissal, diminishing, and denial of Black discomfort and pain during presentation to L&D triage is a pervasive problem. Subsequently, the delayed and/or inappropriate clinical response to an initially non-urgent yet valid clinical concern evolves into an emergent situation, as demonstrated in Kiara's account of showing up to L&D triage in a local hospital in Oakland with her mother, who was also a doula.

> I think also being more understanding towards your patients is something I feel like that—so being more understanding—like make sure I'm saying the right word. Okay. Yeah, I'll describe it. So, when I went in, so my doctor had me scheduled for my C-section while it's night. I ended up going into labor. I had a doctor's appointment August 1st. I ended up going into labor August 2nd and had her that night. When I went in, my contractions were five minutes apart but I had no pain. So, all I knew is I couldn't talk through a contraction. It wasn't painful, I just was short of breath. And the lady—they took forever. The nurse. The nurse took forever because she felt like—Took forever to come into the room to check me. She felt like, oh, well, the chart says you're only—you're seven minutes apart so it's not bad, it's not bad, she's still—oh, it's not bad, you're good. Being that I'm—I have a breech baby and I'm telling you that I'm in labor and I—my mom is a doula. She'd been counting like at the time and everything. I was five minutes apart, even shot to three sometimes. And so finally she came like I want to say an hour or two hours later and checked me and was like, oh, because you would send me home being, I had a breech baby. And she was like, oh, wow, you're 3, 3-1/2 centimeters and complete [completely effaced means the cervix is paper-thin], so yeah, we're going to see what we're going to do. My mom said, oh, she's not going home being complete [completely effaced], she's going to dilate every hour—and which I did by—I went in at 4:00—I went in at 4:00 p.m. and I had her at 9:50 that night. So, if I would have went back home, I would have delivered a breech baby and anything could have happened, you know. And it's just the fact that she didn't trust me.

Kiara's reported experience of not being seen, heard, believed, and trusted by the L&D triage nurse represents a broader, pervasive problem of inaction in the face of need. The lack of appropriate clinical recognition and response from the L&D triage nurse reproduces the following four dimensions of obstetric racism: diagnostic lapses, neglect, dismissiveness, and disrespect, intentionally causing pain and medical abuse (Davis 2018; Davis 2019; Davis 2020; Davis, Varner, and Dill 2021). In addition to reproducing acts of obstetric racism, the L&D triage nurse's responses also violate all six domains of quality as defined first by the Institute of Medicine (IOM), now called the National Academy of Medicine (NAM) (and presently endorsed by the AHRQ (IOM 2001; AHRQ 2022). As described in chapter 1, operationalizing the six-domain quality framework served as a systemic approach for health care organizations to increase the likelihood of simultaneously reducing errors and improving the overall quality of health care provision. The second benefit included the design of a communication tool for patients to evaluate care quality and satisfaction with the care they received. Given the second benefit, the quality of care provided to Kiara by the L&D triage nurse violated all six quality domains as defined and utilized by NAM and AHRQ. When operationalizing the six-domain framework with Black women's patient-reported experiences of obstetric care, one better appreciates the violations of quality by meaning-making of text within the narrative.

NARRATIVE ANALYSIS: DUAL APPLICATION OF NAM-AHRQ'S SIX-DOMAIN QUALITY FRAMEWORK AND DAVIS' SIX DIMENSIONS OF OBSTETRIC RACISM

As a strategy for building the capacity of licensed health care professionals, specifically physicians and surgeons in obstetrics, neonatology, pediatrics, and anesthesiology and nurses, including advanced practice nurses in women's health, obstetrics, neonatology, midwifery, and anesthesiology, Dána-Ain Davis and I started a journey and praxis of accepting invited presentations from academic health centers and training programs together. As co-presenters, we developed and implemented online presentations in 2020, the inaugural year of the COVID-19 pandemic (Davis and Scott 2020). The primary goal was to offer a different framework and methodology for evaluating obstetric quality and patient safety. We organized the presentation content and talking points around Black birthing narratives from Davis' book, R*eproductive Injustice: Racism, Pregnancy, and Premature Birth* (Davis 2019). Our combined vision was to compel decision-makers and stakeholders who design, provide, fund, and evaluate childbirth in hospital settings to endorse obstetric racism as the more accurate and precise obstetric quality and patient safety framework by which to better understand, characterize, and justify the disparate, preventable, predictable, and unfair rates of maternal and infant mortality and morbidity impacting Black women and their babies (Scott and Davis 2020).

Using illustrative narratives, audio narratives, and written narratives, we elucidated the meanings and manifestations of obstetric racism by demonstrating real-time live mapping of specific examples of language, practices, behaviors, interactions, non-verbal and verbal communications, consent and decision-making approaches, and documentation and dissemination of healthcare information in patient handoffs, patient sign-outs, and electronic health records onto the six dimensions of obstetric and the original six (now seven) theorized, patient-identified quality domains of the SACKRED Birth framework. This framework evolved into the domains of the patient-reported experiences measure of obstetric racism©, the PREM-OB Scale® suite (Scott 2018; Scott 2019a; Scott 2019b; Davis and Scott 2020; Scott and Davis 2021; White VanGompel et al. 2022; Lett et al. 2023). SACKRED Birth quality domains are based on narratives collected in 2019 during four focus groups with thirty-six Black mothers in Oakland, February 2019, and then in Los

Angeles, March 2019 (Scott 2018; Scott 2019a; Scott 2019b), presented in this existing Black feminist hermeneutic phenomenology of childbirth hospitalization, influenced by Davis' original two publications on obstetric racism (Davis 2018; Davis 2019), and her incredible mentorship, guidance, teaching, consultation, collaboration, and sister-soulship since meeting her in October 2018, at Decolonizing Birth, the brainchild of Chanel Portia-Albert, Founder and Executive Director of Ancient Song Doula Services (Ancient Song Doula Services n.d.). Davis' delineation of the six dimensions of obstetric racism is based on Davis' ethnographic research from 2011 to 2019, during which time she collected and analyzed U.S. based Black women's narratives and documented the manifestations of obstetric racism in their interactions with hospital physicians, nurses, and staff (Davis 2019). Davis expanded the dimensions of obstetric racism to include a seventh dimension, a wild card, for use when Black women's narratives of medical care during pregnancy cannot be mapped onto the existing topology of obstetric racism (Davis 2020; Davis, Varner, and Dill 2021; Davis 2022a; Davis 2022b).

For comparative purposes, table 2.1 lists the names of three different conceptual frameworks available for use in evaluating quality of care and patient safety. In maintaining fidelity to the design and utility of obstetric racism and SACKRED Birth, one must gain access to narratives of care, with the most accurate and precise application to U.S.-based Black women's interactions with any health care professional or health system, for any pregnancy-related care, concern, or condition. From top to bottom, the individual domains or dimensions are entered in the order listed by the author in existing

Table 2.1 Three Different Conceptual Frameworks for Evaluating Quality and Patient Care Experiences (Institute of Medicine 2001; Agency of Healthcare Research and Quality 2022; Davis 2018; Davis 2019; Davis 2020; Davis 2022a; Davis 2022b; Scott 2018; Scott 2019a; Scott 2019b; Davis and Scott 2020; Scott and Davis 2021)

	NAM-AHRQ Quality Domains	*Davis' Obstetric Racism Dimensions*	*Scott's SACKRED Birth Quality Domains*
1	Safe	Neglect, dismissiveness, and disrespect	Safety and Accountability
2	Effective	Diagnostic Lapse	Autonomy
3	Patient-centered	Intentionally Causing Pain	Communication and Information Exchange
4	Timely	Ceremonies of Degradation	Kinship
5	Efficient	Medical Abusee	Racism (anti-Black medical racism and medical misogynoir)
6	Equitable	Coercion	Empathy and Humanity
7	N/A	Wild Card	Dignity in Blackness and Holistic Care

publications. SACKRED is an acronym where each letter corresponds to the name of the patient-identified quality domain. For each row, there is no meaning or significance to the order of domains or dimensions from left to right.

To demonstrate the narrative analysis methodology in practice, with dual application of NAM-AHRQ's six quality domain framework and Davis' six dimensions of obstetric racism, I returned to Kiara's harmful experience with the L&D triage nurse in a local Oakland hospital. In examining Kiara's narrative, one must follow four steps: (1) Identify the perpetrator(s) of harm and their role on the health care team assigned to the patient; (2) Describe the harm(s) as specific quality violations across one or more of the following components of care: interactions, communication, consent, decision-making, and documentation and dissemination of healthcare information in patient handoff, patient sign-out, or electronic or paper health record; (3) Organize the list of quality violations and the involved care components based on the topology of the chosen framework (map the quality violation onto one or more of the domains or dimensions of the selected framework); (4) Provide the evidential(s) of harm(s) using the exact thoughts, feelings, and words of the index patient and her support person (e.g., caregiver, parent, sibling, friend, doula), avoiding the tendency to use or prioritize hospital knowledge or language over patient and community knowledge, information, expertise, and wisdom; and (5) Describe and explain the impact of the quality of care on the patient from the patient and caregiver/community perspective, and not only based on the system's recognition and interpretation of harm. As explained by my co-authors, including Davis, in *BMJ Quality and Patient Safety,* the prioritization of being safe as defined by traditional or existing quality and patient safety experts and health plans over feeling safe as defined through patient experience and community wisdom creates another hierarchy of human value, truths, and power (Lyndon et al. 2023). Consequently, existing quality and patient safety paradigms and practices reproduce and reiterate epistemic injustice, testimonial injustice, and hermeneutical injustice (Fricker 2007; Scott 2021; Lyndon et al. 2023). Below one will find the application of the narrative analysis methodology to Kiara's account of her hospital birthing experience, starting with the interpretation of Kiara's experiences using NAM-AHRQ's quality domains (IOM 2001; AHRQ 2002) and then adding manifestations of Davis' dimensions of obstetric racism (Davis 2018; Davis 2019; Davis 2020; Davis and Scott 2020; Davis, Varner, and Dill 2021; Scott and Davis):

- *Safe*: avoiding harm to patients from the care that is intended to help them:
    - L&D triage nurse behavior: Harm created by causing the Black mother to fear being admitted with a diagnosis of active labor and with a baby in breech presentation, necessitating communication, consent,

decision-making, and documentation and dissemination of healthcare information in patient handoffs, patient sign-outs, and health records for admission, preparation for, and performance of a cesarean birth.
- Kiara's reported experience: "So, if I would have went back home, I would have delivered a breech baby and anything could have happened, you know. And it's just the fact that she didn't trust me."
- Quality Impact: Provision of unsafe obstetric care and perpetuation of testimonial injustice due to the system's action in not seeing, hearing, believing, and trusting Black women.

- *Effective*: providing services based on scientific knowledge to all who could benefit and refraining from providing services to those not likely to benefit (avoiding underuse and misuse, respectively).
  - L&D triage nurse behavior: Ineffective provision of services given the scientific knowledge of active labor with cervical dilation of 3.5 centimeters, 100% effacement (completely thinned out cervix or cervical length of 0 centimeters, a paper-thin cervix) with a baby in breech presentation.
  - Kiara's reported experience: "She felt like, oh, well, the chart says you're only—you're seven minutes apart so it's not bad, it's not bad, she's still—oh, it's not bad, you're good. Being that I'm—I have a breech baby and I'm telling you that I'm in labor."
  - Kiara's reported experience: "She'd been counting like at the time and everything. I was five minutes apart, even shot to three sometimes. And so finally she came like I want to say an hour or two hours later and checked me and was like, oh, because you would send me home being, I had a breech baby. And she was like, oh, wow, you're 3, 3-1/2 centimeters and complete (completely effaced (paper-thin cervix)), so yeah, we're going to see what we're going to do. My mom said, oh, she's not going home being complete (completely effaced), she's going to dilate every hour—and which I did by—I went in at 4:00—I went in at 4:00 p.m. and I had her at 9:50 that night."
  - Quality impact: Provision of ineffective obstetric services that violates patient and family "emotional" safety, appears to harm, and not benefit, the patient and also harm the patient's caregiver, her mother.
- *Patient-centered*: providing care that is respectful of and responsive to individual patient preferences, needs, and values, and ensuring that patient values guide all clinical decisions:
  - L&D triage nurse behavior: neglectful, dismissive, and disrespectful provision of "nurse-centered" obstetric care with inappropriate clinical and social responses, motivated by validating the nurse's self-worth and upholding her domination over the patient, with no regard for the patient's and the patient's mother's expressed concerns (reproducing two

of Davis' six dimensions of obstetric racism: medical abuse and neglect, dismissiveness, disrespect).
    - Kiara's reported experience: "She felt like, oh, well, the chart says you're only—you're seven minutes apart so it's not bad, it's not bad, she's still—oh, it's not bad, you're good. Being that I'm—I have a breech baby and I'm telling you that I'm in labor and I—my mom is a doula."
    - Quality impact: reproduction of systems-centered and nurse-centered care that reproduces acts of obstetric racism and violates quality.
- *Timely*: reducing waits and sometimes harmful delays for both those who receive and those who give care:
    - L&D triage nurse behavior: neglectful, dismissive, disrespectful behavior, grounded in an uninterrogated harmful belief that Blackness is pathological (e.g., anti-Black racist and anti-Black misogynistic ideologies originating in slavery and proliferating during the antebellum period that Black people are subhuman and wild beasts, and that Black women are mules), causing the nurse to de-emphasize Kiara's symptoms, leading to inappropriate or delayed diagnosis (reproducing Davis' dimension of obstetric racism: diagnostic lapse).
    - Kiara's reported experience: "I went in at 4:00—I went in at 4:00 p.m. and I had her at 9:50 that night."
    - Quality impact: Harmful delay felt and expressed by the patient. Based on Kiara's narrative, one cannot ascertain if the triage nurses and staff communicated effectively to L&D nurses, physicians, and staff, including the surgical team and anesthesiology physicians and staff of the possibility of a cesarean birth, given the arrival of a Black mother in active labor with a baby in breech presentation.
- *Efficient*: avoiding waste, including waste of equipment, supplies, ideas, and energy
    - L&D triage nurse behavior: neglectful, dismissive, disrespectful behavior including medical abuse and diagnostic lapse grounded in the uninterrogated harmful belief that Blackness is pathological (e.g., anti-Black racist and anti-Black misogynistic ideologies originating in slavery and proliferating during the antebellum period that Black people are subhuman and wild beasts, and that Black women are mules), causing the nurse to de-emphasize the Black patient's pain, potentially missing a critical diagnosis that would require communication, coordination, and mobilization of multiple different yet interdependent systems, and patient and caregiver/family level responses for admission, preparation, and participation in an unscheduled cesarean birth in the late afternoon or early evening of a shift change.

  - Kiara's reported experience: "I think also being more understanding towards your patients is something I feel like that—So being more understanding."
  - Kiara's reported experience: "And the lady—they took forever. The nurse. The nurse took forever because she felt like—Took forever to come into the room to check me. She felt like, oh, well, the chart says you're only—you're seven minutes apart so it's not bad, it's not bad, she's still—oh, it's not bad, you're good."
  - Kiara's reported experience: "And so finally she came like I want to say an hour or two hours later and checked me and was like, oh, because you would send me home being, I had a breech baby. And she was like, oh, wow, you're 3, 3-1/2 centimeters and complete [completely effaced (paper-thin cervix)]."
  - Quality impact: Facilitating waste of ideas, energy, and resources.
- *Equitable:* providing care that does not vary in quality because of personal characteristics such as gender, ethnicity, geographic location, or socioeconomic status.
  - L&D triage nurse behavior: neglectful, dismissive, disrespectful behavior including medical abuse and diagnostic lapses grounded in the uninterrogated pathological belief that Blackness is pathological (e.g., anti-Black racist and anti-Black misogynistic ideologies originating in slavery and proliferating during the antebellum period that Black people are subhuman and wild beasts, and that Black women are mules), causing the nurse to de-emphasize the Black patient's pain and potentially missing a critical diagnosis that would require communication, coordination, and mobilization of differential system, patient, and family level responses for admission, preparation, and participation in an unscheduled cesarean birth in the late afternoon or early evening of a shift change.
  - Black woman's reported experience: *"I think also being more understanding towards your patients is something I feel like that—So being more understanding."*
  - Quality impact: Reproduction of anti-Black racist, anti-Black misogynistic, and inequitable care that dismisses Black women's dignity and humanity.

In evaluating the quality of care provided to Kiara using the narrative analysis methodology, first designed and implemented by me and Davis (Davis and Scott 2020), one cannot deny the pattern of inaction in the face of need as institutionalized racism (Jones 2020), demonstrated by the reproduction of all six dimensions obstetric racism and violations of all six domains of healthcare quality.

Another Black mother in Oakland named Gabrielle recounted her experience with a nurse who lacked empathy in the provision of obstetric care and repeatedly asserted her domination over the patient. The pattern of operationalizing anti-Black racist and anti-Black misogynistic ideologies in the provision of obstetric care necessitates ongoing diminishing, degrading, and dehumanizing of Black women's lives and experiences. Consider the focus group dialogue during which a chorus of Black women, including myself, interject in a call and response manner to show support to the narrator, Gabrielle, and to reassure her that Black women believed her and believed in her.

> *Gabrielle:* Can I add on to that. With the—my second son, you know, after your first child, you know when you're in labor. I went in. Well, I got stuck in the shower because my contractions were hitting back to back and I froze up and I couldn't move. So, I was home alone with my oldest son. I called my neighbor. She came and got me out the shower, helped me get dressed, and took me in. And as I said before, my second son, his bones were grinding against my bones as he was dropping down which makes it more painful. And I couldn't sit on the bed. And this nurse, you know, sometimes when you go in there, nurses brag about how long they've been a nurse and this and this and that. And as she's like, well, I'm not going to check you in until you sit down and let me check you. I said I can't right now, I'm in pain, give me a second, let me breathe through these contractions. And she said, well, this is the last time I'm coming in here. I said I'm telling you I'm in labor. I said I know I'm in labor. She said, well, I'm not going to do—I'm not going to go by what you say, you need to sit down so I can check you. And I said, well, I'll sit down in a minute. Like at this point, I'm in pain, then you're pissing me off because you're trying to tell me like you're not in labor, you're fine. And then you're going to tell me that if I don't let you check me right now, you're going to send me home. Well, eventually after having a meltdown, the contractions subsided a little bit. I sat down. And she checked, she's like, oh, you're right, you are in labor. Well, hello. And so, she goes, okay, well, I'm going to check you in and then she told me to walk down the hallway to my room. Mind you my contractions are still going up and down and it's still painful. And so, I walked to the room. I'm holding onto the rail walking, because you know the walls have a little railing thing. So, I'm walking myself down. I get in there, she checks me in, she's like, oh, yeah, you're right, that's why it's probably painful, your son's bones are grinding on your bones so I know it's intense. And I just looked at her like...
>
> *Tiffany:* Have you listened to anything I've been throwing out?
>
> *Garbielle:* Exactly. And then they gave me—I forgot what they gave me, but it was like a slight pain medicine before an epidural to help with the pain, and then I started, you know, smiling and everything. She's like, oh, you are a happy person.

Brianna: Damn girl, they be judging you.

Tiffany: She judged you.

Gabrielle: She was—yeah. She was an older woman.

Dr. Scott: She looked different than you?

Garbielle: Oh, she did. She did. She did. She was an older White nurse.

Dr. Scott: Yeah.

Brianna: Yeah.

Jada: And that's how it is.

Gabrielle: I wasn't too happy with her.

As previously described in chapter 1, cultural rigor sits at the intersection of scientific rigor, as defined by the National Institutes of Health (National Institutes of Health n.d.; Lauer 2016), and cultural humility, as defined by two Black women physician scientists and public health scholars (Murray-García and Tervalon 2014). Cultural rigor simultaneously operationalizes reproductive justice, Black feminism, and research justice across four modalities: analytic framework, social movement, vision, and praxis (Scott 2019a; Scott 2019b; Scott, Bray, and McLemore 2020; Scott 2021; VanGompel et al. 2022; Lett et al. 2023). In the application of cultural rigor, patient, community, and content experts and expertise are equally prioritized, as explained through research justice.

Likewise, cultural rigor situates gender and race at the center of knowledge production, as defined in Black feminism. The hierarchy of knowledge and knowing in traditional quality and patient safety paradigm deprioritizes patient experiential, cultural, and spiritual knowledge, relegating the title (and corresponding compensation) of experts to individuals with formal education and researcher to individuals who acquired formal skills and training (Scott 2018; Scott 2019a; Scott 2019b; Davis and Scott 2020; Scott, Bray, and McLemore 2020; Scott and Davis 2021; Scott 2021; White VanGompel et al. 2022; Lett et al. 2023). Thus, research justice requires a re-imagining of the researched as the researcher and the experts with cultural, spiritual, experiential, and mainstream (or institutional) knowledge. Research justice offers a strategic vision with principles and practices to acknowledge, affirm, activate, and amplify the political power and legitimacy of structurally marginalized and minoritized communities as valid knowledge incubators and producers (Jolivétte 2015; Scott 2018; Scott 2019a; Scott 2019b; Davis and Scott 2020; Scott, Bray, and McLemore 2020; Scott and Davis 2021; Scott 2021; White VanGompel et al. 2022; Lett et al. 2023). Consequently, research justice situates patient and community experts in a position to leverage all three types of knowledge to drive policymaking decisions in rectifying historical and contemporary power inequities and advancing social justice (Jolivétte 2015).

Weaving cultural rigor throughout the obstetric quality and patient safety paradigm also supports women and gender-expansive individuals to the right to have children, the right not to have children, and the right to nourish and nurture their existing children in safe and healthy environments as outlined in the tenets of reproductive justice (Ross and Solinger 2017; Ross et al. 2017; Scott 2019a; Scott 2019b; Scott, Bray, and McLemore 2020; Scott 2021; Scott and Davis 2021; White VanGompel et al. 2022; Lett et al. 2023).

As a social movement, cultural rigor catalyzes a new obstetric quality and patient safety paradigm that is continuously dismantling the hierarchy of knowing and knowledge production and its consequences, including structural arrogance and absence of empathy. As Rhonda reflected on her hospital birthing experience in Oakland, in the larger context of Black women's birthing experiences within hospitals, she offered a meaningful critique of the role of nurses and other support staff in perpetuating harm against patients. Her critique highlighted how some nurses assume a certain level of knowledge possessed by patients, particularly Black pregnant and postpartum patients, and how nurses exploit a perceived knowledge to reassert their authority over patients, including hospital workers with racial and/or sociocultural concordance with Black patients.

> I think they come in—a lot of nurses come in with these assumptions of like, our knowledge, they automatically assume there's lack of knowledge in certain things, they can tell us whatever. They automatically assume that we're dramatic because we're portrayed as dramatic. One minute we're you're saying that this hurts, they don't necessarily believe you all the way. And so, I think they need to come in with an open mind. There's not an open mindedness when it comes to Black women because we are not empowered to be the—you know, we're not all that stereotypical Black woman that they assume. Because I just heard that there's lactation consultants that would pass on a Black woman's room because they assume she's not going to breastfeed. So, they'll go to another mom's room. And that's coming from an actual African American lactation consultant hearing them say that. They're assuming this. And so, they make all these assumptions and so then we don't get the kind of care that we need or deserve because they assume you're overexaggerating or they assume that you don't know what you're talking about when you're asking questions and, you know, things like that. So, they're just—they need to be more open-minded when it comes to us and like there's no telling, you know, who they're sending in.

As thoughtfully and clearly explained by Rhonda, some, if not many, nurses go out of their way to repeat behaviors during service provision that undermine patient experiential knowledge, perpetuating testimonial injustice (Fricker 2007; Scott 2021; Lyndon et al. 2023). In doing so, the nurses assert their domination over Black pregnant and postpartum patients, reproducing medical abuse, one of six dimensions of obstetric racism (Davis 2018; Davis 2019; Davis 2020; Davis 2021). When a nurse holds and operates under an uninterrogated belief that Blackness is pathological, including acting on a problematic bias that Black women avoid or dislike breastfeeding, then the nurse de-emphasizes or ignores a Black patient's interest, desire, autonomy (freedom to choose without external control or approval), agency (ability to take action or choose what action to take based on available options and resources), and self-efficacy (confidence in one's self to make a decision or successfully achieve a goal) to breast-, chest-, or body-feed their infant or children. The inappropriate avoidant behavior grounded in the uninterrogated belief that Black women avoid or dislike breastfeeding reproduces diagnostic lapses, another dimension of obstetric racism (Davis 2018; Davis 2019; Davis 2020; Davis 2021).

A primary mechanism for reproductions of unmitigated harms is to curate and sustain an institutional culture void of empathy and motivation to end Black suffering, which is intentionally causing pain as elucidated by Davis' obstetric racism (Davis 2018; Davis 2019; Davis 2020; Davis, Varner, and Dill 2021). Sustaining an institutional culture in obstetrics care that is void of empathy for Black women's suffering and regard for Black women's dignity and humanity requires the maintenance of hierarchies of human value, knowing, and knowledge that advantages white cisgender heterosexual women over all other women and gender-expansive individuals. In U.S. obstetric care, systems and structures maintain, protect, and amplify the goodness of the worthy white woman. In contrast, systems and structures excel in degrading and dehumanizing Black lives at every point of care. The assault on Black women's knowing and knowledge, including Black women's autonomy, agency, and self-efficacy in making decisions for themselves, their bodies, their babies, and their families, seems orchestrated and executed in plain sight. During focus group dialogue among three Black mothers in Los Angeles, one learns more about their perceptions and perspectives of health care professionals in relationship to (mis)treating Black patients, particularly Black pregnant and postpartum patients.

> *Aaliyah:* I don't know what the right word is, but I think what ends up happening is what a lot of healthcare providers is the implicit bias. They—they—and they don't—the reason they think they respect us is because they don't understand that they're disrespecting us. They don't—they act without realizing what they're actually doing. I think sometimes—I think if you go and ask them, hey, do you respect your—your black patient moms, they would tell you yes. I don't think they have enough—they don't experience what we go through. So it's in their blind box. They don't have enough self-awareness to know that what they're doing is wrong.

Jasmine: It's disrespectful, yes. And I'm going to piggyback on my sister downstairs what she went through when we went to the BIH—this program, black infant health or whatever. We went there to learn that stress—there's a lot of stress on black moms, which creates this high infertility rate amongst babies. And my sister doctor at Hospital #7 told her stress doesn't affect the baby. My sister immediately switched doctors. So that's—some of them are ignorant. . .. It doesn't make it right, and I'm not trying to [defend] them or anything like that, but they're ignorant.

Ebony: Incredibly ignorant.

Jasmine: You know, and some of them—that example right there is like what—what do you mean stress doesn't affect the baby.

Ebony: I think mothers are treated as if they don't know. Like, they don't know what's best for their babies. They don't know like we—because we don't have the degree. Because we didn't spend, you know, 12, 8 years in school, because we didn't do X, Y, and Z that we don't know so we don't get to be a part, we don't get to be a part of our birthing experience. Like, a lot of times we're told what's going to happen instead of being asked are you okay with this.

The focus group dialogue among Black mothers, Aaliyah, Jasmine, and Ebony, builds the case for an aggressively oppressive obstetric system of care designed to undermine Black women's knowing and knowledge as part of a broader strategic vision and plan to deny Black women's right to bodily and decisional autonomy. As a result, the obstetric model of care justifies the subjugation of Black women, Black bodies, Black births, and Black babies using mechanisms of action that track along histories of anti-Black racism, eugenics, chattel slavery, and antebellum ideologies of Black people existing as subhumans and nonhumans. Consequently, securing continuous consent throughout the provision of obstetric care in hospital settings feels abnormal and unnecessary to hospital administrators, clinicians, and staff when they see Black women as mules or inanimate objects without consciousness, feelings, or free will.

One Black mother in Los Angeles, Nia, shared how she felt pressured by physicians and nurses to comply with their clinical recommendations. She provided insight into feeling coerced or forced to accept clinical guidance compared to feeling free to choose clinical therapies based on the opportunities, options, and optimal conditions for actualizing her free will and achieving the highest level of care and health, as determined for, by, and with herself.

Doctor comes in. Oh, you're not progressing. We're going to give you Pitocin. No, you're not going to give me Pitocin. Even after I delivered, they're like,

> okay, well, we're going to give you Pitocin to deliver the placenta. No, you're not going to give me Pitocin. I don't want Pitocin. I've said this more than once. So instead of asking me or even—even explaining. Because I know there are black midwives who came back and said, oh, well, because of hemorrhaging that you're supposed to blah, blah, blah. But that wasn't explained. You could have said, hey, this is because of the risk of hemorrhaging post-partum and delivering the placenta, we typically give moms Pitocin. Is that something you're comfortable with? And then I get to say yes or no. But because you think you know better, I don't get—I don't get to be a part of [the decision].

The internalization of anti-Black racism and misogynoir by obstetric physicians, nurses, social workers, and other support staff fuels their beliefs that the safest place for a Black baby is in the possession of the state. The disproportionate and inappropriate use of CPS to coerce or force Black mothers and their given and chosen kin to comply with medical care is merely a symptom of the larger problem, as examined through the scholarship of Roberts and Goodwin, respectively (Roberts 1997; Goodwin 2017; Goodwin 2020; Roberts 2022). The threat or actual use of CPS to subjugate Black women, to revoke their right to make decisions about their body and the safety and well-being of their child, and to facilitate parent-child separation and family destabilization is obstetric racism, as described in the dimension, ceremonies of degradation (Davis 2018; Davis 2019; Davis 2020). During the Oakland focus group, Dominique opened up about being forced to accept a cesarean birth under the threat of CPS,

> it was no, they was like you're either going to have a C-section or we're going to have—they even threatened with CPS like we'll have to call CPS. And so, I had to switch my regular doctor, yeah. I had to switch the C-section doctor. Because Doctor #2 wasn't in the one that—but, yeah, so, basically, I was forced to have a C-section. Which they wasn't answering none of my questions. Because it was like their way or no way. So, I really had to talk to my other doctor and then we switched around. But I ended up having a C-section because they just made it no other way.

Another consequence of the proliferation of anti-Black racist and anti-Black misogynist antebellum ideologies in the U.S. systems of obstetric care is the assertion of our subhuman and nonhuman characteristics. Such horrific ideologies manifest as denying our innate capability to speak up for ourselves or make our own autonomous decisions. The infantilization, degradation, and dehumanization of Black people, particularly Black women, during the provision of obstetric care is fundamental to maintaining a hierarchy of human value, knowing, and knowledge based on anti-Black medical racism and misogynoir. In Los Angeles, one of the Black mothers, Tamara, shared her perception and perspective on why physicians, nurses, and other health care professionals frequently (mis)treat Black pregnant and postpartum women.

> *Tamara:* I think it's very stereotypical.
>
> *Dr. Scott:* Tell me what you mean by that.
>
> *Tamara:* Hey—they look at us as we're dumb, we don't know, so therefore, we're going to tell you what you're going to do. Everything is costly now. So automatically, it's like, oh, no, you're high risk because you're black. You have to get a C-section automatically. Surgery and then how long you have to stay in there. That's all money. Versus you're having a vaginal birth. You're out, what, the next day? I was also going to say I feel they should explain or give you that option of having a birthing plan from the beginning. Do I want a cesarean in the beginning, why do I want a cesarean, give me the risk of a cesarean? Do I want a vaginal birth? Why do I want a vaginal birth? Give me the risks of a vaginal birth. Run the testing for—for everybody. Like is it—would it be okay for me to have a cesarean because I could actually, you know, I would rather not.

In the next Black hospital narrative, a Black mother in Los Angeles, Kenya, recalled an experience during her childbirth hospitalization when she expressed discomfort repeatedly while her boyfriend and mother also expressed concerns for the explicit violations in quality, manifesting as acts of medical abuse and intentionally causing pain during a cervical exam. For clinical context, the cervical exam offers valuable information about labor status or progress in order to advance clinical care during childbirth, independent of birth setting or attendant. Despite the intent of the cervical exam, Kenya declined the cervical exam. However, the nurse's response to Kenya's valid act of refusal or resistance aligned with acts of retaliation that displaced the nurse's onus of ending Black suffering onto the patient and her kinship. According to Davis' ceremonies of degradation, the nurse's response to Kenya, her boyfriend, and her mother represents a series of ritualistic ways designed to humiliate and shame Black patients and their families. Over and above that, the ritualistic ways include a process for assigning a value to Black lives and determining the worthiness of the patient or support person(s) who may be viewed as a threat. When the physician, nurse, or institution views Black patients and their families as a threat, hospital clinicians and staff may deploy security, police, social services, CPS, hospital administration, or psychiatry to achieve compliance with clinical recommendations or to remove the "threatening" person. Ritualistic practices to threaten or actualize family destabilization, separation, or disruption demonstrate a heinous abuse of power that always favors the healthcare system and workforce over protecting Black patients and their given and chosen families.

Kenya: And they were just so, like, after she made that comment, she's all, like, well I'm going to have to clear the room, because now I have to ask you if you've ever been raped, or if you've ever been a victim of sexual assault—

Dr. Scott: Because of—

Kenya: Because she was rough—

Dr. Scott: But you told her she was rough, and now she needs to ask you if you were raped?

Kenya: Yes. She cleared the room—she made my boyfriend leave, she made my mom leave, and she was just, like, I need to ask, you know, these series of questions—if you've ever been sexually assaulted, are you a victim of domestic violence, because—

Michelle: Is this the nurse?

Kenya:—it was [Hospital #6]

Michelle: Okay, [Hospital #1] asked me the same set of questions, so I know what you're talking about.

Kenya: And it's not—it's not . . ..

Dr. Scott: The questions can be asked, but my thing is, like, because you expressed discomfort with your exam, doesn't mean you were raped, or—

Kenya: Right, at all—right.

Michelle: The questions were a scapegoat for her.

Kenya: For her—for her, right, right. Because I was literally in tears, and my boyfriend was, like, on the—you know, he's, like, what are you doing to her?

Focus group dialogue between Black mothers, and also between me and Black mothers, demonstrated how the obstetrics model of care is grounded in the erosion and erasure of Black voices and Black lives. The diminishing of the dignity and humanity of Black patients and their given and chosen family by the medical industrial complex originates in antebellum ideologies of anti-Black medical racism and misogynoir. Performing the cervical exam serves as a primary lever utilized by physicians, nurses, resident physicians, and clinical fellows to facilitate medical abuse and intentionally causing pain. Performing a cervical exam also serves as a lever to assert domination over the patient and reinforce power inequities between the patient and hospital clinician, and patient and the entire health system. Knowledge of the labor status and progress depends on two key sources: trusting the experiential knowledge of a patient in her body about a phenomenon happening in her body and performing a cervical exam by anyone who is not the patient.

Hospital nurses repeatedly choose violence by refusing to see, hear, believe, trust, and help Black pregnant or postpartum women in need.

The next birth narrative centers on a Black mother in Los Angeles, Shante, who shared her experience with a hospital nurse who also ignored her concerns for the changes happening in her body. Shante's story is another example of a nurse willfully choosing to ignore a pregnant Black mother in increasing discomfort, as well as the Black mother's expressed request to the hospital nurse to respond in an appropriate and timely manner and provide optimal, equitable obstetric care to her daughter.

> Well, I have a crazy story, so that's why I'm kind of holding off, but—I had the—I wanted a water birth, as well—that was my plan. But I had my son premature at 26 weeks. He's a micro-preemie. But he's fine now, thank God. He's two—he just turned two. But, so I had my baby at the hospital because of that, and it wasn't planned—obviously—he came early. So I had to be rushed there. But I felt like—once I got there—because I knew that I wasn't going to have the birthing experience that I planned, I just surrendered, you know. It was just, like, whatever they want to do—because I didn't want to fight while I was in that situation. I did everything up until that point to prepare to not have that birthing experience, and it all happened because I had him early. So—but while I was there, right before giving birth, I was shaking—like, shaking really hard. And I kept telling the nurses to check me. My mom was there, so she kind of advocated for me. But I was shaking uncontrollably, and they were, like, oh, it's normal, you know, don't worry about it. You know, it's—it's a normal thing. And I'm, like, okay, but I don't think this is—you know, like, this is—it just feels too crazy. So I'm, like, Mom, tell them—this is like an hour later—I'm, like, tell them to check me because, like, I know something is wrong, like, I don't—this just doesn't feel right. And it's, like, literally, like, I—I can't stop. And I—I feel like I have the mental strength and capacity to, you know, stop it, but I—I literally couldn't, like, no matter what I did. So they finally came and checked me, and then, you know, she checked me, and she's like, oh, you're complete. I'm, like, what does that mean—what is complete? And she's like, you're 10 centimeters dilated. I'm, like, oh, well, if you guys would've came, you know, before while I'm asking you to check me, you know, I—I just knew something was up. So, you know, they started prepping and everybody's rushing in, and I had him. But I—I just didn't feel heard because I was asking them for about an hour, hour and a half to check me and they never—they never did."

Based on the lived experiences of Black women, the standard of U.S. obstetric care provided to Black women is denial, dismissiveness, or delay. The preeminent dimensions of obstetric racism emerging from the individual texts and focus group dialogue is medical abuse and intentionally causing pain, with an emphasis on failing to alleviate Black people's suffering. The pattern of persistent cries for help without acknowledgment and reassurance from the bedside nurse speaks volumes about the epidemic of failed or limited empathy. When Black mothers verbalize that they feel birth is imminent, triage and L&D nurses respond in an inhumane, apathetic, and condescending manner. During one of the Oakland focus groups, Imani shared more details about her hospital birth experience beyond being repeatedly asked by hospital physicians and nurses if all her children had the same father.

> I feel like I had a different [experience] but I feel like I have to speak up. I had her natural but it's like I kept asking them, could they come check me. Because I knew that she was low and that I was ready to push. But every time they would say oh, we don't want to check because it's more of a cause of infection, the more we stick our hands up there. And then, eventually, I just felt her too low. I was like you need to come because I'm about to have this baby. You need to come put your hand in here. And, you know, they put their hand in there. And they're like okay, yeah, it's time to push. And they rushed like five nurses in there. It was like I had to tell you all I'm ready to push this baby out. They didn't understand.

If, at that point in the labor, there were no overt signs of clinical or subclinical infection, what did the nurse gain from refusing to perform a cervical exam? In that moment, the L&D nurse prioritized prevention of an adverse physical outcome (when there were no subclinical signs of infection) over the manifestation of a patient-reported experience of emotional safety and connectedness. Deciding to withhold compassionate care warrants an immediate investigation of a nurse's performance by supervisors and the impacted patient and family. The repeated and persistent patterns of quality violations consistent with the dimensions of obstetric racism need to be formally and explicitly named, recognized, and reported to hospital leadership, human resources, risk and liability professionals, credentialing and licensure-granting organizations, and insurance companies.

A Black mother in Los Angeles, Regina, summarized her experience with an L&D triage nurse whose behavior and language reinforced several dimensions of obstetric racism.

> That—or even—so I think I knew when I first got there because he came two weeks early. Literally my first day of maternity leave. I was going to get my hair done, and I had like a mini-panic attack. I need to go to the hospital. So like when I get to the hospital, they kind of just, like, you don't look like you're in labor. So I was like—yeah, so they, like, took me to the room. And she's [the hospital nurse] like telling me—because I had just previously just threw up. So I was kind of feeling a little better. So she was, like, you know, when was the last time you saw your doctor. I was like Thursday. She said I wasn't dilated at all. So she kind of gave me a look like, why are you here kind of thing. And I'm like because I've been having, like, these contractions. I thought they were

> Braxton-Hicks because she said I wasn't dilated. So, I was like, maybe, these fake contractions. So she was looking at me, kind of like how she's responding is just, like, girl, you're not in labor. Like, why are you here? She was, like, since you're here, I'll get some [vital signs] and we'll check you. And she ends up checking me or someone else checks me. And then she kind of comes back like, oh, I heard you're three centimeters dilated. She said, well, you didn't look like you were in labor. She was like—I was just, like, oh my God. I walked into triage, and they're like, oh, yeah, we're probably not going to admit you. And I'm like why? From the beginning it's kind of like—like, what is this experience going to be, you know.

As a result of the L&D triage nurse's harmful language and behavior, Regina began to doubt her experiential knowledge of painful contractions as well as her own account of her bodily experiences. When the cervical exam supported the Black mother's bodily experience and her testimony of her bodily experience, then the nurse offered a snarky response, "*And then she kind of comes back like, oh, I heard you're three centimeters dilated. She said, well, you didn't look like you were in labor.*" The absence of empathy, dignity, and humanity in the provision of obstetric care by the L&D triage nurse characterizes the current culture and conditions of hospital-based obstetrics beyond California maternity-birthing hospitals, extending across many hospitals across the United States.

The use of focus group dialogue further reveals a pattern of medical abuse and intentionally causing pain within the same and across different birthing hospitals that centers the nurse as the lead actor and lever for reproducing obstetric racism. At the same time, the focus group dialogue shows a conformity of thought in which one Black mother activates a new self-efficacy belief in her right and capacity to refuse medical care, specifically cervical exams. The second self-efficacy belief is her right, capacity, option, and choice to resist systemic behaviors that perpetuate medical abuse and intentionally causing pain during cervical exams.

> *Regina:* And another thing—if I could just add—they were so rough, like, when they were checking for, like, the dilation. Did anybody else experience, like—
>
> *Kenya:* Yes.
>
> *Michelle:* Yes.
>
> *Zaria:* I wouldn't let them check.
>
> *Shanice:* Oh, my god.
>
> *Zaria:* Oh, my girlfriend, I could not—

Regina: I wish I knew—I wish I knew to deny. I found out that you could deny the check after I had the baby. I—I wish I had known, because—It was hurting too much. Man, what are you doing? I cried—

Kenya: Yeah.

Regina:—like, she hurt me so much I cried.

Michelle: Yeah.

Regina: And she's just, like, well you got pregnant, like—it—my two fingers—right—she's like if my two fingers are going to hurt you, imagine what your baby's head is going to feel like.

Kenya: Oh my—

Shanice: Oh no, no.

Zaria: She would've had to leave the room—

Michelle: Right, right.

Regina: And she did—and she did. She had to do a staff change. I'm, like, oh no, she cannot do anything for me or my baby, because I'm about to fight her, okay—in labor, everything. You know, it's just—not to make it violent, but don't do that.

In choosing to make meaning of focus group dialogue instead of individual excerpts, one observes a swelling of peer support, reassurance, and empathy, as well as shared rage, as responses to obstetric racism. The current typologies of responses to obstetric racism demonstrated by five Black mothers in the narrative include acts of refusal (declining to participate in the medicalization of birth, including medical abuse, coercion, disrespect, medical intervention, and domination) and resistance (applying experiential knowledge to mobilize against the systems and structures of obstetric care). An elaboration of Davis' three responses takes into account a righteous rage in response to patterns of neglect, dismissiveness, disrespect, intentionally causing pain, medical abuse, coercion, ceremonies of degradation, and diagnostic lapse.

Instead of rage, many Black women expressed hurt, disappointment, or shock at the magnitude of harm they experienced while hospital clinicians and staff withheld compassionate and responsive care. In the case of Mariah, one learns about the horror and agony of laboring with an inadequate epidural and a hospital birth team that was non-responsive to the suffering of a Black reproducing body in labor with inappropriate and inadequate pain control. For context, Mariah is a Black mother married to a Black man in Los Angeles, with a history of two prior normal and healthy vaginal births, and then pregnant for the third time with their first twin pregnancy. Mariah shared her harmful experience,

> I know I was carrying twins, but I imagined that it would be just like my first two children. I would get the epidural, push the out when the babies were ready, and that be the end of it. Unfortunately, I brought—well, I brought my exercise ball there. So I was bouncing around. They—you know, they were okay with that. They didn't want me to walk around. So the only way I could sneak and walk around was I have to go to the bathroom. I have to go to the bathroom. I have to go to the bathroom. I have to go to the bathroom. And so I would take that opportunity to walk back and forth. Walk back and forth. And then when I was inside the bathroom, I would walk a little bit. And then walk back and forth. So—but once I got the epidural, and the doctor—the first doctor said we can't break your water, C-section. Finally, the specialist comes, and he's, like, we have to give your body a fighting chance. Otherwise, you could bleed to death if you [choose a cesarean birth]. So they break my water in the surgery room, but they were not prepared to transport me from the regular birthing bed to the small metal bed. So I had to scoot. They helped me, but I had to scoot. So I really believe that in that scooting, it knocked the—the tubing for the epidural out of place because when it was time to push, I felt absolutely everything. I felt everything. And the—I'm pressing the little button to give me extra doses. Nothing was working. I literally lost all of my breath and started to hyperventilate and shake out of control because of how painful it was. I mean, and so to the point where—and I don't—I would consider myself a pretty, you know, mentally stable person. And I was losing my breath to the point where I was hyperventilating. And I'm not one for drama, you know. So I'm, like, what is happening to me. And they're [h hospital clinicians and staff] just—complete shock. Complete shock. So I'm losing my breath. I felt like I'm about to pass out. Thank God I got through that contraction. And they just couldn't understand it. They're—you know, it's—you know, there isn't any way that we can control where the anesthesia—where the anesthesia goes. I mean, we can do it—I felt like his ego [the anesthesiologist] was challenged. We can do it again [epidural placement number two], but you're just feeling pressure. And who can argue when you're nine centimeters dilated? I'm pregnant with twins. Thank God my husband was there, kind of going toe to toe with him, but I mean, it was ridiculous. It was absolutely ridiculous. And I felt like I was completely overlooked, probably could have died. I probably could have passed out. Do you need oxygen? Yeah, I need oxygen. I can't breathe.
>
> *Dr. Scott:* Did someone ever look at your back to see if the catheter was still there [connect to her back in the epidural space of her vertebral column]?
>
> *Mariah:* No, I don't believe so.

A simple and quick visual inspection of Mariah's back and the bedsheets to check for an intact epidural catheter could have addressed Mariah's reported experience of an abrupt onset of severe pain. Instead, the hospital birthing team of nurses, physicians, and support staff activated their uninterrogated belief that Blackness is pathological, permitting the hospital team to deemphasize, diminish, or ignore the Black mother's symptoms. Ultimately, the hospital team's denial of Mariah's pain, as well as their lack of motivation to explore different possibilities for identifying the problem and activating a solution to end Mariah's suffering, resulted in an inappropriate or lapsed diagnosis (e.g., displacement of the epidural catheter). The callous responses from the anesthesiologist and L&D nursing staff reproduced neglect, dismissiveness, disrespect and intentionally caused ongoing pain, with no expressed desire or motivation to end Mariah's suffering. Once again, the pattern of dismissing Black suffering reinforces the manifestations of nineteenth century antebellum anti-Black racist and anti-Black misogynistic ideologies in twenty-first century contemporary models of obstetric care practices, policies, and procedures.

The lack of righteous rage is more obvious nearly five years after the collection of Black women's narratives of pregnancy, childbirth, and postpartum in Oakland and Los Angeles, in community partnership and with participation by the African American BCOT and BWW. A few times, Black mothers policed their own language, behaviors, and attitudes in real time as a method to prioritize the comfort of hospital clinicians and staff during their own physical and emotional suffering. This self-induced policing could be interpreted as a form of racial reconnaissance, which Davis describes as the Herculean effort made by Black women to avoid or mitigate racist encounters, including being hypervigilant about procedures and finding providers. In the above narrative, Mariah described a very challenging and painful experience of severe pain while pushing the patient-controlled anesthesia or handheld device to manage the administration of epidural doses.

During her severely painful contractions, Mariah policed her own attitude, behavior, and language to avoid being seen as a threat, an angry Black woman, or an angry and crazy Black woman. The internalization of medical misogynoir and ableism emerged from the shadows of the text, highlighting Mariah's fear of being labeled and treated as a stereotype, "I mean, and so to the point where—and I don't—I would consider myself a pretty, you know, mentally stable person. And I was losing my breath to the point where I was hyperventilating. And I'm not one for drama, you know." Instead of responding with a valid and appropriate expression of rage, the Black mother chooses to practice self-imposed tone policing, effectively shifting the conversation away from her pain to maintaining peace, decorum, and order with the hospital clinicians. According to Ijeoma Oluo in her book *So You Want To Talk*

About Race, tone policing is when someone (usually a privileged or more powerful person) in a conversation about oppression or violence shifts the conversation from the oppression or violence being discussed to how oppression or violence is being discussed. Tone policing prioritizes the comfort of the privileged (or more powerful person) in the situation over the oppression or violence of the structurally marginalized or minoritized person (Oluo 2019; MacLachlan 2022). Another Black mother in Oakland, Tasha, shared several harmful patient-reported experiences, and yet she felt the need to talk herself into believing the hospital remained a good place to birth despite all of her harmful experiences. "You know, like—and then he—of course, just her reaction and her response to all of that was inappropriate, you know. But I just—I was floored, literally. I had to make it very clear to the hospital staff that she could not do anything for me at all, whatsoever. And my experience with hospital #6 was wonderful, you know, outside of her. You know, and the vitamin K thing, you know, but other than that, I was okay. Like I don't have any other complaints." Black women's decision to shrink themselves while under assault by hospital clinicians and staff, including self-imposed tone policing of expressions and moods, is an example of racial reconnaissance. For the purposes of maintaining psychological, physical, cultural, and emotional safety and securing one's protection, Black women must make choices every moment throughout every day about how to show up in the world to prevent or mitigate any further harm.

In reflecting on the lived experiences of Black mothers navigating the U.S. maternity health systems and birthing hospitals in California and beyond, the overall goal of contemporary obstetric care is to pathologize, medicalize, and monetize pregnancy and Blackness. By assigning numerical and monetary values to each medical diagnosis, visit type, and medical procedure including laboratory tests and imaging studies, the erosion of empathy, humanity, and dignity is a natural progression in the evolution of care. The entire system of care from conception to postpartum at design, implementation, expansion, evaluation, sustainability, financing, and dissemination feels anti-Black woman. Ebony, in Los Angeles, offered a rationale for the collective anti-Black woman practices and overt culture of medical misogynoir permeating birthing hospitals,

> Right. Exactly. Because she was saying like you're just a number. So, is it just the business part if like, okay, well you just need the new—the new bed. And, you know—this is your policy, this is what was in writing, this is what you signed. Or is it, we're just kind of like cutting you off and, you know, not providing you with continuity of care because you're African American.

The business of birth relies on the commodification of the womb.

When contextualizing the current financialization of obstetric, one cannot help but draw parallels between the commodification of the womb with chattel slavery and the commodification of enslaved Black lives, bodies, labor, and sexual and reproductive labor. According to 2021 data, one in three live births in U.S. hospitals occurred by way of a cesarean birth (Hamilton, Martin, and Osterman 2022). Nearly 32 percent of all live births in the United States required longer hospitalization, higher intensive care, higher staffing, and more for both the birthing parent and newborn. A big data analysis published in 2022 examined the association between patient race/ethnicity and the odds of a hospital performing a cesarean surgery in one of the largest health systems in the country that also serves as a supplier of private insurance. Study findings demonstrated that hospitals throughout this California-based health system and supplier of private insurance were more likely to perform a cesarean surgery on Black women, despite white women being the most represented in the study sample (Black participants 5.32 percent, white participants 41.62 percent) (Okwandu et al. 2022).

The critical questions raised by Ebony in Los Angeles highlight existing concerns for the medicalization, pathologization, criminalization, and commodification of Black bodies, Black wombs, and Black motherhood (Roberts 1997; Sharp 2000; Roberts 2011; Roberts 2012; Cooper 2015; Goodwin 2017; Goodwin 2020; Roberts 2022).

> Well, it makes me think about like, is the value associated with just—is it just the business side of it or is it the fact that we're African American? That's what comes to mind. I mean, I don't know the answer to that. But it just makes me think like the cutoff, how it's just like, okay, you are no longer in our care. And you're just—it's just like abrupt cutoff. I'm wondering is that abrupt cutoff because it's business or because we're African American and we're being treated that way. And I wish I could get an answer for that.

What happens when an OBGYN cannot profit from the pathologization, medicalization, and commodification of Black wombs? How does an OBGYN within the broader systems and structures of obstetric care react to a full-bodied pregnant Black woman with no pre-existing medical co-morbidities? The absence of perinatal pathology does not guarantee the presence of perinatal equity, quality, and safety. Anti-Black racism and misogynoir serve as the foundation and pillars upon which the institution and profession of obstetrics and gynecology were built (Roberts 1997; Eichelberger et al. 2016; Owens 2017; Davis 2018; Davis 2019; Scott, Britton, and McLemore 2019; Scott 2019a; Scott 2019b; Davis 2020; Davis, Varner, and Hill 2021; Khabele et al. 2021; Scott 2021; Scott and Davis 2021; Chambers et al. 2022; Scott and Davis 2022; White VanGompel et al. 2022; Lett et al. 2023; Edmonds, Tucker, and Walker 2023; Scott and Lusero 2023).

When a full-bodied pregnant Black woman screened negative for most medical conditions, the OBGYN responded in shock, doubting the master's tools and science, then one can only surmise that their disbelief is informed by the uninterrogated belief that Blackness is pathological. Introducing Felicia, a Black mother in Los Angeles, who shared her interactions with an Asian woman OBGYN physician as her first Black pregnant patient and the impact of anti-Black racist and anti-Black misogynistic ideologies, interactions, and practices.

Felicia: I had the doctor—so I was in this space or group called Melanin Moms. That kind of, like, helped me with, like, just a lot of the information because I actually went through two doctors because I learned that I don't have to just stick with a doctor that I don't feel is for me. If I know this doctor isn't giving me the care that I need, I don't have to just put up with this doctor. And I didn't know that at first. So I literally switched when I was about 26 weeks because when I found that out, I said, okay, yeah. No, well, we'll be getting another doctor then. Because it was—I wasn't getting the treatment that I needed. And then—so switching that late, I got another doctor that kind of, you know, didn't really know me, and going over—and then I learned that this was—through my experience, I learned this was her first African-American mother that she had treated.

Dr. Scott: You?

Felicia: Yes. So I was tested for every possible—anything that any black woman has ever had—I kid you not, I kid you not.

Dr. Scott: Tell me more about that, please. Like, what did she test you for?

Felicia: I can't even think. The first one, she tested me for something with an S.

Dr. Scott: Like, in general, was it a chronic condition, a disease, STI?

Felicia: A condition that African women—African-American women have.

Dr. Scott: For your blood?

Felicia: Yes.

Dr. Scott: Sickle cell?

Felicia: Yes. Sickle cell. She tested me for that. And she tested me—and I am a bigger woman. So she tested me for diabetes and was shocked that I did not have diabetes.

Michelle: Not shocked.

Felicia: She was shocked. She was, like, oh, okay. Not diabetes. I was—I was tested for everything. And she was in shock when the results were not what she thought they were, and—

Dr. Scott: I got to ask you. How did you know she was in shock?

Felicia: Her reaction.

Dr. Scott: Her words?

Felicia: She came back—yeah, her words. Her words and the way she—it was—you can tell it was shock. She was like, oh okay, no—okay. Okay—

Dr. Scott: You're healthy, and she wasn't ready for that.

Felicia: Yes. So I ended up kind of getting stuck with the last Ob-Gyn who was kind of like a—this is the way I do it. No, we're not—she literally would tell me, no, no, this is how we do it. No, no—it was like a—I don't want to use her."

Felicia experienced and endured an uninterrogated belief in the pathologization of Blackness combined with an uninterrogated disbelief in Black vitality and wellness with the Asian OBGYN physician. Based on the OBGYN's approach to caring for a full-bodied Black woman, the physician demonstrated multiple gaps in clinical cognition and responsiveness to historical and contemporary intersecting systems and structures that inform and control access to, utilization of, and distribution of structural and social determinants of health and wealth, particularly for Black women in Los Angeles, the United States, and the world. Clinical cognition includes processes such as problem-solving, reasoning, decision-making, comprehension, memory retrieval, perception, interpretation, and synthesis of patient findings, and rationale for diagnostic and therapeutic decisions (Cimino, Li, and Weng 2018). According to Metzl and Roberts, the response of the Asian OBGYN physician and the other OBGYNs to Felicia would be identified as structural incompetency in clinician recognition of the social and structural needs of Felicia and communities of Black women, and the relationship between social and structural needs and race and racism, gender and gender oppression, and race plus gender and misogynoir (Metzl and Roberts 2014). Structural incompetency to structural racism leads to "impaired clinician recognition of the health-related influences of institutions, markets, and health care delivery systems" (Metzl and Roberts 2014, 675). Consequently, impaired clinician recognition of structural racism and other oppressive structures and systems on health care funding, resource allocation, and delivery system will likely prompt suboptimal use of medical knowledge by physicians to determine diagnostic and therapeutic options and decision-making (Metzl and Roberts 2014).

Each failure to establish psychological and sociocultural safety and connectedness between Felicia and a prenatal care team of health professionals represented a missed opportunity to actualize Felicia's autonomy, agency, and self-efficacy in care exploration, utilization, communication, consent, and decision-making. Instead, Felicia encountered an OBGYN whose uninterrogated beliefs, practices, and behaviors led the OBGYN to de-emphasize or ignore normality, or normal pregnancy physiology in a full-bodied Black woman, not only in test results but in Black pregnancy. Subsequently, the OBGYN's uninterrogated beliefs and behaviors resulted in a lapsed diagnosis of a healthy and free Black woman choosing pregnancy and parenting. And that is the unintended consequences of uninterrogated obstetric racism—adopting assumptions that Blackness is inferior, and a positive outcome suggests a positive experience of care. Therefore, my Black feminist hermeneutic phenomenology of Black pregnancy, labor, birth, and postpartum mandates the dismantling of the hypocrisies of quality and safety in contemporary U.S. obstetric care in hospital settings.

Chapter 3

Safety and Accountability

Tasha: So, I felt like they wasn't hearing me, especially in the operating room. So, I thought why they were doing it and why then—like the room was cold but they were pushing to make—keep pushing to, you know, get the baby out. So, they were pushing me and pushing me. All of that I like really felt sick, light-headed, the room started spinning. I was like throwing up. And I kept telling her I feel sick, I feel sick, I feel sick. He put a vomit had thing up. And then, you know, they were like oh, no one ever feels sick. Like how could you be feeling sick. And I'm telling her like it's, you know, because it's a nurse by here. And whoever you have in the room is over here. And so, I'm telling the nurse who was holding my hand is that I feel sick, I feel sick, I feel sick. Like wake me up or lift me up, give me that thing. She wasn't giving nothing. She said no. She was like no one ever complains about feeling sick. You're the first one ever. I've never heard that in all my years of working. And I'm like but I feel sick. I feel real sick. The room was spinning. And then like I had to tell myself like to just close my eyes and try to breathe. But I just couldn't. And then all of a sudden, the throw up came up. And, of course, that was a whole big old thing. And I'm like I told you. I made sure of it this way. Admit it. She, by the way, was mad but I'm like I told you. And she told me like after it was over—after the baby came out, they put me in a room and I was trying to breast feed her. And they said—and I'm telling her like my whole upper region is numb. Everything—my neck. I just felt numb. And she told me like oh, you're not supposed to be feeling that. Nobody can be feeling that. Your supposed to numb from this, you know, from the abdomen all the way down. And she was like if anything your feet would be numb and this and that. And I'm telling her like my breast feels numb. They was tingling and stuff was going on. And she was just like you can't be numb up there. And I said I am. I don't feel the baby sucking. Like she's sucking, I can hear her.

Dr. Scott: You could see her, yeah.

Tasha: But I couldn't feel her because it was just, I felt like all the nerves, I was just tingling. I just remember it was tingling.

Dr. Scott: So, what was her response?

Participant Speaker: Her response was you couldn't be numb. She said you couldn't be numb

Dr. Scott: Did anything happen as a follow up or they just basically dismissed what you were saying.

Tasha: No, she dismissed it and it was no like follow up. When the physician came to check on me, I did tell him that I was feeling numb. And it was like okay, well give it about an hour or two and if it doesn't get better then tell your nurse again. And I was like okay. But it did go away the next day. But—

Jada: That's a long time.

Tasha:—still—right. I was just scared because, you know, you have to lactate and I'm like am I having an allergic reaction or. You know, I wasn't feeling no itchiness. It was just constantly tingle, tingle, tingle, tingle. But it was a painful tingle. It was like a hurt tingle.

Dr. Scott: And it was all over?

Tasha: Just from the neck down here to my breasts. Like I wasn't feeling nothing down here.

Dr. Scott: So, you had no acknowledgement and no real response to what you're saying. Just dismissing you?

Tasha: Yeah

Black mothers defined safety as protection and security from unintended, unwanted, unplanned, unwelcomed harm, injury, or malicious event, experience, or outcome. The loss of protection and security from harm, injury, or malice threatens a Black mother's sense of innate human worth, or dignity. With the loss of protection and security to preserving the dignity of Black mothers, then the health system violates Black mothers' right to decisional autonomy and optimal and equitable care. The safety violation combined with the lack of accountability (accepting responsibility for one's own actions) and oversight (accepting responsibility for the monitoring of others' actions) in keeping Black mothers safe, undermines a Black mother's sense of belonging (psychological safety, and connectedness) and dignity (innate human worth) as an autonomous patient, as an active participant in the provider-patient dyad, and as a credible patient expert within the medical industrial complex. A single safety violation or a series of safety violations within an episode of care can erode a Black mother's trust and perceived self-efficacy in accepting, believing, trusting, understanding, and sharing her truths, and then having her truths be both easily understood and believed by others.

When a Black mother reports the occurrence of an event or a series of events happening within her body to one or more hospital clinicians and staff, and the immediate initial and follow-up hospital response consists of denial and dismissiveness, the hospital commits epistemic injustice (Fricker 2007). Epistemic injustice occurs when systems, structures, institutions, groups of individuals, or an individual denies the capacity of another individual to act as a knower and fundamentally, unfairly denies the human value, or dignity, of the individual (Fricker 2007). According to Fricker, two fundamental epistemic practices include gaining knowledge by being told and making sense of social experiences. Thus, epistemic practices in the provision of health care services require collecting information from the patient about the nature, onset, frequency, duration, exacerbating or alleviating factors, intensity, timing, location, or radiating factors of symptoms or bodily events.

In the above Black birthing narrative about Tasha, a Black mother in Oakland, she repeatedly communicated the occurrence of different bodily events (e.g., nausea with urge to vomit and numbness and tingling in her upper body/breast area including areolas and nipples) while the hospital nurse responded with neglect, dismissiveness, and disrespect, one of six dimensions of obstetric racism (Davis 2018; Davis 2019; Davis 2020). According to Davis, the act of ignoring or dismissing a person's expressed need for reproductive help or care and/or treating them with disdain is defined as neglect, dismissiveness, or disrespect. The evidence of denial of Tasha's expressed need for help and care by the hospital nurse in the operating room and later in the postpartum room manifested in nursing communication. In those moments, epistemic injustice describes the form of unfair treatment stemming from the nurse's decision to deny Tasha's knowledge, understanding, and participation in communicative practices about events occurring in her body. Consequently, the nurse denied Tasha's autonomy (free will), agency (power to make decisions with available options and resources), and self-efficacy (one's belief and confidence in making decisions or achieving goals) in meaning-making and knowledge-generating practices about clinical symptoms and disease manifestation (Kidd, Medina, and Pohlhaus 2017).

Epistemic injustice creates two byproducts, testimonial injustice and hermeneutical injustice. Testimonial injustice occurs when the system or the individual health care professional combines prejudice with exploitation of power differentials and dynamics, exerts dominance over the patient, and undermines the patient's credibility in meaning-making and knowledge production about events in their own body. When a health care discipline, system, or individual denies patients and their communities of origin full participation in meaning-making and knowledge-producing practices about events in their individual and collective bodies, the phenomenon is called hermeneutical injustice. As a result, hermeneutical injustice renders patients, their family members, and their communities of origin incapable of making sense of their own experiences, and of having those experiences understood by others (Fricker 2007; Kidd, Medina, and Pohlhaus 2017; Scott 2021; Lyndon et al. 2023).

The implications of epistemic injustice result in having one's meanings or knowledge contributions distorted, misheard, or misrepresented by structures, systems, or disciplines that weaponize exclusion and erasure, being silent and silenced, or invisibility and inaudibility (Kidd, Medina, and Pohlhaus 2017). Based on Vivian May's scholarship that explores feminist theory and epistemology, including Black feminist thought, she asserted that Black feminist civil rights activist and public intellectual Anna Julia Cooper anticipated the concept of epistemic injustice during the 1890s by claiming that Black women are denied full and equal recognition as knowers (May 2014). The systematic and structural failure to include Black women as knowers in the development and operationalization of broader, more inclusive, patient- and community-focused safety meanings and measures facilitates testimonial and hermeneutical injustice.

Existing literature describes the persistence of significant problems in the reporting of patient safety incidents. One specific reporting barrier includes the lack of shared language and meaning to facilitate the accurate identification and measurement of harm. Additional challenges include the lack of alternative and complementary methods for data gathering about patient safety and the utilization of these data to catalyze organizational transformation (Rodziewicz et al. 2024). At the close of the nineteenth century, patient safety focused on medical errors. The Institute of Medicine (IOM), now referred to as The National Academy of Medicine (NAM), endorsed the following definition of a medical error, "the failure of a planned action to be completed as intended or the use of a wrong plan to achieve an aim" (Institute of Medicine Committee on Quality of Health Care in America 2020, 2). Adoption of a limited definition of safety resulted in systems denial of and/or accountability for patient harm as a possible consequence of medical errors, independent of structural or institutional intention (Grober and Bohnen 2005; Oyebode 2013; Kapaki and Souliotis 2018). Subsequent research then focused on adverse events defined as an injury resulting from a medical intervention. The Institute for Healthcare Improvement (IHI) equates adverse events with harm and offers the following definition of an adverse event, an "unintended physical injury resulting from or contributed to by medical care that requires additional monitoring, treatment, or hospitalization or that results in death" (Griffin and Rezar 2009, 2). However, the different definitions and perspectives create differential assumptions and approaches to preventability, mitigation, and accountability, ultimately confounding safety measurement research in healthcare (Hooker et al. 2019). According to the IOM, all errors are preventable, unlike adverse events, which can be either preventable or not preventable. Interestingly, injury to healthcare workers has been included in the broader definitions of healthcare safety (de Bienassis, Slawomirski and Klazinga 2021).

Despite the proliferation of scholarly articles related to patient safety, with most work addressing the measurement of specific phenomena such as inserting central lines, patient and worker falls, needlesticks, medication safety, and hospital-acquired infections, there has been little to no significant effort to incorporate patient perspectives and priorities in safety definitions and measurements (de Bienassis, Slawomirski and Klazinga 2021). If given the opportunity, we know that patients will provide feedback on the quality, safety, and impact of care using their own lived experiences and offer novel and nuanced details about specific types of medical errors and adverse events that might be missed or underestimated using traditional reporting systems, mechanisms, and platforms. For example, patient-reported events or experiences are often not expressed using the limited lexicon of clinical safety. Therefore, patient involvement in safety definition and measurements can provide more robust insights and accounts of the nature of the problem as well as potential solutions for mitigating the onset, frequency, duration, magnitudes, and reoccurrence (Scott 2019a, 2019b, 2021; Scott et al. 2021; Scott and Davis 2021; Lyndon et al. 2023; Scott and Lusero 2023).

While the obstetric patient safety literature recognized the engagement of administrative and clinical leadership, particularly nursing leadership, substantial progress in the standardization and documentation of critical processes, establishment of national quality benchmarks, reduction in elective deliveries less than 39 weeks' gestation, and reduction in fatal post-cesarean pulmonary embolism (Pronovost 2011; Grobman 2012; ACOG 2003), there are no safety meanings or measures in hospital-based obstetrics as defined for, by, or with Black mothers and birthing people. Organizations such as the National Quality Forum (NQF), the World Health Organization (WHO), the National Patient Safety Foundation (NPSF), AHRQ, and IOM have endorsed many different definitions of patient safety. In summary, different organizations defined patient safety in different ways:

- "*a discipline in the health care sector that applies safety science methods toward the goal of achieving a trustworthy system of health care delivery. Patient safety is also an attribute of health care systems; it minimizes the incidence and impact of, and maximizes recovery from, adverse events,*" according to AHRQ (Emanuel et al. 2008, 1);
- "*the prevention and mitigation of harm caused by errors of omission or commission that are associated with healthcare, and involving the establishment of operational systems and processes that minimize the likelihood*

of errors and maximize the likelihood of intercepting them when they occur," according to NQF (Angood et al. 2009, 4);
- "*the absence of preventable harm to a patient during the process of health care. The discipline of patient safety is the coordinated effort to prevent harm, caused by the process of health care itself, from occurring to patients,*" according to the WHO (WHO 2009, 14);
- "*the avoidance, prevention and amelioration of adverse outcomes or injuries stemming from the processes of health care including errors, deviations and accidents. Safety emerges from the proper interaction of the components of the health care system,*" according to the NPSF (Cooper et al. 2024, 3); and
- "the prevention of harm caused by errors of commission and omission," according to the IOM (Institute of Medicine (US) Committee on Data Standards for Patient Safety 2004, 2–3).

My overall impression of the various patient safety definitions is the atheoretical and ahistorical approach to developing meanings of safety in the provision of health care to human beings. The exclusion or erasure of the influence of racism in creating and exacerbating differences in safety responses and outcomes, considering the 2000 publication of "Levels of Racism" by Dr. Camara Jones, MD, PhD, MPH, former president of the American Public Health Association (APHA) (Jones 2000) and the IOM 2003 report titled, *Unequal Treatment* (Institute of Medicine (US) Committee on Understanding and Eliminating Racial and Ethnic Disparities in Health Care 2003). Dr. Jones provided an ecological framework for naming and recognizing levels of racism using the allegory of the Gardener's Tale in 2000 (Jones 2000).

In 2003, the IOM provided substantive evidence to confirm the existence of racial and ethnic disparities (more aptly defined as inequities and injustices) and identified many drivers of racial inequities in health care systems, health care providers, and patient and utilization managers (Betacourt and Maina 2004). Given the plethora of evidence of discrimination in the provision of health care, including intersectional drivers such as racial capitalism, gendered racism, misogynoir, and transmisogynoir, the existing patient safety meanings create a myopic approach that feels callous, irrelevant, inhumane, mechanical, and irresponsible. Even when searching the literature for a well-developed consensus on the definition of obstetric patient safety, one finds the same rhetoric shaped by the IOM definition of patient safety. Obstetric patient safety is defined as "the absence of the potential for, or the occurrence of, healthcare-associated injury to the patient, contributing to the larger paradigm and discussion on health care quality" (Grobman 2012, 3). By focusing on obstetric morbidity and mortality, obstetric patient safety applies a dichotomous framework for characterizing an obstetric quality problem as an adverse event, an outcome due to health care management as opposed to the progression of natural disease, or a potential adverse event, an outcome resulting from defective processes in health care provision and management that have a high likelihood of causing harm (Grobman 2012). Increasing concerns for protection from potential liability fueled by obstetricians, combined with rates of perinatal morbidity and mortality, shaped the development and refinement of the obstetric patient safety paradigm, according to Grobman. Yet, the patient's expectations, experiences, and expressions of care remain excluded from known definitions of patient safety. The individuals and communities most impacted by the people, processes, procedures, practices, and policies that design, implement, evaluate, govern, and fund health care remain the least involved in safety meaning development, measurement selection, monitoring strategies, and accountability and oversight mechanisms.

In listening to and learning from and with thirty-six Black mothers who gave birth in hospital settings in Oakland and Los Angeles, we developed seven patient-identified quality domains. The first domain in the SACKRED Birth framework is Safety and Accountability. Black mothers developed a shared meaning of safety during the provision of hospital-based obstetrics as the state of feeling unconditional love whereby a Black mother is not always being in a state of fear, which then generates stressful feelings and stress responses as manifested by fight, flight, freeze, or fawn as a daily reality, reaction, or response to hospital clinicians and staff. The feeling of unconditional love in obstetric patient safety also conjures feelings of comfort, relaxation, and peace because of the protection and security from unintended, unwanted, unplanned, unwelcomed harm, injury, or malicious events, experiences, or outcome. According to the intellectual thoughts about Black mothers' expectations, experiences, and expressions of care by Black mothers, obstetric patient safety is determined by access to and utilization of rich and robust resources and assets (i.e., finances, education, training, health, well-being, stability, wisdom, transgenerational kinship ties) that activate and amplify the inclusion and integration of partners, especially Black men, in care, communication, interactions, and decision-making. A primary driver of obstetric patient safety as defined for, by, and with Black mothers is the active acknowledgment and affirmation of Black given and chosen kinships in care provision. Space-making for Black given and chosen kinships throughout any hospital setting and across all phases of childbirth hospitalization (e.g., triage, admission, labor, birth, and immediate postpartum) leads to increased perceptions and experience of safety and trust for Black mothers and birthing people.

Black mothers also expanded the application of the definition of obstetric patient safety to Black community and neighborhood safety and well-being. The expanded definition of obstetric patient safety holds hospitals accountable for curating environments of safety within hospital settings that honor the context and conditions of feeling, knowing, and being a Black woman or person first, within and outside of the hospital, and beyond pregnancy and birth. By including the context and conditions of feeling, thinking, knowing, and being a Black woman within the definition of obstetric patient safety, Black women feel they have more self-efficacy in controlling their future based on present-day actions, opportunities, options, and resources to secure safety in birthing while Black in U.S. hospitals.

Black mothers and birthing feel safety show up in eight core behaviors that can be measured, monitored, and managed in hospital-based obstetric policies, processes, procedures, and practices as:

1. Feeling love and loved as manifested by hospitals caring for, supporting, consoling, reassuring, and comforting Black mothers through gentle, affirming, mindful, motivating, and patient attitudes, language, and behavior;
2. Curating a hospital culture of belonging (psychological safety, and connectedness) during social and clinical interactions in hospital settings where Black mothers, birthing people, and their loved ones *feel seen, heard, affirmed, desired, valued, and included* in the health care provision and decision-making by a hospital system and team that is accessible, approachable, appropriate, accepting, attentive, available, accommodating, and responsive (Levesque et al. 2013);
3. Avoiding hospital systems, teams, or individual attitudes, language, or behaviors that result in Black mothers feeling rushed, dismissed, ignored, neglected, not listened to, or not having their questions and concerns addressed during clinical encounters and interactions, inciting and exacerbating psychological or emotional vulnerability combined with feelings of insecurity and unreliability toward hospital systems, teams, and individual clinicians and staff;
4. Acknowledging, affirming, activating, and amplifying the presence and participation of the social network or kinship ties between the Black mother and her newborn, her partner, her parent, her existing children, her siblings, and her loved ones;
5. Protecting, securing, and activating patient autonomy (free will), agency (power to make a decision or achieve a goal with optimal options, opportunities, and resources), and self-efficacy (one's belief and confidence in one's ability to make a decision or achieve a goal);
6. Facilitating consistent communication and information exchange among patient, primary physician, specialist physician, hospital team, and given and chosen kin for the purposes of activating, actualizing, and

amplifying the power of the patient in meaning-making and knowledge production;
7. Prioritizing infant well-being as maternal/parental welling and maternal/parental well-being as infant well-being by avoiding the dissociation of mother/birthing person from the fetus/child in social and clinical interactions, communication, counseling, and decision-making; and
8. Facilitating transparency and accountability at the level of the hospital systems, teams, or individual workers.

Black mothers identified accountability as a solution to mitigate the onset, frequency, duration, and magnitude of obstetric racism and described the following as proposed change actions: hospital culture, structures, mechanisms (i.e., policies, practices, protocols, procedures, people, power) that elicit feedback in formal and informal ways from patients about their hospital experience, and then require clinicians and staff to report, explain, or justify their actions in response to patient-reported experiences to patients or the public. The synthesis of the shared meanings and measures for safety and accountability established two overarching themes or manifestations: demonstration of love or feeling loved; and multiple levels of accountability for assuring the presence and integration of love or loving attitudes, language, and behaviors in the care provision (e.g., hospital system, hospital team, individual hospital worker, individual patient).

Multiple times, Black mothers expressed feeling safe in the presence of nurses whose attitude, language, or behavior embodied love during the provision of hospital-based obstetrics care. Consider the lived experiences of Brianna, a Black mother in Oakland, who explains feeling safe throughout her first overnight stay in the hospital, an admission to induce, or start, her labor by first preparing her cervix by administering a medication taken by mouth. The purpose of the oral medication, or pill, is to soften and thin the cervix, a cervical ripening agent, as the preferred initial medication for her induction.

> But my triage nurses and my doctor, they were all Black women. So, I felt really comfortable. They took their time and explained all of the steps. And then they even took the time throughout the night to explain all my options for induction. Because they knew that if I stayed, I was going to be induced. They explained—I wanted to have a natural birth. I didn't want any meds, or anything. And so, I just explained that to them. But I had a whole night to kind of explain that to them. And they took their time to explain to me all my options about how to do that. Not to start with Pitocin but to do the [pills first]—I did everything. It was three days. And all of my [care]—every shift was full of Black women.

In the above individual excerpt, Brianna shared her lived experience of obstetric patient safety because she felt comfortable. Three phenomena occurred during her lived experience of obstetric care that created her comfort: racial and gender concordance, patience, and consistent communication and information exchange. Seeing herself in her entire team caused an immediate sense of psychological safety and connectedness. Then the entire team of Black women facilitated consistent communication and information exchange among the patient, primary physician, specialist physician, hospital team, and given and chosen kin for the purposes of activating and amplifying the power of the patient in meaning-making and knowledge production. Brianna, a Black mother, felt love and loved because the hospital team offered her continuous support and comfort in the form of relevant and responsive communication and information exchange throughout the night in a patient, deliberate manner. The hospital team of Black women curated acts of love by protecting, securing, and activating Brianna's autonomy (free will), agency (power to make a decision or achieve a goal with opportunities, resources, and options), and self-efficacy (one's belief and confidence in one's ability to make a decision or achieve a goal) by offering and explaining all care options related to the labor induction or physician-nurse midwife-initiated onset of labor. The attitude, language, and behavior of the hospital team of Black women facilitated transparency and accountability at the level of the hospital systems, teams, and individual workers. Thus, Brianna, a Black mother, felt safe based on the interactions, communication and information exchange, consent, and decision-making approaches embodied by the hospital team of Black women.

Black mothers described particular kinds of behaviors, nonverbal gestures, and language choices that curated feelings or a spirit of comfort, peace, and relaxation throughout the provision of services and supports. Black mothers conceptualized patient safety as the ever-presence of unconditional love for Blackness, Black people, Black reproducing bodies, Black mothers, Black parents, Black babies, and Black given and chosen kinship as conveyed in every clinical encounter and experience. Safety as a demonstration of love or feeling loved is described by Black mothers as being cared for, supported, consoled, reassured, and comforted throughout their care. Safety as love is manifested by social and clinical behaviors from hospital clinicians and staff that demonstrate gentleness, patience, and mindfulness from staff. Safety as a demonstration of love or feeling loved was exemplified by a labor and delivery (L&D) nurse who visited the patient on her day off or made a special effort to return to the patient's room to say good-bye after the end-of-shift patient hand-off. For Mariah, a Black mother in Los Angeles, safety as love manifested itself in the role of the nurse as cheerleader,

> the last nurse on my team that actually delivered the twins, I call her my personal cheerleader. I pushed both of the babies [eight pound twins] out within a ten-minute time frame, and she's like this is unheard of. She just—I'll never forget—she locked eyes with me, and she was like you can do this. And she was just like this is just one moment in time. You have the rest of your lives about these babies. Give it all you got. Push. And I was like okay. And I pushed. So she was amazing.

In the above Black birth narrative, the nurse fulfilled Mariah's patient expectation of safety by serving as the ultimate pushing coach, showing customized energy and enthusiasm for Mariah's positionality, power, and potential as giver and caretaker of a new life. The nurse fostered safety as love with and for the patient, as demonstrated by "locking eyes" with the Black mother, reassuring the patient with her presence and her direct connection with the patient's needs. Safety as love or feeling loved inspired Black mothers to expand the definition of patient safety beyond the absence of medical errors, adverse events, or near misses. The broader definition of patient safety centers and amplifies social, cultural, emotional, and physical safety in which hospital behaviors, language, images, or messaging cultivate a spirit or culture of belonging. Safety as love and belonging, as defined by Black mothers and birthing people, feels seen, heard, affirmed, and included in the health care team. A Black mother in Los Angeles, Zaria, shared the experience of when she requested a switch from a man nurse to a woman nurse, resulting in a Black nurse at her bedside who honored her autonomy and agency when she declined a cervical exam. Zaria's narrative demonstrated how hospital clinicians and staff can remain engaged, connected, and attentive to patient needs even within the context of informed refusal.

> she was amazing. Like -She checked on me a lot. Even though I told her, no, you can't check me [my cervix], it's [contractions] hurting, but she still was like how are you feeling, are you in pain, what do you need, how can I help you. She literally came and sat in the room like basically her whole entire shift. Like, I went to sleep, I woke up, she was there. She was, like, I'm not going anywhere. Like, if you need anything, let me know. And when I was ready to push, the doctor wasn't there, and they had to page the doctor. And she was, like, the doctor is going to be coming in, like, ten minutes, but you can start pushing now. Like, I'm going to help you. Like, she didn't make me wait for the doctor to get there and start pushing.

Hospitals can sustain patient safety as love and belonging even when patients, especially Black pregnant mothers in labor, decline one cervical exam. Black mothers also described feeling love or loved when hospital clinicians and staff, particularly nurses, show up to work being fully present, passionate, and purposive in their provision of care. One nurse came back to the hospital to visit Ayana, a Black mother in Oakland, on their day off.

> I had a Black woman. She was with me the time that I checked in and then her shift was over at around 5:30. And she was so sad because right when her shift ended like everything started happening. I was starting to push—everything. So, she clocked out, she came back to my room, and she stayed for two hours off the clock. And then she was off the next day and she came up here to visit me on her off day just to meet this baby girl and, you know, just to say hi to my family. Because she was like really involved in my family all day. So, she was so nice.

The expectation for nurses to return to the hospital on their days off to visit previously assigned patients is unrealistic. The more crucial element of the nurse's behavior in Ayana's narrative is contextualizing the meaning and impact of the gracious gesture. For Ayana, she felt psychologically safe and connected to the nurse based on how the nurse cared for her and her family during her labor prior to the birth. The nurse acknowledged, affirmed, activated, and amplified the presence and participation of kinship ties between Ayana, a Black mother, and her family during hospital-based obstetrics. A primary driver of obstetric patient safety as defined for, by, and with Black mothers is the active acknowledgment and affirmation of Black given and chosen kinships in care provision. Space-making for Black given and chosen kinships throughout any hospital setting and across all phases of childbirth hospitalization (e.g., triage, admission, labor, birth, and immediate postpartum) leads to increased perceptions and experiences of safety and trust for Black mothers and birthing people.

Authentic recognition and inclusion of kinship during the provision of hospital-based obstetrics create a love-filled environment. Inclusion and integration of partners, especially Black men, in care communication, interactions, and decision-making, leads to increased perceptions and experiences of safety and trust for Black mothers and birthing people, and the Black men in their lives, independent of kinship ties. Black mothers feel love or loved when the hospital system, team, or individual team members promote belonging for the Black mother and her given and chosen kin.

> I want them to be more supportive of the dads. I didn't like when I had her, I did bonding for like five minutes. And then my son's dad was like really excited about this baby, you know. So, he wanted her, so I gave her to him. And he took off his shirt. You know, he was so ready [for skin-to-skin daddy-baby bonding]. It [the hospital system] was just like we need her to be with the mom right now and just like wrenched her out of his hands to give her back to me. And I was offended because I wanted him to, you know [bond] Yes, you know, he is just as much part of this baby as me. So, give him his time, you know."

From Jada, a Black mother in Oakland, one learns about a nurse dismissing the value and benefit of skin-to-skin daddy-baby bonding. The consequence of the nurse's dismissal led to disrupting the physical connection between a Black father and his newborn. The nurse's decision to separate the Black father from his baby undermined and diminished kinship identity, attachment, and bonding within and across the entire family triad of a Black mother, a Black father, and their Black baby. No excuse or explanation supported the nurse's actions, which reminded Jada and her family that their celebration and new existence of Black love as a Black family they chose to build mattered very little to this nurse.

In general, the impact of a nurse's behavior while "on and off the clock" curated a culture of belonging during social and clinical interactions in hospital settings, where Black mothers and their loved ones, including the newest addition to the expanding family, feel seen, heard, affirmed, and included in the health care team. Many Black mothers repeatedly discussed the role of Black nurses and Black travel nurses in generating love in the provision of care. The expectation for a hospital birth team to exclusively consist of Black physicians and nurse midwives is also unrealistic, given that 7.3 percent of American Midwifery Certification Board (AMCB)-certified nurse midwives and 5.7 percent of active physicians identified as Black or African American based on 2021 workforce demographics, respectively (American Midwifery Certification Board 2021; Harrison et al. 2023; Boyle 2023). Likewise, the assumption that racial and gender concordance (e.g., sociocultural) is inherently protective and life-affirming is unrealistic and naive. Independent of workforce demographics, most Black physicians and nurse midwives in the U.S. obtained education, training, licensure, and certification in the U.S. Therefore, most Black physicians and nurse midwives adopted professional standards of being and knowing that maintain or expand imperialist capitalist white heteropatriarchal supremacy. Consequently, their behaviors, attitudes, and language sometimes reinforce norms and narratives whereby reproductive, partnership, parenting, pleasure-seeking, and family planning choices, options, opportunities, and incentives to imagine a future fall along racialized, gendered, and commodified roles, identities, intimacies, and performances dating back to U.S. chattel slavery and the antebellum era.

Two Black mothers in Oakland, Simone and Imani, exchanged insights in a conversation that reflects the colloquial saying in Black communities, first quoted by Zora Neale Hurston, "All skin folk ain't kin folk." One must be mindful in thinking or believing that sharing similar or same skin hues or shared histories, or culture translates into mutually shared values, visions, and behaviors around Black emancipation, liberation, pleasure, joy, power, or sovereignty.

Simone: And then I had another overnight nurse. She was Black as well but she didn't even really interact with me. She checked on the baby like twice and that's it. She was like in and out. Some of the nurses be like be ready to go. Like they wouldn't want to have a relationship with you, you know.

Imani: Yeah, they were just ready to just do the job but not being—like why would you get a job like that and not love your job. Not—

Simone: Exactly.

Imani:-- care about your job. Not really just that's—it just sometimes it makes you feel it's all for just a paycheck—the nice paycheck."

Any nurse, independent of race, including a Black nurse, can behave in a manner that feels psychologically unsafe and disconnected to a Black mother during the provision of hospital-based obstetric care. Instead of feeling love or loved by the nurse's professional behavior, Simone experienced apathy as manifested by the nurse's practice of exclusion or isolation of the patient in the culture of practice or as a participant in the health care team. Simone then internalized the apathy as the Black nurse's only motivation to work as a nurse is to collect a sizable paycheck. The absence of tender loving care, support, reassurance, comfort, encouragement, patience, mindfulness, affirmations, or meaningful time spent with the patient and her newborn at the bedside fostered feelings of insecurity and worthlessness. Independent of the nurse's motivation, intention, mood, or prior stellar bedside manners, the nurse's performance in that moment elicited feelings of isolation, disconnectedness, and insignificance within the Black mother during one of the most pivotal moments in human life and development.

Simone: Well when you love your job you come in with a whole different persona, a whole different—

Dr. Scott: What is that persona? Describe it.

Simone: Like you're smiling.

Dr. Scott: Okay.

Simone: You're asking questions, you're very attentive, you are just present. You're there. Anything—you're even looking into a person's eyes like when they going through—like you really want to understand. Understand the pain and understand are you in pain. Is there anything—ask other questions afterwards. And [if] you just don't get that. Like okay, bye.

Imani: If you're going to be there love your job and be into your job. Just basically be there. If you're going to have that like in those type of jobs—if you're going to have that kind of job where you're working with people with pain

> medication, you need to really love your job and really do your job the right way. Not just having a paying job and you take a paycheck.

Focus group dialogue between Simone and Imani revealed shared sentiments among the Black mothers in Oakland about the idealistic nurse, a nurse who loves her job and subsequently translates that love into attitudes, language, and behaviors that make Black mothers feel love or loved. Black mothers feel safe when nurses demonstrate genuine interest and concern for Black mother's desires and priorities. Black mothers perceived authentic curiosity and concern as a nurse paying close attention, asking questions, and looking into the eyes of Black mothers to better understand what Black mothers feel, think, know, and desire. Black mothers also explained how they feel when being centered and listened to during the provision of hospital-based obstetrics, particularly across multiple shifts. Brianna's experience at a safety net hospital in Oakland illuminated the importance and impact of feeling love and loved from midwives working their Midwifery Magic on L&D.

> How I felt I was heard? Like a couple things. For one, at Hospital 2 there's a whole staff of midwives that actually run the labor and delivery. Which is amazing because the nurses aren't overworked. The nurses just can come in and check and kind of assist. But the midwives, they have a lot more time I feel like. So, when the shifts would change like I felt like a celebrity. Like the whole staff—the new staff would come in, introduce themselves, get back on the same page about what I want, what we're doing, what the last people did. The prior shift would introduce the new shift. And it was crazy like. Like it was just like I couldn't believe it. I was like is this real like. And they all looked like me too. So, it was like I'm home. They could have been horrible but like I can't complain because everyone is so amazing. Like I was crying like the whole time just happy like—I felt safe because everybody would explain everything. Nobody—I never felt like anyone was being rushed. Like they needed to go and see someone else or talk to someone else. Everyone was talking to me. Like they were present and in the moment.

The implementation of a safety huddle at each shift change in hospital settings, especially throughout different units in a birthing hospital, strengthens team communication. A safety huddle during the provision of hospital-based obstetric and perinatal services is a brief meeting consisting of interdisciplinary members of the hospital team that facilitates coordinated, collaborative, and coherent approaches to care, focusing on patient safety and facilitating team communication (Shaikh 2020). Safety huddles activate the participation among, partnership with, and power of hospital teams to effectively and efficiently share information, review their performance, identify and prioritize safety concerns, increase transparency and accountability, and embed safety interventions throughout care (Shaikh 2020). For Brianna, active and continuous involvement by the hospital team during the safety huddles curated a hospital culture of belonging (psychological safety, and connectedness). Without patient-focused and patient-involved, or participatory, safety huddles, hospital systems, teams, and individual clinicians and staff can induce feelings of neglect, dismissiveness, and disrespect, one of the dimensions of Davis' obstetric racism. According to Black mothers' definition of safety, system-centered or team-centered safety huddles result in Black mothers feeling rushed, isolated, dismissed, ignored, neglected, not listened to, or not having their questions and concerns addressed during the provision of hospital-based obstetrics. Patient experiences of dismissiveness, denial, or delay incite and exacerbate psychological or emotional vulnerability combined with feelings of insecurity and unreliability toward hospital systems, teams, and individual clinicians and staff. Tasha, a Black mother in Oakland, shared more details about her feeling ignored and dismissed while also feeling misled by her hospital regarding the true indication for her cesarean birth.

> For me, I think that during my—well, during the stay there was I had a high fever and there's so many people in there. And just don't think they wanted to hear me. Like I would be lying in bed and I'm sick—high fever. They'll be conversing with their own selves instead of like hey, I'm over here. But I really didn't have the strength to—I was sick probably before that, having a really, really bad sickness. Sick probably before that so, I didn't have the strength to even be yelling at ya'll. You know what I mean. They really, like I said, they wasn't attentive to me. They weren't like trying to see what I wanted, how you wanted. And, like I said, with the C-section it was like okay, you need a C-section. And when I get to ask a question—yes, you definitely need it. It wasn't really—like I found out that the—supposedly the baby's umbilical cord was wrapped around [the neck] on the way to the room. Like on the way there. Like I don't understand how they get away with that. But, you know, certain stuff like that.

The unspoken patient benefits of mandating patient access and participation in safety huddles materialize as patients *feeling seen, heard, affirmed, desired, valued, and included* in health care provision and decision-making by a hospital system and team that is accessible, approachable, appropriate, accepting, attentive, available, and accommodating (Levesque et al. 2013). Additionally, Black mothers feel love or loved during a patient-focused safety huddle because of consistent communication and information exchange, which then produces trust, transparency, and accountability. Patient-focused safety huddles that involve patient participation affirm, activate, and amplify the power of the patient in meaning-making and knowledge production in hospital-based obstetrics. In chapter 2, Rhonda, a Black mother in Oakland, shared her analysis of how some nurses interact and communicate with pregnant and postpartum patients, specifically Black mothers, in a manner that diminishes and undermines Black patient experiential knowledge, perpetuating testimonial injustice. In her reflection of nurses below, Rhonda offered a more favorable perception and perspective on the role and impact of nurses.

> And then—so some of the nurses that was there, they just kept giving me all this information and it worked out fine because one of my nurses was one of my friends from elementary school, so—and she was pregnant as well too. So, like she got to help me a lot and then I got to help her too to get ready for her son and it was cool. It made me [having a nurse who was a childhood friend]—it made me not feel worried anymore versus like I said I didn't know who was going to be in the room and I didn't want like his family and my family like all fighting to be in there because like this was his first girl on their side and it was the first girl on our side in 17 years.

Rhonda felt love or loved during care provision due to continuous communication and information between her and her nurse. The second driver of feeling love or loved was having a bedside nurse that was a childhood friend. The third factor was the reciprocity of care and support, given that the Black mother and her nurse were both experiencing pregnancy together. The intersection of these factors during one episode of care created an experience whereby a Black mother felt protection and security from unintended, unwanted, unplanned, unwelcomed harm, injury, or malicious events, experiences, or outcome. In the absence of worry and fear, the nurse created multiple opportunities for a Black mother to feel comfort, peace, and relaxation. Feeling love or loved during the provision of hospital-based obstetrics care prevents Black mothers from experiencing feelings of stress and navigating stress responses such as "fight, flight, freeze, or fawn" as a daily reality and reaction. Curating belonging (psychological safety and connectedness) in hospital culture through diversification, inclusion, and democratization of the hospital birth workforce simultaneously benefits the workforce, Black mothers as patients, and their families and communities of origin.

> So, like everybody wanted to be there and I just—one of the nurses that I had, she was a travel nurse, but she became so loving to me. Like I loved her to death. I can't even remember the lady name, but she was an older lady. She was more so like a mom to me. She came in every time I called, every time like my stuff was beeping or I—just anything like and it was more—what made me even more loving about her is because like she wasn't even my nurse on some of the days, and she would come in and ask me do I need this, do I—you know, do I want to take a shower, do I need shower stuff. So that made me feel good because I wasn't prepared to have her. And just knowing that they actually cared

> that much to, you know, ask me every day do I want to take a shower, to ask me every day do I need help like changing my bottoms because I was having an illness crisis as well as having my daughter. All that love made me feel really good to know that I had them as a backbone if anything to go wrong.

Destiny, a Black mother in Oakland, shared her experiences of love or feeling loved by the nurse. Destiny's testimony of safety as love offered a blueprint for defining the role of nurses in responding to acts of obstetric racism. Davis describes three responses to the six defined dimensions of obstetric racism: racial reconnaissance, refusal, and resistance (Davis 2018; Davis 2019; Davis 2020; Davis, Varner, and Dill 2021; Davis 2022a; Davis 2022b). Regarding the above testimony, Destiny's explanation of how the nurse curating safety offers the opportunity to expand responses to obstetric racism and add a fourth response, restoration. Restoration includes attitudes, language, or behavior utilized by the patient, given or chosen kin, a community support person (with no hospital affiliation or alignment), or the hospital workforce choosing to disrupt the pathologization, commodification, dehumanization, and disconnection that dominate and shape the beliefs (ethos) about and behaviors (ethics) toward the Black reproducing body during hospital-based obstetric care.

Deeper reflection and analysis of the metaphors used by Destiny to describe how the nurse made her feel align with acts of restoration to facilitate love or feeling loved. In this narrative, one can more clearly imagine feeling love and feeling loved as strategies to prevent or mitigate obstetric racism and facilitate safety. First, the Black mother felt the impact of the nurse in the role and responsibility of a mother and a backbone. The mother metaphor suggested the role of the nurse as a caretaker who nurtures, nourishes, teaches, guides, listens, heals, loves, and protects with familial or kinship ties. The backbone metaphor suggested the role of the nurse as a source of support, structure, and strength. When reflecting on the function, a backbone offers support, protection, and infrastructure to the spinal cord, the nervous system, and the entire body. The backbone also facilitates free bodily movement, flexibility, balance, and stability to the body. The backbone serves another critical function by protecting the spinal cord, which provides the communication and information hardware and highways, connecting the brain with the body. As a mother and a backbone, the role and responsibilities of the nurse can violate safety or prevent and mitigate obstetric racism through the restoration of humanity, psychological safety, connectedness, and empathy in the provision of hospital-based obstetrics. Destiny felt love and loved by simple gestures of the nurse, such as being fully present and attentive, and offering support to Destiny in preserving and celebrating the innate human value or dignity of the Black reproducing body. Offering continuous support to a Black mother to maintain a level of cleanliness as determined by a Black mother, and not the nurse's expectations, demonstrates the fourth response to obstetric racism, restoration of a Black mother's humanity as validation of a Black mother's dignity. Acts of restoration at the level of the nurse, the hospital team, and the hospital system facilitate experiences of feeling love and loved among Black mothers, and thereby promote safety and accountability during the provision of hospital-based obstetrics care.

According to the testimony of Chantelle, a Black married mother in Oakland who experienced birth in a community (as the local birthing center led by midwives) and in a hospital setting, acts of restoration occur with greater frequency and ease in community births. By design, community births, particularly when led by Black midwives, offer different options, opportunities, and conditions that restore the humanity, honor the dignity of Black mothers, and curate experiences of feeling love and being loved.

> Like one, the opportunity and the privilege to have who you want in your birthing experience. Like if you wanted your children or your mother or your husband or whatever, best friend, a priest, whatever you wanted, you know what I'm saying, you could have it and there's no restrictions about that. It's not even no issue, conversation like, oh, okay, sure. You can have music, you can have a whole list of things like, you know, if you need the lighting a certain kind of way, if you need certain type of comfort measures, you want to use the ball and you want to use the stretchers. And then the people that are going to help you deliver are really connected to you and your family. So, at the birthing center, you know, the midwives met with us several times before, you know, the day came. So, it was almost like they became family. And so even though your ass is out and, you know, you may be looking some kind of way, you don't feel no kind of way. You feel loved. And that they want to see your birthing experience be what you imagined it to be and that's what they're there for. They're just there to support. And then whereas like in a hospital, you have caring people that work in a hospital, yes, but sometimes those caring people get caught up in the culture of how hospitals operate and they just kind of go with the flow of things and maybe that's not the best thing you needed to do. So, having control versus not having control, having option to have people there or not have people there, the option to not have medication or to have medication, but it not being like forced on you, right. And then the patience, there was just a lot of patience, like, okay, you want to stand up, oh, okay, you want to sit down, oh, you want to lay down, oh, you need some tea, okay, well, you think you're ready to push, oh, you want to get in the water now, oh, okay, well, let's go, and it was just like that whatever I said.

Birthing in the community reproduces and reinforces all eight core practices or behaviors identified by Black mothers as measures of safety. Birthing in community facilitates the manifestation of all eight meanings and measures of safety: (1) feeling love or feeling loved; (2) culture of belonging; (3) timely clinical recognition and responsiveness; (4) inclusion and integration of given and social kinship; (5) actualization and protection of patient autonomy, agency, and self-efficacy; (6) consistent communication and information exchange; (7) prioritization of infant well-being as maternal/parental well-being and maternal/parental well-being as infant well-being; and (8) transparency and accountability. Feeling love or loved is possible in the presence of nurses who intentionally acknowledge and affirm the humanity and dignity of Black women as Black women, and not as only as the assigned pregnant or postpartum patient on their roster of patients for the shift.

Many of the testimonies of feeling love or loved included the role of Black travel nurses in curating a hospital culture of belonging (psychological safety, and connectedness) whereby Black mothers, birthing people, and their loved ones *feel seen, heard, affirmed, desired, valued, and included* in care provision and decision-making.

> —and I'll say with Hospital 3, they were good. I had traveling nurses, two Black sisters from Atlanta. I loved them, Nurse 1 and Nurse 2. I called them Nurse 1 and Nurse 2 from Atlanta. And I just remember them. It was like they was like my big sisters or something. You know, it's like they had been knowing me. But just that they were my color—you know, they were—they knew what—they knew what I come from because they came from similar so we could just relate. You know, if I was saying something, I feel like that was very important because these are moments that only happen when they happen and you can't rewrite the moment. And so, to have people of your culture or your—or you share some similar background, it just make you feel safe, comfortable, received, accepted, no judgment. Yeah, and it was just a lot of laughter in the Hospital 3 birth.

In Chapter 2, Maya, a Black mother in Oakland, offered insights into why hospital nurses failed to provide care in a way that more closely aligned with Black women's dreams and desires for their birth. When reflecting on her own experiences, she named sociocultural concordance, based on shared histories that track along race, gender, and community of origin, as a mechanism for facilitating nurse-patient interactions and relations, including the establishment of chosen sister kinship ties. The byproduct of chosen sisterhood between Maya and two Black travel nurses created a milieu of safety, comfort, acceptance, and unconditional love. Extending the role of nurses in responding to obstetric racism as a big sister to Black mothers reinforces the restoration of humanity of Black women and the dignity of Black life, Black women, and Black sisterhood. According to a Black woman's blog, sisterhood is a unique bond established between women with shared stories, expectations, expressions, or experiences, including common goals, who mobilize each other to obtain respective and collective goals (Pennycoke n.d.). Sisterhood is also the mechanism by which women show authentic, radical, and unconditional love, empathy, grace, and support to each other. The metaphor of a big sister suggests the role and responsibility to provide both shield and shelter from the hurt and harm caused by hospital individual workers, teams, and systems. The Black travel nurses as big sister offer safe(r) spaces for Black mothers to be and feel vulnerable, curious, strong, and silly, honoring the full expression of a Black mother's humanity.

When considering which hospital to select as the preferred birthing hospital, a Black mother in Oakland, Tiffany, admitted to having very strong notions about a local hospital. Her testimony demonstrated the transformative power of high-quality, person-focused or personalized nursing care in disrupting negative norms and narratives about community hospitals or safety net hospitals that disproportionately serve large numbers of structurally minoritized or marginalized patient populations.

> Can I chime in on that real quick? So, like I said I gave birth at Hospital 2 and I was totally anti against Hospital 2. Like I cried for like three hours because I didn't want to give birth at Hospital 2, but like I said from the time I got there, they was like so supportive for me. I felt like they was more so my family than my actual family. Like I said, when my 37 weeks hit that day and they started my induction, they gave me so many different options. They told me I could walk around. They told me I could go where I wanted to go in the hospital, I just needed to be back at the checking times. They also told me that if I felt like I had a boo-boo and I'm like down the hall, to don't like try to walk back, like stop the nearest nurse or whatever and just get a wheelchair so that they could wheel me back. They also told me like—because a lot of people be like you can't eat, you can't eat. She was like no, eat what you want to eat, don't listen to everyone.

Like Tiffany, Black mothers determined the quality of obstetric patient safety based on access to and utilization of rich and robust resources and assets that expand options and then choices for optimal care. The provision of a menu of options and choices during care provision engendered Black mothers to believe they have more self-efficacy in controlling their future based on present-day actions and opportunities to actualize their autonomy and agency. Multiple experiences of safety as feeling love or loved with several nurses at Hospital 2 compelled Tiffany to change her positionality from antagonist to advocate of Hospital 2.

> here was a—one—there was another nurse, a travel nurse, too, she was my age too, and me and her had became cool because she was my night nurse for the last couple days. And she wasn't even like on my side, but she came over to help me and I felt really loved for that too. And she just kept saying, you'll be okay, like

you'll be okay. On the day of my induction it felt really, really well and really good for me because like my family wasn't there. My mom had came because she took off work, but the baby didn't come. And I didn't want to my mom to take off the second day and then she didn't come again. So, my mom was on the phone the whole time while I was giving birth, but just having that—having her there and like those two nurses for the—for the most part was like everything. And they told me like, you know, don't—whatever way she come is the way she come, because I was begging like just please give me a C-section, like I don't want to do this no more. And she was just like, no, you're going to be fine, just keep breathing, things going to work out, you know. And she just kept saying keep praying, God got you, and all of that and all of that. I was playing my gospel music, and every time they came in, it was just, you know, wonderful. And Nurse 3 came in and was dancing and stuff like trying to make me laugh and just trying to take all my stress away. So, like all of that made me feel really, really good, especially because I didn't have my family there. So, it was more so—and I was totally anti against Hospital 2, but I support Hospital 2.

For Black mothers, feeling safety was achieved by the reproduction of the highest attributes and conditions of being a mother, big sister, and backbone within the role and responsibilities of a hospital obstetric and perinatal nurse. The metaphors of mother, big sister, and backbone reveal the desires and expectations of Black mothers to experience protection, prevention, and security from unintended, unwanted, unplanned, unwelcomed harm, injury, or malicious event, experience, or outcome. The dominant source of support, comfort, reassurance, peace, and unconditional love was a nurse, specifically a Black nurse. Black mothers rarely named physicians as architects or curators of patient experiences of feeling love or loved.

Simone: So, my—is it an anesthesiologist? He was a Black male. He definitely—he assured me everything was going to be fine. He would touch me, say can you feel here, can you feel there, can you breathe, and I'm like I can breathe. He asked me—you know, they were like do you need blankets, are you cold, feel warm. When they did the spinal, they held me because my mom couldn't be in there with me and her father wasn't there, so I was already really scared being that my mom couldn't be in the room with me. So, the nurses hugged me as they did the spinal. So, I just—in that way I guess I felt cared for, loved, and safe in that way. They surrounded me with love and care. And they asked me if I wanted to—because now Hospital 1 offers an option to where the drape can drop clear—so you can see your baby get pulled out. So, they offered that to me, if I wanted to see her getting pulled out and—sorry if I get a little emotional too. But yeah, and yeah, they like offered that to me, so—it like—it definitely made my experience a little better.

Dr. Scott: You can cry. It's your birth story.

> *Simone:* I know, but it just gets—it's like always emotional. But yeah, like them being able to just give me that option because I already was just sad that—I would say naturally, but I was sad that I couldn't have her vaginally."

Even when childbirth occurs in the operating room by way of the Black mother's abdomen (e.g., cesarean birth), efforts by the hospital clinicians and staff to curate a culture of unconditional love, protection, and support must be intentional, coordinated, collaborative, accurate, precise, and explicit. The gentle touch combined with concern, curiosity, and care by the Black male anesthesiologist and comforting hugs from the nurses served as a restorative action that recognized the humanity and dignity of a Black mother. In Simone's own words, "*in that way I guess I felt cared for, loved, and safe in that way. They surrounded me with love and care.*"

Even when an intervention is needed to facilitate any aspect of care, Black mothers' experiences and expressions of childbirth hospitalization confirmed the possibility of curating love and safety in hospital spaces. An Oakland Black mother, Brianna, shared a moving testimony of a gentle, facilitated vaginal birth that continuously actualized and honored Brianna's humanity and power.

> *Brianna:* And I went 8-1/2 centimeters natural all the way up until that point. So, it was just like knowing—she was almost there and I just couldn't complete it that way. But with them just reassuring me with the safety and the love and given that option to say, here, you can just watch us pull her out, that was like the best experience ever. And then plus they put her on me first, so that was—
>
> *Dr. Scott:* Nice. So, skin-to-skin, yes?
>
> *Brianna Yeah. And she latched right away.*

Providing a menu of birthing options while seeking continuous consent throughout care upholds Brianna's bodily and decisional autonomy. Honoring the Black reproducing body while honoring a Black woman's agency over her Black reproducing body prevents and mitigates acts of obstetric racism and curates feeling loved and protected. The acts of giving the Black mother the option of facilitating the birth of her baby and seeking continuous consent revealed the nurse's commitment and decision not to comply with the medicalization or pathologization of birth, as a phenomenon, and birthing, as a process. By choosing a pathway that promoted the participation of and partnership with the Black mother during childbirth with patient consent, the nurse then deployed her own will as a bystander against a system of control and the demands of consent. The nurse's alignment with the ethical and legal principle and practice of respecting a patient's autonomy and inclusion in decision-making is an act of refusal that rejects the possibility of coercion, forced medical intervention, abuse, disrespect, and the power that is used to exert reproductive and birthing dominance over Black reproducing bodies. The refusal of the medicalization of birth also served as a mechanism of action that prevented both the dehumanization of birth and the de-prioritization of the Black mother and her reproducing body as the stars of the hospital birth. The nurse's alignment with centering Brianna, a Black mother, during childbirth, even with hospital assistance, served as an act of restoration of humanity and dignity in the human experience of childbirth in hospital settings. As the newest addition to Davis' existing three responses to obstetric racism, restoration induces feelings of love and being loved, reassuring a Black mother of her humanity and dignity in the world, particularly during the sacred moment of childbirth. Black mothers desire and deserve the right to design and experience their sacred birth, independent of birth settings, modalities, technologies, or attendants.

In reflecting upon the patient experiential knowledge and wisdom of a Black mother in Oakland, Chantelle, who participated in a prior community and hospital birth, one can see the potential for transforming hospital quality of childbirth practices and investing in existing or new community-based resources in preparation for the life beyond birth in the postpartum period.

> *Chantelle:* Once—it's like, you know, at the hospital, it's like, oh, you know, you didn't have these warm, fuzzy connections. You know, you might have these real cool conversations with the nurses and the doctors and the people that you interact with while—in you're—during your stay, but it's just like, oh, okay, well, you know, good luck to you, blessing or whatever, or they might not even be on shift when you leave—and the relationship—that's just—that's it. It's done. Whereas with the birthing center, I still have a relationship with them like—and they even—we did like a birthing testimonial. They uploaded it onto their website so like other people could share that. You can—they got classes that you can go to for—
>
> *Dr. Scott:* So, you still have interactions that they—any opportunities or events, they're still offering things for people after their birth?
>
> *Chantelle:* Yes.
>
> *Dr. Scott:* Got it.
>
> *Chantelle:* And then my midwives actually extended themselves outside of their work and they are coming to my son's first birthday. I just feel like at the birthing center every aspect about giving birth is what the focus is. And the mother is the main focus because she is the one that is going to get this baby here. Yes, we're exterior supports, but actually it's going to come from within. And the birthing center, it was just like a magical experience from beginning to

> end and I can't say that at the hospital I felt I was in a magical place. I just felt like I was in a place of business and they was doing what they do. And I was another number. They let you bond with your baby more so than the hospital versus you having to like bring the whole—My baby never went nowhere. Like they let you bond.

In lifting up the growing 2 percent of all mothers, birthing people, and families across racial lines, that birthed in community (NASEM 2020), outside of hospitals, birthing centers serve as political, structural, institutional, and disciplinary acts of refusal, resistance, restoration, and racial reconnaissance, manifesting all four responses to obstetric racism. According to 2019 to 2020 and 2020 to 2021 vital statistics, the number of community births, defined as births occurring in community birthing centers or at home, increased by 22 percent and 12 percent, the highest rate since 1990 (MacDorman and Declercq 2010; NASEM 2020; CDC National Center for Health Statistics (NCHS) 2022; National Partnership for Women and Families n.d.). More importantly, the spike in community births, with the dramatic shift led by the decisions of Black and Brown communities, happened during the context of rising rates of maternal deaths yearly from 2019 to 2022 (Hoyert 2023). Infant deaths spiked in 2022 for the first time in thirty years. (Hagen 2023). Likewise, preterm births (occurring at less than 37 weeks pregnancy age) in the U.S. earned a grade D+ from the March of Dimes for the second consecutive year (March of Dimes n.d.). Disproportionate, predictable, preventable, and unfair rates continue to be manifested in Black and Brown communities.

With respect to rising rates of community births, the percentage increased by 36 percent among Black women and 30 percent among Hispanic women from 2019 to 2020, compared to a 21 percent and 22 percent increase among white women and the national rate (CDC, NCHS 2022). While birth justice involves the removal or reduction of political, structural, institutional, and disciplinary barriers and burdens to access and utilization of birthing centers, interest and investments in community and home births cannot occur in isolation of simultaneously securing birth justice and accountability for the remaining 98 percent of mothers and gender-expansive individuals dependent on hospital births, by choice, force, or coercion.

Through the experiential, spiritual, and cultural knowledge of Black mothers and mainstream knowledge from national organizations, one can no longer refute the need for massive disruption, innovation, and transformation of existing harmful birthing options, opportunities, settings, attendants, and conditions in the U.S. Divestment from "unsafe and accountability free" and investment in SACKRED births engenders acts of racial reconnaissance, refusal, resistance, and restoration. In 2018, I first defined and presented SACRED (without the letter k) Birth as a Black women-person focused model of care for re-imagining quality improvement and improvement for, by, and with Black mothers and birthing people, Black women-led community-based organizations, and Black academic and independent content experts and scholars, and the Black workforce, within and beyond the hospital health system (Scott 2018; Scott 2019a; Scott 2019b). By 2019, I defined SACRED birth as a theorizing framework built upon guiding principles that shape attitudes, values, intentions, skills, conditions, practices, and behavior impacting Black Mamas and Black birth across all settings, spaces, technologies, modalities, and attendants, independent of birth outcomes (Scott 2019a; Scott 2019b). SACKRED Birth is a radical attitude toward human births, specifically Blackness, Black bodies, and Black births, that regards all birth activities as fundamentally normal, healthy, spiritual, familial, magical, transformative, erotic, communal, emancipatory, and power-activating. SACKRED birth encourages diverse and inclusive birth pleasure, practices, care, spaces, options, partners, communities, and experiences. The SACKRED birth movement advocates for safer, respectful, dignified, high-quality "participatory" birth care, conditions, experiences, and outcomes, and improved workforce diversification, development, sustainability, and restoration of Black Midwifery care and Black Doula support models as part of its campaign (Scott 2018; Scott 2019a; Scott 2019b).

A SACKRED birth in hospital or community settings engenders feelings of love and being loved and promotes social, cultural, emotional, and mental safety within the context of clinical safety. SACKRED birth curates a culture of belonging during social and clinical interactions in hospital settings where Black mothers and birthing people, in the presence of their loved ones, *feel seen, heard, affirmed, and included* in the health care team. For some Black mothers, safety is directly related to the capacity to connect and form healthy attachments and bonds with the hospital system, team, or individual hospital clinicians and staff. For many of the Christian fundamentalists who sit in positions of political, structural, institutional, and disciplinary influence, I often think of the amount of fear and terror engendered by the application of their Christian ethics, ethos, and leadership in the U.S. sexual, reproductive, and perinatal matrix of care. Yet in the King James Bible, 1 John Chapter 4, verse 18 reads, "There is no fear in love; but perfect love casteth out fear: because fear hath torment. He that feareth is not made perfect in love" (Biblegateway n.d.). When Black mothers define obstetric patient safety as feeling love or loved, then birthing while Black in the U.S., independent of birth setting, position, technology, or attendant, must occur without anticipated or actual fear.

In Los Angeles, Charlene shared how she prepared herself for birth by watching a documentary and naming her birth expectation with intentionality: to give birth without fear.

Charlene: Oh no—like, am I going to end up in a Caesarean—like, I don't want to do this, you know, like. I was so afraid, which was also something that was against my plan, like, I wanted to birth without fear. Like, that was my major goal, was—

Dr. Scott: You're the reason why I kept saying fear today.

Charlene: Yes, and when you said that I was, like, oh, she's reading me. Yeah, but that was my major goal—I was just—I want to do this with no fears—my first baby, you know. And of course it's scary, you know. But—

Jasmine: Yeah.

Ebony: Right.

Charlene:—at the same time, you have to relax, and the situation was just—it was heightened, you know. And like I said, that documentary really helped me take—take control, you know. I can't, like, pinpoint, like, you know, too much more about what it was in the documentary, but just knowing that I had the option to deny—

Dr. Scott: Yes, yes.

Charlene:-- and say, like, I have—no, this is my birth, like, you know. Yes, I'm in your facility, but it's my body, it's my baby, you know.

The focus group dialogue involving Charlene, Jasmine, and Ebony in Los Angeles expanded safety as a paradigm and measure by which to improve quality. If Black mothers define safety as feeling love or loved, and the manifestation of love is the absence of fear, then the anticipation or actualization of fear during childbirth hospitalization is a violation of obstetric patient safety and quality. Birthing in love without fear is a fundamental right for all pregnant women and gender-expansive individuals, and their given and chosen kin. Informed refusal is also an ethical and legal principle and practice in providing health care. Accordingly, culturally and scientifically relevant and responsive and communication and information exchange about birth options, opportunities, optimal conditions, risks, and resources causes Black mothers to feel safer, cared for, protected, and more prepared during care. When exploring the role and responsibilities of birthing hospitals in curating a culture of safety as a mitigating strategy against poor quality of care during childbirth hospitalization (and for any pregnancy-related concern or condition), one effective, responsive, relevant, and patient-identified solution is to better prepare Black pregnant and postpartum women and individuals to equitably participate in clinical practice, decision-making, and care delivery. Building hospital system, team, and individual hospital clinician and staff capacity and self-efficacy in meaningful person-focused communication and information exchange that then activates and actualizes patient autonomy, agency, and self-efficacy would likely prevent and/or mitigate fear in childbirth hospitalization, advance safety, and improve quality.

From the perspective of Patrice, a Black mother in Los Angeles, a barrier to a safe hospital birth experience is lack of adequate and relevant information available to Black mothers about the various potential clinical risks and adverse events (e.g., hemorrhage) and how the hospital team's current or changing capacities to recognize, respond, and resolve the possible emergent or urgent clinical events.

> In regard to like making it harder—again, I feel like it's a lack of information. You know, like they ask you, oh, do you have any questions. It's like, [I] never done this before. I don't know what questions I have. And then, so, I feel like they don't prepare you or tell you what happens if you tear. Or if you hemorrhage or—you know, like that information is not readily available. They just take action. So, when it happens, it's very scary and like and traumatic. But I feel like if doctors and OB's [obstetricians] and PA's [physician assistants] and like if they were all just a little bit more considerate—of, I don't want to scare you, but this is what could happen. At least—you'd be a little bit better prepared.

Absent or inadequate communication and information compromises Black mother's trust in the hospital systems, teams, or individual team members, as in the case with Patrice. Moreover, suboptimal communication violates bodily and decisional autonomy. In the next Black birth narrative from Oakland, constrained, delayed, or diminished autonomy or agency in birthing positions, spaces, and mobility resulted in coerced or forced birthing positions that violated Gabrielle's sense of safety, trust, and security in herself and those around her. Birthing on one's back seems focused on facilitating access to the mother and the baby for the birth attendant and staff, and not on the most physiological and patient and baby focused positions to facilitate an optimal birth.

> Okay. So, you got the water births, you've got the squatting. You got the Lotus birth. You got—and I just want to say the last reasons I'm saying that is I got in the water because I was ready to give birth. I felt like I was ready to push. And in my mind and in my birthing plan, I was going to get in the water and be positioned a certain kind of way. I got in there and it was just like I was stuck for a minute and I was stuck in a forced position. Like I was on my knuckles and my knees. But what I needed to do was get on my feet and be in a squatting position. So eventually they kept saying like he's right there but you need—you know, so basically, she was like just get your right leg up. She kept saying get your right leg up. I couldn't get the right one up. My brain got the left one up. And then boom, he came out as soon as I got in that squatting position. So, I also feel like for women in general being told to lay down on your back and push

is not the best way at all to give birth in a hospital versus at home or a hospital versus birthing center. You have that option.

A meaningful consequence of re-reading Black mothers' lived experiences of birthing in U.S. hospitals is that one begins to see deeper connections between safety and autonomy, and love and liberation. Safety is greatly influenced by access to and utilization of rich and robust resources and assets (i.e., finances, education, training, health, well-being, stability, wisdom, transgenerational kinship ties) to achieve the birth of a Black mother's desires and dreams. The withholding of a diverse and inclusive array of birth information, options, opportunities, and optimal conditions to achieve the highest quality of birth health controls and constrains birth choices. Limiting birth options and choices undermines patient autonomy and facilitates coerced or forced birth experiences and outcomes. Consequently, hospital systems, teams, and individual hospital workers enact acts of obstetric racism against Black mothers such as coercion, medical abuse, medical intervention, and neglect. Davis asserts obstetric racism is a threat to positive birth outcomes (Davis 2018; Davis 2019; Davis 2020; Davis, Varner, and Dill 2021). Fundamentally, obstetric racism erodes all interests, intentions, and initiatives to engender an experience of childbirth hospitalization grounded in unconditional and radical love and liberation. According to the focus group discussion in Oakland, Angie and LaToya expressed the overwhelming feelings of derailed dreams and unfulfilled desires during childbirth.

Angie: And I would say that they need to be more open to giving other options other than going straight to the epidural or some type of pain meds. Like—so I didn't really—my first birth was at Hospital 4. They pretty much—I was overdue. They told me basically once I sat on the table, I hadn't had any meds yet. After I sat on the table and they had to hold me, it was you can't get back up. And I was like, well, what if I have to use the bathroom. We're going to give you a bag. My second pregnancy, they allowed me to walk around until I got to five centimeters, and then they were like, no, we're going to have you lay on the bed, you know, we don't know how this is going to go. And then my son was bone on bone, so then that made it more painful and they're like we don't want you to like fall out or anything to happen. And then her, they didn't give me no options. They didn't say, oh, you want to go walk around. They didn't offer the ball. They didn't offer none of that. And actually, with her I wanted to do a water birth, but unfortunately Hospital 1's only water tub or something is towards Sacramento and they were like, oh, that's not an option. I was like okay, that's not an option.

Latoya: Not just assume that you were going to give birth the way they thought you were going to give birth.

Angie: But I had already told my doctor that because she originally asked me if, you know, there was something that I had specifically wanted. I said I want to do a water birth, like, you know, I presumed this was going to be my last baby, you know I was like I want to do a water birth and I want to get my tubes tied. She completely ignored the tubes tying.

Political, structural, institutional, systematic, departmental, and disciplinary acts of obstetric racism, independent of awareness, intention, positionality, or demography, serve one unified purpose: reproductive dominance of the Black reproducing body and her progeny. The nature and progression of unmitigated obstetric racism leaves no space for generating a safety and accountability paradigm with meaning, measures, monitoring, prevention, and mitigation strategies. At one point during the focus group discussions in Los Angeles, I asked Black mothers to reflect and then elaborate upon their role as Black mothers within the health care system. Their lived experiences deserve national recognition and responses from the various actors, including architects, administrators, gatekeepers, and financiers of the obstetric and perinatal matrix.

Tiara: I'm just I'm a product. I'm a number. I'm not a person. I'm money. I was somebody when you all wanted to cut on me. Because I feel like the cesareans, I heard a doctor is paid more for cesareans—

Shanice: Yeah.

Zaria: Of course. It's surgery.

Tiara:—so, than a natural birth. It seemed like they were kind of more edging that on. I was walking and swimming and everything to try to push. Like, I thought that was going to be the plan. But I ended up having preeclampsia at the very end at that last little appointment. On like August 25th. No, no. August 27th. And then, they made me stay in the hospital and they delivered her on August 29th. And I wasn't due until September 22nd.

Despite maternal indications for facilitating birth prior to the estimated due date, Black mothers continue to feel a sense of manipulation and betrayal by the hospital system and team. One must then interrogate the quality of communication, consent, decision-making, and documentation and dissemination of health care information about the indication, processes, and procedures for an induction of labor or cesarean birth in patient handoffs, patient sign-outs, and health records. During focus group interactions and influence, Black mothers explored the difference between venting to family and friends and reporting harmful experiences for the purposes of facilitating transparency and accountability at the level of the hospital systems, teams, or individual hospital or health care worker. Black mothers and birthing people identified accountability as a solution to mitigate the onset, frequency, duration, and magnitude of obstetric racism. Black mothers offered the proposed change actions as part of patient and community-driven accountability (accepting responsibility for your own actions) and oversight (accepting responsibility for monitoring the actions of others) strategies. Black mothers demand that hospital culture and structures mandate recognition, reporting, and response mechanisms of actions (i.e., policies, practices, protocols, procedures, people, power) that elicit feedback in formal and informal ways from patients about their hospital experience. Upon receipt and review of patient and community-reported experiences of obstetric racism, the hospital system would then require administrators, clinicians, and staff to report, explain, or justify their actions to the patient, to their family and communities of origin, or to the public.

The synthesis of the shared meanings and measures for safety and accountability established two overarching themes: feeling love or loved and multiple levels of accountability. The multiple levels of accountability are organized into four categories:

(1) hospital system—the institutional or organizational policies and processes in place that facilitate recognition, measurement, and monitoring strategies, reporting, and response to any imaging, messaging, language, or behavior that violates physical, emotional, cultural, and social safety;
(2) hospital team—2 or more hospital clinicians and staff are held responsible for their actions, leading to an interrogation of hospital culture, structures, and mechanisms (i.e., policies, practices, protocols, procedures, people, power) that govern how administrators, clinicians, and staff take responsibility for the assurance of physical, emotional, cultural, and social safety in clinical practices, decision-making, and care delivery;
(3) individual hospital administrators, clinicians, and staff members—Black mothers describe variations in the quality of care based on the presence or absence of an individual woman OBGYN physician, a clinician, or a staff that advocates for the Black mother to optimize birth conditions, experiences, and outcomes. Examples include variations in care quality that deviate more toward high or poor quality based on the individual lead clinician (e.g., OBGYN attending physician, Anesthesiology attending physician, Nursing Administrative Supervisor, Charge Nurse);
(4) individual patient actions—Black mothers/birthing people describe different barriers and facilitators that affect their personal role in hospital

systems, clinicians and staff responsibility for the provision of "safe, effective, timely, efficient, equitable, and people centered care" that is culturally and clinically competent, timely, appropriate, relevant, and responsive. Examples include filing a formal grievance, reporting to nurse managers, finding resources, and making their own appointments.

The narrative below highlights the lack of hospital accountability for recommending dietary changes to a Black mother, Dominique, in the Oakland focus group. Dominique restricted her food intake in terms of food selection and calories. As a result of complying with medical advice, Dominique's baby's weight at birth was recognized as low birth weight, prompting a protocol that recommends obtaining a baseline serum glucose level, or blood sugar check, in the newborn. Dominique's baby's serum glucose level was found to be lower than normal (clinically defined as neonatal hypoglycemia). The unintentional harm imposed by the OBGYN prenatal physician onto Dominique and her baby girl as well as the subsequent regret and grief that overshadowed Dominique at the time of her birth and nearly two years later during the focus group.

> I want to say to let them just be mindful that not every birth is the same and it doesn't go by the books that they study. And, yeah, just every birth is different and it's not going to always go as planned. And so be flexible and show sympathy and compassion especially the ones [hospital clinicians and staff] who have birthed themselves. Like you know how it is. I think they need to explain the information they give out. Why did they tell me to go on a diet and then when my daughter don't got no sugar, explain to me why was that diet necessary? Or take fault for the issues of what you just caused. Because now my daughter is suffering and your all not giving me no answers.

Black mothers desire and deserve hospital systems to take responsibility for their actions when medical advice or interventions produce undesired side effects. These side effects and risks associated with medical interventions are called iatrogenesis (Peer and Shabir 2018). In 1972, the WHO defined iatrogenesis as "any noxious, unintended, and undesired effect of a drug, which occurs at doses used in humans for prophylaxis, diagnosis, or therapy" (WHO 1972). In comparison, the Joint Commission on the Accreditation of Healthcare Organizations defined these side effects as adverse drug reactions (ADRs), an undesired effect of a medication that either increases toxicity, decreases the desired therapeutic effect, or both (Lazarou 1998). A critique of the WHO definition of iatrogenesis revealed the exclusion or erasure of therapeutic failures, intentional and accidental poisoning, drug abuse, incorrect drug administration, and noncompliance (Peer and Sabir 2018). The WHO definition also underestimated ADRs and incidences such as diagnostic procedures including mechanical and radiological procedures, the therapeutic regimen which includes drugs, surgery, invasive procedures, hospitalizations, and the actual treating doctor himself/herself (Lazarou et al. 1998; WHO 1969; Krishnan and Kasthuri 2005; Singh et al. 2015).

Based on the WHO definition of iatrogenesis (WHO 1969; WHO 1972), the hospital system would not be held accountable for mandating Dominique to maintain a restricted diet to control her blood sugars, which then led to hypoglycemia of her newborn at birth and sequent admission to the neonatal intensive care unit (NICU). Dominique carried much guilt for following the medical advice that led to iatrogenic newborn hypoglycemia and NICU admission. She also felt the hospital systems, teams, and individual clinicians owed her an explanation for recommending an intervention that protected her and subsequently harmed her newborn. She felt the hospital undermined her bodily and decisional autonomy in protecting and securing optimal health and safety for herself and her newborn.

Based on the pioneering work of Ivan Illich in expanding the nomenclature and determinants of iatrogenesis, the hospital system, team, and individual obstetrician owe Dominique an explanation and an apology. Ivan Illich is cited as a prolific critic of modern medicine. In 1974, he published *Medical Nemesis* which opened with the following statement: "The medical establishment has become a major threat to health" (O'Mahony 2016, 134; Illich 1974; Illich 2023). Illich argued that scientific progress and advancements in medicine had little effect on the overall health of populations. In fact, he asserted that the medicalization of Western society and the impact of physicians and the pharmaceutical industry contributed very little to population health, and likely created more harm than good. Illich's critique of modern medicine shares many parallels with the analyses of the medicalization, professionalization, and commodification of birth (O'Mahony 2016, 134; Illich 2023).

For the purposes of this book and chapter, introducing Illich's scholarship provides an additional interpretative framework to further support the demand from Black mothers that hospital systems, teams, and individual clinicians take responsibility for maternal or infant morbidity or harm resulting from health policies or practices imposed on Black reproducing bodies and Black babies. His transformative scholarship generated a re-classification of iatrogenesis into a binary phenomenon: "direct, caused by the medical care which can cause death, pain or sickness and indirect, wherein health policies themselves are responsible for illness, death, or disease" (Peer and Shabir 2018, 310). Additional readings demonstrated that Illich described three types of iatrogenesis: (1) clinical, the direct harm done by various medical treatments; (2) social, the medicalization of ordinary life; and (3) cultural, the loss of traditional ways of dealing with and making sense of suffering, death, pain, and sickness (Peer and Shabir 2018; O'Mahony 2016; Smith 2003).

In reflecting on Dominique's expressed concerns, the application of Illich's topology of iatrogenesis to the lived experience of a Black mother reveals a violation of safety due to clinical and cultural iatrogenesis. The safety violation eroded Dominique's autonomy (free will), agency (power to make decisions or achieve a desired goal), and self-efficacy (belief in one's capacity to make decisions or achieve a goal) in making decisions about how to care for her Black reproducing body, her prenatal health, and the prenatal development and health of her Black baby girl. As Illich explained in his book, iatrogenesis is a structural form of violence that undermines people's agency and competence to deal with their own disease (Smith 2003).

Another Black mother from the Oakland focus group, Yolanda, discussed her experience of structural violence as manifested by clinical iatrogenesis during her childbirth hospitalization.

> *Yolanda:* I feel like the labor and delivery should have had a little more communication with them after post-partum—just because the IV that I—what is it called? The IV but it's not the IV attached to it.
>
> *Dr. Scott:* Oh, the saline lock [a thin, flexible tube placed in a vein in your hard or arm, sticks out a few inches, for easy access to administer medicines through a vein]
>
> *Yolanda:* Yeah, the little thing that you stick in. That was the same one that they gave me for six days. So, I got two final transfusions. Everything I got was through this—pain meds—So, my arm before I left swelled up like crazy. And like they was like oh, you got this on the day you arrived. I'm like yeah. They're like oh, we're supposed to change it every two days. I'm like I've had it in for now almost seven days. Like why didn't they—that should have never happened. Like something terrible could happen. And I was like something terrible did happen. They were just like oh, that shouldn't have happened. All right, okay. So, that could have been a little better. And that way I felt like I was neglected like. And how did that happen? How did no one stop that [from] happening. I don't know, you know.

The retention of the saline lock in Yolanda's arm and the subsequent suffering violated physical and emotional safety. Multiple individual nurses and physicians failed to comply with institutional standards, failing to protect Yolanda. As a result of neglect and delayed recognition and response to removing the saline lock, the hospital system and team are actively complicit in intentionally causing pain, one of six dimensions of obstetric racism (Davis 2018; Davis 2019; Davis 2020; Davis, Varner, and Dill 2021). The absence of empathy in the face of Black people's physical suffering and lack of motivation to end Black suffering reproduces anti-Black racist and anti-Black misogynistic ideologies and practices dating back to the antebellum era as previously explained in chapter 2. Thus, race and gender-based discrimination fuels the institutionalized disdain for the humanity and dignity of Black women, which is a manifestation of misogynoir (Bailey 2016; Bailey and Trudy 2018; Bailey 2021). The failure to change the saline lock represents another example of clinical iatrogenesis without any accountability or oversight at the hospital system, team, or individual clinical or staff level (Smith 2003).

Black mothers also shared examples of system levels of accountability to achieving and advancing patient safety. Facilitating consistent and clear communication and information exchange among patients, primary physicians, specialist physicians, hospital teams, and given and chosen kinship is one strategic action to achieve and improve safety. Optimal patient and kinship focused, participatory communication also activates and amplifies the power of the patient in meaning-making and knowledge production during the provision of hospital-based obstetric care. Brianna, from the Oakland focus group, emphasized the intentional inclusion and integration of her presence and participation in every aspect of care.

> I think the most important part of my experience was that every medical professional took their time to explain every step, every procedure that was happening, every medication that was administered, all of my options and I never felt rushed. Those things were like the key. Those were the things that made me feel safe. There was no talking amongst themselves and me not being having been included.

Optimal communication and information exchange can also be extended to Black mothers and birthing people to secure and sustain a culture of safety for themselves in real-time or for themselves and other Black mothers and birthing people during future childbirth hospitalizations. During one focus group session in Oakland, Angie explained the difference between complaining (i.e., sharing stories of safety violations with family and friends or posting on online platforms) and reporting (i.e., filing a formal grievance or complaint to the hospital or medical or nursing board). Angie's full excerpt can be found in chapter 2. For the purposes of this chapter, I focus more on the different meanings and manifestations of complaining and the motivations associated with the different manifestations. Distinguishing between complaining to loved ones or venting on social media and filing a formal complaint is crucial to understanding motivations and desired goals for communication. Complaining or venting may serve to garner support, attention, and/or empathy. In contrast, filing a report may elicit support, attention, and empathy and a commitment to investigate, monitor, and reconcile the harm by addressing immediate concerns and implementing processes to prevent or mitigate future harms. Complaining may achieve awareness, whereas reporting may elicit awareness combined with actions toward accountability, oversight, and justice.

The challenge for some Black mothers is how to reconcile and report harm enacted by Black or Brown administrators, clinicians, or staff. An important mistruth is that obstetric racism only occurs in the presence of non-Black clinicians and staff. According to Davis, acts of obstetric racism can be performed by any medical personnel or health care professional, independent of race, gender, affluence, or positionality (Davis 2018; Davis 2019). Black mothers, their given and chosen kins, and their communities of origin would benefit from political, structural, and organizational sources of support to address the power relations, dynamics, and differentials in reporting any health care professional or health care system for violating safety, with additional empathy and care when the perpetrators are Black or Brown individuals or Black or Brown-led teams and hospital systems.

In the same manner, political, structural, and organizational support is needed for Black mothers and their given and chosen kin to report quality and safety violations that occur because of clinical iatrogenesis driven by acts of obstetric racism. A Black mother in Los Angeles, Vanessa, explained her birthing experience in which hospital clinicians and staff communicated to her and her husband that an emergency cesarean birth was necessary. As the expert of her body, Vanessa immediately identified a potentially serious adverse event, dislocation of her jaw during induction for general anesthesia and endotracheal intubation due to a pre-existing diagnosis of temporomandibular joint disorder (TMD). She also explained that her blood levels were too low (i.e., platelet count) to utilize epidural anesthesia for labor pain management.

> You and the baby are in danger. We need to go now. So, they wheel me into the OR to deliver. I have TMJ....So, I'm yelling to the anesthesiologist, I've got TMJ. I know my life—I know my life is more important than my jaw. But I'm telling you, I have TMJ. So, my blood levels are too low for me to get an epidural. So, you have to intubate which means you have to give me [general] anesthesia. What does that mean? You have to put a tube down my throat. So, I'm yelling, I have TMJ. What does he do? He pops my jaw. He dislocates my jaw. It's Mother's Day weekend. They don't want to get sued. So, they won't touch my jaw. The specialist doesn't come in till 16 hours later. So, my jaw is—dislocated for 16 hours.

The anesthesiologist, as an individual physician, and the entire team perpetuated multiple acts of obstetric racism, reproducing the antithesis of love in the provision of hospital-based obstetrics. In the context of having a pre-existing TMD and being pregnant, the prenatal health team (outpatient pregnancy team) and the intrapartum team (inpatient labor team) missed a critical opportunity to evaluate other forms of pain control, including different forms of intubation for an emergency cesarean birth, especially given the inability to utilize epidural or spinal anesthesia. Medical literature suggests that general anesthesia with orotracheal intubation poses a risk factor for the development or exacerbation of TMJ disorders (Martin et al. 2007). As the second most common musculoskeletal pain after low back pain, at least one TMD symptom affects about 33 percent of the population. Approximately 4.8 percent of the population suffers from severe TMD (NASEM 2020b). In 2002, Argó et al. demonstrated the incidence of TMD after intubation to be 5 percent, while the worsening of a previous TMD was reported in 44 percent of patients (Argó et al. 2003). Additional epidemiological data demonstrated that temporomandibular joint (TMJ) injuries represent 10 percent of airway trauma claims, with TMJ pain and dislocation being the most common complications (Toufeeq et al. 2019). To prevent or mitigate TMJ complications, the individual clinician must perform an appropriate and comprehensive TMJ assessment before and after anesthesia (Manfredini et al. 2011). Furthermore, the American Society of Anesthesiologist practice guidelines recommend an evaluation of the TMJ as part of the preoperative airway examination (Apfelbaum et al. 2022). According to Argó et al, a preoperative airway examination that includes a TMJ evaluation will permit the anesthesiologist or nurse anesthetist to identify the best intubation technique and simultaneously reduce the risk of the new onset of TMJ issues or the exacerbation of misdiagnosed or undiagnosed TMD after intubation (Argó et al. 2003). Unfortunately, obstetric racism eroded the possibility of permeating obstetric care with unconditional love.

The outpatient and inpatient teams' uninterrogated belief that Blackness is pathological led them to deemphasize and ignore the Black mother's pre-existing TMD and her screams for the anesthesiologist or anyone on the team to validate her diagnosis and act accordingly. Because of the diagnostic lapse, both teams violated obstetric patient safety. When the intrapartum team, including the anesthesiologist and operating room (OR) team, ignored and dismissed the Black mothers' shouts for help and care, the hospital treated her with disdain, reproducing a second dimension of obstetric racism, neglect, dismissiveness, and disrespect (Davis 2018; Davis 2019; Davis 2020; Davis, Varner, and Dill 2021). When the hospital labor, OR, and post-operative teams failed to appropriately manage the Black mother's pain and dislocated jaw for sixteen hours, then one can only determine that the motivation for such cruelty may be rooted in racialized beliefs about pain immunity. Additionally, the cruelty of the entire hospital system is facilitated and fueled by the absence of empathy for Black people's physical suffering, leading to an institutional lack of internal motivation to alleviate or reduce Black suffering. As discussed in chapter 2, inaction in the face of need is institutionalized racism (Jones 2020).

Black mothers and birthing people need ongoing reassurance that a culture and practice of safety will be both achieved and sustained through various security measures, checks, and balances, regardless of changes in hospital administrators, clinicians, and staff over time (i.e., shift changes) and space (i.e., transfer to different units). In fact, Black mothers deserve and demand accountability to prevent the loss or erosion of safety and to facilitate the activation of unconditional love. They assert that control of future events (i.e., health care and experience) is determined by present-day actions and opportunities to secure and sustain a culture and practice of safety. Black mothers described variations in the quality of care based on the presence or absence of a Black women hospital clinician or staff member as a safety violation. Thus, some Black mothers held an expectation that higher quality of service provision and care required the presence and subsequent individual-level intervention by or advocacy, of a Black clinician or team of Black clinicians and staff, to ensure optimal birth experiences based on safety.

Racial reconnaissance, one of three responses to obstetric racism, describes the Herculean effort made by Black women to avoid or mitigate racist encounters, including being hypervigilant about procedures and finding providers (Davis 2018; Davis 2019; Davis 2020; Davis, Varner, and Dill 2021; Davis 2022a; Davis 2022b). In this instance, a Black mother in the Oakland focus group, Yolanda, recognized significant variations in the quality of care based on the absence or presence of her Black woman obstetrician, and therefore expressed concerns for her safety and that of her baby. Upon recognition that the presence of her Black woman obstetrician added a level of accountability in mitigating the onset, duration, and magnitude of obstetric racism in her medical experiences, she took on the "emotional and practical labor of avoiding it" and bypassed the hospital in-person team by calling her physician directly using her personal number.

> But when she [Black woman OBGYN] who supported participant during hospital birth] was there, the nurses—everybody was on their toes. But when she left it was a different story. So, I had a different experience when she was there. So, I kept on calling her because I had her personal number. So, I had to text her a couple of times so I can get the help that I need.

The fact that the Black woman obstetrician shared her personal number with her Black woman patient demonstrated a form of individual physician-level racial reconnaissance. The insider within the health system utilized her hidden insights about obstetric racism embedded in the system and enacted an individual-level intervention to protect her patients from the harm of obstetric racism during childbirth hospitalization. This specific mitigation step is common among Black women physicians in private or hospital-based practices, which ultimately benefits a select group of patients who experience a form of privilege and protection from unsafe care. The individual physician level of accountability is a workaround protective solution for implementation in immediate unsafe circumstances or conditions. However, work-arounds are not equitably extended to all Black mothers and birthing people seeking help or care for childbirth hospitalization across the entire system. Individual-level interventions ultimately reinforce structural and institutional incompetencies and inequities, as the population level harms in the form of obstetric racism imposed on Black reproducing bodies and Black babies go unchecked and unresolved.

Black mothers consistently define obstetric patient safety as unconditional love in the context of protection and security from unintended, unwanted, unplanned, unwelcomed harm, injury, or malicious events, experiences, or outcomes. The ongoing denials and delays of protection and security from harm, injury, or malice during childbirth hospitalization in U.S. hospitals threaten the innate human worth, or dignity, of Black mothers and the futures of Black lives. Without political, structural, institutional, and disciplinary accountability and oversight in preserving the dignity of Black lives and the human right to bodily and decisional autonomy and safety, genocide is inevitable.

Chapter 4

Bodily and Decisional Autonomy

> So I was completely terrified thinking I'm going to have a three pound baby, then they kept saying, like, oh, your baby's going to be too small to come through the birth canal, like, he's going to be too tired, he's not going to have enough strength to get through, so because he was so small. So we should do a C-section . . . .I was, like, I don't even want to be induced, let alone have a C-section. But that was one thing they kept pushing, like, oh, you should get the C-section because he's too small and he's not going to have the strength to get through the birth canal because it's very tiring for him because he's so little. [Kendra, a Black mother in Los Angeles, who birthed her baby into the world through her vaginal birth canal, weighing five pounds and six ounces].

A common violation of care quality enacted against Black mothers by hospital systems, teams, and individual obstetric physicians, nurses, and staff during childbirth hospitalization is the use of medical coercion, abuse, and ceremonies of degradation, manifestations of obstetric racism—to undermine Black women's free will or autonomy (Davis 2018; Davis 2019; Davis 2020; Davis, Varner, and Dill 2021; Scott and Davis 2021). The most dominant scenario explored during the focus groups in Oakland and Los Angeles was repeated violations of Black mothers' autonomy over their bodies during care provision and decision-making about cesarean births. Most Black mothers shared narratives of perpetual attempts and successes in eroding their agency (the free will or power to make decisions or successfully achieve a desired goal with optimal options, resources, and conditions) or self-efficacy (belief in one's capacity to make decisions or achieve a desired goal) in securing the actual birth and birth experience they desire and expect. In the process of examining how well or how poorly hospital physicians and nurses in obstetrics safeguard patient autonomy through the expressions and experiences of thirty-six Black mothers, I uncover the dominant practice of coerced or forced inductions and cesarean births through a careful orchestration of hospital team language and behaviors and manipulation of communication grounded in obstetric racism. First, hospital physicians identify a suspected, but not always definitive, pathological diagnosis during the antepartum or prenatal period prior to labor, which may or may not increase the risk for an adverse outcome impacting the Black mother, fetus, and/or placenta. Second, the hospital obstetricians and maternal-fetal medicine specialists document and disseminate health care information about the suspected pathology and its potential clinical sequelae during patient sign-outs and handoffs and throughout electronic health records. The consequence of the second step is the mobilization of powerful hospital personnel, policies, practices, protocols, and procedures to synchronize all their efforts in the weaponization of the fears of Black mothers as being seen and treated as unfit and incapable of protecting their children, particularly the unborn developing and dependent Black baby inside their Black wombs.

One primary catalyst facilitating the insidious chain of medically coercive, abusive, and forced processes and chain of events is the racist praxis of biological determinism. The unchecked practice of disproportionately recommending and performing labor inductions or cesarean births by hospital-based obstetricians and perinatal nurses reinforces the trope that the most dangerous place for a Black baby is inside the womb of a Black mother. On Friday, February 18, 2011, an anti-abortion group based in Dallas, Texas, Life Always, set up a billboard in SoHo on the corner of Avenue of the Americas and Watts Street, a half mile from a Planned Parenthood center. The anti-abortion billboard stood "several stories high outside of the Holland Tunnel declaring, "The Most Dangerous Place for an African American Is in the Womb," featuring a young Black girl in a pink dress with a bow in her hair beneath its message" (Bowie 2011, 1; Robbins 2011). Life Always initiated the campaign in New York in February, with intentionality, coordination, and clarity of purpose, during the simultaneous local and national observations of Black History Month, to highlight the disproportionate number of abortions among Black women and gender-expansive individuals. The malicious, feckless, and myopic interpretation of the statistics and use of the anti-abortion billboard, without historical and structural context, extend beyond the purposes of this book. What must be addressed in this chapter and throughout the book is the presence and permeation of anti-Black racism and misogynoir embedded in and behind the message (Bailey 2016; Bailey and Trudy 2018; Bailey 2021) and movement spearheaded by the far-right religious dogmatic conservatives to control, constrain, and revoke the human right to bodily and decisional autonomy of all people, particularly Black women. Prior to the events in

New York City, the Georgia Right to Life and Radiance Foundation spent $20,000 to post sixty-five anti-Black racist and anti-Black sexist anti-abortion billboards in predominantly Black neighborhoods in Atlanta on February 5, 2010, with the image of a sad-looking Black male child and the message "Black Children are an Endangered Species" (Trust Black Women, n.d). SisterSong, a Southern-based, national membership organization that builds and strengthens capacities and strategic, coordinated actions of an effective network of individuals and organizations to improve institutional policies and systems that impact the reproductive lives of marginalized communities (SisterSong n.d.), immediately took action, analyzed the current political movement, convened a partnership of Black women's organizations, and formed the national Trust Black Women partnership in 2010 to combat the accusations and lies blaming Black women for genocide by obtaining abortions. Within the first year of existence, the Trust Black Women partnership defeated the billboards and a concomitant bill to restrict abortion. By joining the Black Lives Matter Movement, the Trust Black Women partnership continues to mobilize the Reproductive Justice movement through training, capacity building, advocacy, and organizing of Black women and people and active allies to disrupt norms and narratives rooted in misogynoir and create and spread power-affirming, activating, and actualizing images and messages of Black women (Trust Black Women n.d.).

One must wrestle with the reality that hospital administrators, physicians, nurses, clinical administrative leaders, and staff represent members of society who hold particular values and beliefs that then influence how they socialize, organize, and move about within and across various formal and informal sociocultural, religious, and political groups. Consequently, hospital teams of administrators, physicians, and nurses engage in a pattern of coordinated, unrelenting, and pernicious language and behavior consistent with undermining patient autonomy, agency, and self-efficacy by first causing Black women to doubt their innate power and potential to birth based on their desires and dreams. The medical-industrial complex pathologizes birthing while Black by translating the physiology of Black birth into processes of risk identification, stratification, and mitigation. In the medicalization and pathologization of Black reproducing bodies and Black births, hospital teams and individual nurses and physicians work in concert as a system to offer one cure to the "peculiar disease" of Black pregnancy, a medical intervention that disrupts the duration of the pregnancy with a labor induction or cesarean birth. Thus, Blackness becomes synonymous with death and dying in narratives created and controlled by academic centers, hospital systems, public health departments, insurance companies, medical and nursing professional organizations, and the media whereby physicians and nurses play the heroes in a war against the villains, emancipated and liberated Black reproducing bodies.

Reading, re-reading, and interpreting the text of hospital birth narratives shared by thirty-six Black mothers in Oakland and Los Angeles reads more like movie scripts that mix genres of horror and war. In making sense of the lived experiences of Black mothers through text, the battleground is the mind or free will of Black mothers. In health care, every patient possesses the human right to bodily and decisional autonomy, based on the ethical, legal, and biomedical principal of autonomy, the authority over decision-making about what happens to, through, within, and about one's body (Braun et al. 2010; Beauchamp 2007). Autonomy is characterized by the processes of communication, comprehension, voluntariness, and consent or refusal of the recommended clinical plan (Braun et al. 2010), which is examined in detail in chapter 5. For this chapter's purpose, I examine the rhetoric and reality of protecting and pursuing bodily and decisional autonomy through textual analysis of the lived experiences of Black mothers navigating childbirth hospitalization.

According to thirty-six Black mothers in Oakland and Los Angeles, the shared meaning of autonomy is having the right to make independent decisions about one's body, pregnancy, baby, and care based on having access to comprehensive, accurate, and scientifically and culturally relevant, rigorous, robust, and responsive information, options, resources, choices, and optimal conditions. A Black mother's autonomy is shaped and strengthened by self-efficacy (the individual belief in one's capacity to achieve a desired goal or make a decision). Black mothers also feel that autonomy also includes the right for their expressed desires, expectations, concerns, and needs to be acknowledged and fulfilled by the healthcare profession, system, teams, and individual clinicians and staff. For autonomy to be optimally actualized, Black mothers expect health systems, teams, and individual clinicians and staff members to recognize and include their peers, partners, and support persons in the care provision, interactions, communications, decision-making, and consent or refusal of clinical advice and treatment. Black mothers view their community support persons, any person without hospital affiliation or alignment, as advocates, shields, and negotiators who can ensure that their birth experiences align with birth expectations, prevent or mitigate any potential harm, and address social isolation, neglect, and abandonment (White VanGompel et al. 2022; Lett et al. 2023).

Black mothers identified three core behaviors or conditions that actualize, protect, or optimize their autonomy, which can be measured, monitored, and managed in hospital-based obstetric policies, processes, procedures, and practices:

- Knowing about, having access to, and utilizing a full array of laboring, birthing, and postpartum options and choices, including diverse and inclusive information, education, and direct care services and supports;
- Independently giving permission to participate as the patient along each step of the way during care provision about one's body and baby during pregnancy, labor, and the immediate postpartum;
- Being an active participant with voice, lived experience, wisdom, and power in every social and clinical interaction, communication, counseling, decision-making, and documentation and dissemination of care information in patient sign-outs, patient handoffs, safety huddles, and paper and electronic health records.

The synthesis of the shared meanings and measures for bodily and decisional autonomy in the provision of hospital-based obstetrics care established five overarching themes or manifestations of activating or violating Black mothers' autonomy:

1. Seeking information outside of the hospital/health system or medical industrial complex as a practice of advocacy, protection, and preservation of self as a Black woman during care access and utilization;
2. Obtaining written or oral communication about birth preferences, expectations, visions, options, and opportunities for chosen birth attendants, spaces, places, positions, partners, and practices;
3. Navigating coerced or forced care;
4. Activating or amplifying agency or self-efficacy;
5. Questioning or rejecting the presence and/or participation of learners in care provision.

Black mothers explained the various strategies they implemented to protect and preserve their humanity during anticipated or actual threats to their autonomy. For example, they asked clarifying questions, sought out the professional support and protection of a doula, or utilized assertive communication when feeling unsure, neglected, ignored, or dismissed during care provision and decision-making throughout pregnancy, labor, birth, and immediate postpartum. In Chapter 2, the reader learned about Felicia, a Black mother in the Los Angeles focus group, who previously encountered and navigated the uninterrogated belief held by an Asian woman OBGYN physician, with no prior experience caring for Black women in her practice, that Blackness is pathological and that the combination of Blackness and pregnancy leads to death and dying or disease and disability. At the time of her pregnancy, Felicia described herself as a full-bodied Black woman, existing and thriving with no pre-existing social or medical co-morbidities common to pregnancy and Black women during pregnancy (e.g., hypertensive disorders of pregnancy, pre-pregnancy or pregnancy-induced diabetes, sickle cell trait or disorder, sexually transmitted infections (STIs), including HIV).

> *Felicia:* Okay. This is an Asian woman [OBGYN physician] who was like—just—she literally just kept telling me, no. And I'm like, how do you tell me no. I'm pretty sure I'm in control still. This is the way I want to do things. So she was pushing the C-section. So I looked up her C-section rates, and they were extremely high. And I read a lot of reviews regarding to, like—and it was like—because I actually did research, but the doctor that I asked for wouldn't take me because I was so far along. So they gave me this person that I ended up delivering with.
>
> *Dr. Scott:* How did you know to look up her C-section rate?
>
> *Shanice:* That's so good.
>
> *Felicia:* The Melanin Moms group. Once I give the information on how to, you know—that you don't have to put up with the—like, the situation that you're in, you can, you know, kind of do research for the doctor that you want and kind of try to [leave, find a new doctor], you know—as long as you're within your insurance. Like, so I have private insurance with my job.

When Felicia felt ignored, dismissed, and disrespected, one of Davis' six dimensions of obstetric racism (Davis 2018; Davis 2019; Davis 2020; Davis, Varner, and Dill 2021; Scott and Davis 2021), she decided to seek out and gather additional information about the professional conduct and reputation of the Asian OBGYN physician. The persistent violations of decisional autonomy prompted Felicia to investigate whether the Asian OBGYN physician had a prior history of violating the autonomy and agency of other patients. The acts of looking up cesarean birth rates and patient reviews of individual OBGYN physicians revealed clinical behaviors and practices that misaligned with Felicia's expectations. Likewise, seeking additional support and guidance from the Melanin Moms group further activated and strengthened Felicia's autonomy, agency, and self-efficacy. In response to anticipated and actual violations of her bodily and decisional autonomy, Felicia gathered information from multiple sources outside of the health system and changed physicians. Her response perfectly aligns with one of three responses to obstetric racism, as defined by Davis (Davis 2018; Davis 2019; Davis 2020; Davis, Varner, and Dill 2021; Scott and Davis 2021; Davis 2022a; Davis 2022b), racial reconnaissance, which describes the Herculean efforts made by Black women to avoid or mitigate racist encounters, including being hypervigilant about procedures and finding providers.

In chapters 2 and 3, the reader learns about Rhonda, a Black mother in the Oakland focus group, through her critique of overall nursing care, with a focus on the role, responsibilities, and impact of the nurse on obstetric quality of care. In the narrative below, Rhonda shared her disappointment in not being able to experience a home birth due to high-risk identification, as well as her gratitude and relief for meeting doulas and having the option to choose a doula part of her hospital birth, if she desired.

> I believe because I was high risk come to find out, I couldn't really—I couldn't do it and they were like half managing me. So, I was kind of sad, but I learned something new for other moms who wanted to, you know, maybe want [a home birth]—because I really wanted like a home birth, you know, and I couldn't do that. So yeah, we got to meet different doulas and doulas that operate differently, some were holistically all the way and the other ones that, you know—so I was thankful to have just those if I needed. I never actually had a doula or hired a doula or anything, but I was actually supposed to do doula training before I had him, but I got sick right before. But yeah, just I was thankful for all the other different resources and information I was given this fourth time around.

Black mothers shared that they sought professional information, advocacy, support, and protection from doulas. For Rhonda, knowing about, having access to, and utilizing a full array of laboring, birthing, and postpartum options and choices, including diverse and inclusive informational, educational, and direct care services and supports, activated and actualized her autonomy. For both Felicia and Rhonda, Black mothers actualized their autonomy, agency, and self-efficacy in refusing to participate in the medicalization, pathologization, and commodification of birth. As explained by Davis (Davis 2018; Davis 2019; Davis 2020; Davis, Varner, and Dill 2021; Davis 2022a; Davis 2022b), both Black mothers responded to obstetric racism by deploying their own will against a system of control and the demands of consent to harmful care. In both scenarios, the refusal of Black mothers demonstrated a firm understanding and choice to reject the possibility of coercion, medical intervention, abuse, disrespect, and the power that hospital systems, teams, and individual clinicians and staff members use to exert dominance over Black reproducing bodies and Black mothers' decisions.

Another strategy to protect and actualize Black mothers' bodily and decisional autonomy during the provision of hospital-based obstetrics is the development and dissemination of a birth plan. With a birth plan, Black mothers, partners, and given and chosen families have the opportunity, option, capacity, and capability to speak up and share their birth desires, dreams, expectations, and non-negotiables. Angie, a Black mother in the Oakland focus group, introduced a colloquial expression that means the person is in possession of a weapon (e.g.,) and they are prepared to use said weapon for protection.

> *Angie:* I came locked and loaded.
>
> *Dr. Scott:* In case a person listening doesn't know what "locked and loaded" means tell us what locked and loaded means.
>
> *Angie:* I came with my birth plan.

For Angie, childbirth hospitalization was warfare, and her birth plan was her weapon of choice. Developing and sharing a written or oral communication about one's birth vision, priorities, preferences, and needs is essential in activating one's authority over the decisions impacting their body, baby, and placenta, including the birth space, hospital attendants, and community support persons. Pregnant women usually utilize the birth plan to specify the procedural elements of care, determining if, when, and how hospital teams place the intravenous (IV) lines, initiate any fluids or medications, or implement other medical interventions such as cervical exams, fetal monitoring, breaking the amniotic sac, and so on. Additionally, pregnant women alone or with support and guidance from their partners, kin, or community support persons (e.g., community doula, community midwife, community perinatal worker) utilize an oral or written birth plan to determine their birth modality preference, prioritizing a non-operative vaginal birth (without assistance of forceps or vacuum operated by a trained obstetrician physician). Beyond the mechanics of birth, Black mothers and their partners expressed the need for greater workforce diversification and inclusion in hospital settings that involve Black birth workers.

Dominque, one of many Black mothers in the Oakland focus group who felt forced into having a cesarean birth, provided additional details about her hospital birth experiences through her white husband's perceptions and perspectives.

> *Dominique:* I just wanted a natural birth and I just really feel like it wasn't necessary for a C-section.
>
> *Dr. Scott:* And tell me what you mean by natural. So, because that can mean different things. What is a natural birth to you?
>
> *Domnique:* A vaginal birth. Support. My husband was really mad. And he's like not even, you know, our color. He's from Europe, or whatever. And he was even mad like, you know, about the whole—there was. . . he was mad about there was no Black people. He was like there was no support. And he kept saying my wife's Black. So, you know, it's just I don't know. I wanted it to be a little

> bit—my pregnancy was awesome compared to the last pregnancy. This pregnancy was like awesome, no problems, none of that. But I just dreamed that the whole way through would have been better. Like from pregnancy to birth, you know, to after birth, and stuff like that.

Developing and sharing a written or oral communication about one's birth vision, priorities, preferences, and needs is essential in activating one's authority over the decisions impacting their body, baby, and placenta including the birth space and birth attendants. Several Black mothers envisioned a hospital birth experience with a midwife or doula, specifically a Black midwife or doula. Black mothers also envisioned a birth experience that included the presence and participation of their partner or parent. Unfortunately, the lack of diversification, democratization, destigmatization, and inclusion in the hospital birth workforce constrains the capacity, choices, and conditions for Black mothers to actualize their autonomy and manifest their birthright to a SACKRED Birth, defined for, by, and with Black mothers.

Previously in chapter 2, the Oakland Black mothers Angie and LaToya engaged in a conversation of shared feelings of disappointment from unfulfilled expectations and stolen moments during their childbirth hospitalization. Another unfulfilled desire for LaToya was not having access to a midwife (for clinical care), a doula (for support and advocacy), or both throughout pregnancy, labor, and postpartum. "I asked [about access to Black midwife or doula in Oakland/Bay area]. And I got nothing. I was so disappointed because I wanted one. Yeah, nothing. I wanted a midwife or a doula to go through my pregnancy with. And I got no information." Although LaToya possessed free will to choose (autonomy) and design her perinatal support team, the existing systems and structures of health care delivery, financing, and training robbed her of options, resources, and optimal conditions by which to utilize her free will to choose and decide (agency). Similarly, in Oakland, hospital policies and/or practices between 2017 to 2019, prior to the widespread 2020 COVID-19 mitigation strategies, violated Chantelle's autonomy and agency in curating her desired birth experience. Chantelle envisioned birthing in the presence of her husband and her mother, surrounded by love. Instead, a hospital policy or practice (maybe even a decision made by her team without prior consent or deliberation) shattered her birth dream, "I wanted my mom there but they said only one person could be in the room."

The SACKRED Birth framework is a radical attitude toward *human births*, specifically *Blackness, Black bodies, and Black births*, that regards all birth activities as fundamentally normal, healthy, spiritual, familial, magical, transformative, erotic, communal, emancipatory, and power-activating. In action, SACKRED Birth movement affirms, activates, and amplifies diverse and inclusive birth pleasure, practices, care, spaces, options, partners, communities, and experiences. The SACKRED movement advocates for safer, respectful, dignified, high-quality "participatory" birth care, conditions, experiences, and outcomes, and improved workforce diversification, development, and sustainability. More importantly, the SACKRED Birth movement calls for the restoration of Black Midwifery care and Black Doula support models as part of its campaign to prevent and mitigate acts of obstetric racism and to manifest birth justice and accountability. Thus, the SACKRED Birth movement supports the actualization of Black mothers' autonomy, agency, and self-efficacy in determining their birth experience, independent of birth settings and attendants, especially when choosing one's birth companions and support team (Scott 2018; Scott 2019a; Scott 2019b; Davis and Scott 2020).

Being transformed by the experiential knowledge, bravery, boldness, and brilliance of the thirty-six Black mothers in Oakland and Los Angeles, I started offering different guidance on developing a birth plan for pregnant Black women and gender-expansive individuals and their given and chosen kin.

> In this era of fragmented health care, I would encourage folks to think beyond just, 'I don't want an I.V.' What birth experience do you want? What are the traditions you want to continue? What does birth mean to you? It's helpful to define that on your birth plan. 'This birth is a symbol of this…' People don't know what birth means to most communities, but particularly to a community where the narratives and norms of humanity have been so contorted and degraded and devalued. Is this birth a sign of liberation or resistance? Is it a renewal of a vow? If there is something traumatic or something triumphant about the experience of pregnancy, I need the birth plan to frame the interaction. I want to know the humanity of your birth as opposed to just the mechanics and management. If I can understand the meaning there, it can shape how I approach my communications, interactions, counseling, and decision-making. —Dr. Scott. (McClain 2019, 7)

Black mothers also sought out resources outside of the medical industrial complex to activate and actualize their bodily and decisional autonomy, such as participation in state and federally funded pro-Black initiatives designed with the goal of addressing drivers of the manufactured Black maternal health crisis. As explained in greater detail in Chapter 7, Black Infant Health (BIH) is a state health equity program of the California Department of Public Health (CDPH) that offers free individual and group support services to Black mothers and birthing people aged sixteen years or older, who are pregnant or up to six months postpartum at the time of enrollment, regardless of income (CDPH n.d.). According to CDPH, the structure and strategies of the BIH program strengthen the life skills of Black mothers and birthing people within the context and conditions of offering a culturally affirming and supportive environment that honors the unique history of Black women and birthing people. BIH aims to make a meaningfully lasting imprint and impact beyond existing participants, extending to future Black women, infants, and families. Based on the lived experience of a Black mother in Los Angeles, BIH provided meaningful information that strengthened her self-efficacy in actualizing her autonomy and agency during her childbirth hospitalization.

Dr Scott: What things made it easier or harder for your birth preferences to be heard or recognized?

Toni: I think Black Infant Health helped with feeding and birthing plan. Now, whether or not that birthing plan was followed, just the initial, you know, preparation of having that and then, being educated on certain things that I think made it a little bit easier in retrospect. Because it's, you know, kind of telling you something that you probably wouldn't otherwise think about. Like, not wanting Pitocin. You know what I mean? Or like, you know, just different like, what medications or what don't you want or what do you want? And I tried to make sure that my husband was aware of this, that and, you know, my mom also. To this day I kind of hate that I kind of don't remember if they followed the birthing plan exactly. I know I gave birth on my back. So, I'm like, well that didn't happen. But I think that that really helped in regard to going in like knowing this is what I absolutely do not want. But something else is okay.

According to Shanice, a Black mother in Los Angeles, a culturally affirming program for her community, operating outside of the hospitals, provided her with the resources and strategies to better negotiate with the hospital system to actualize her birth and infant feeding intentions. Additionally, Shanice identified and described other crucial actors outside of the hospital system that supported her in affirming and activating her autonomy. In the scenario below, Shanice explained how she leveraged kinship ties between her and her husband, and her and her mother, to hold the hospital system, hospital team, and individual clinicians and staff members accountable for protecting her autonomy. When identifying factors that facilitated the transfer of information in the birth plan from the Black mother to the hospital system, hospital team, and individual clinicians and staff, many Black mothers in Oakland and Los Angeles named their husbands.

Shanice: For me, it was my husband. For me, it was my husband. He was my best advocate. And he was like this is what we're going to do. Because like I said, he followed the nurse. And he was like, you give my baby formula, I will hit you. Because they were just—I mean, it was ridiculous how much they was pushing formula because I was gone four hours, five hours. You know—I still hadn't seen my baby. So, we had it written down. And then, of course, my

> birth plan went out the window, you know, a lot of the stuff because it was an emergency for this one. But he was the one that was making sure. But anything that we did have control over—we was able to do. Things that we were communicating.

In several instances, Black mothers describe their husbands as serving in the simultaneous roles of patient shield and birth plan enforcer. The presence and participation of husbands during care provision sometimes manifested as a force field, protecting their laboring, birthing, and postpartum wives and their babies against violations of patient autonomy and agency. Likewise, husbands also served as the enforcers of hospital actions that aligned with their wives' expressed needs, priorities, and preferences, facilitating person-focused care and shared decision-making, particularly for Black mothers (Starfield 2011; Scott and Davis 2022).

> *Mariah:* Let me tell you all, if that man [participant's husband] was not there I probably would be in tiny little pieces. Like, he was like my number one cheerleader—like, you can do it, babe. You're almost there. I was like you're right. I can do it. But he was like everything. And I just I was scared because I only had him. You know, that moment to me, I feel like I needed my mom.
>
> *Regina:* Right.
>
> *Jasmine:* Right.
>
> *Mariah:* Like she's the only one who truly understands. But because I couldn't have her there and, you know, I didn't know how he was going to react. But he—I'm telling you all, he put people in their place. And he was like, this is what you're all going to do. He was in there praying. Like this is what's going to happen. And he's egging me on the entire time, and he made me feel like I wasn't alone. Like and that was so important to me. Because I did feel alone because I was going through everything physical. But he was just—it's like he just go in tune with me and I wanted him in that space, and he was there.

Black mothers also identified another kinship relationship that they leveraged to protect, secure, and actualize their autonomy and agency. Black mothers relied on the presence and participation of their mothers in the provision of hospital-based obstetric care as a strategy to hold the hospital system, team, and individual clinicians and staff accountable for complying with their daughter's birth plan. Based on reading the room in Los Angeles, I asked the question, "Who else had someone else at least try to get what's in the birth plan to the clinician?" to gain a better understanding of Black mothers' intense need and desire for the presence and protection of their own Black mother throughout the childbirth process. Black mothers such as Nia, Regina, and Shante, erupted in unison with "My mom" to highlight the power, beauty, sanctity, necessity, and purpose of multi-generational kinship births.

The experiential knowledge and wisdom of Black mothers birthing in Los Angeles hospitals highlighted the realities of birthing while Black in most U.S. hospitals. Going to a hospital to give birth places Black mothers and birthing people, and their given and chosen kinship, in a battle with the hospital over whose voice and will ultimately determine what happens to, within, through, and about the Black reproducing body and her Black baby. The following depictions of a Black mother in Los Angeles, Nia, navigating the authority and control of hospitals in undermining their bodily and decisional autonomy read like a movie script of the latest war and horror film.

> For me, it was my husband. I don't think that I was heard because like when I was—I went to (inaudible) and I spent with my nurse over and over and I told her that that was my plan. And it was like she disregarded what I said and never put the order in. And so, I never received it. So, now I have to go get it after. And it was like, but when my husband went after and like so, it was long. Like when he went to go speak to someone, it was, you know, they were aggressive about getting whatever he said done that needed to be done. But when I spoke to the nurse that was directly helping me, it was like I (wasn't there]. Unless I told him and he was like we'll see.

Once again, Black mothers leverage the role of their husbands and weaponize patriarchy against the hospital system, team, and individual clinicians and staff in upholding their human right to bodily and decisional autonomy. Black mothers, like Nia and Shanice, deploy multiple strategies to assert, protect, secure, and actualize their ethical, legal, moral, and spiritual right to birth as they desire and deserve with the assurance of safer, respectful, dignified, high-quality "participatory" birth care, conditions, experiences, and outcomes, and full unrestrained access to and utilization of improved workforce diversification, development, and sustainability, along with the restoration of Black Midwifery care and Black Doula support models as part of the SACKRED Birth movement (Scott 2018; Scott 2019a; Scott 2019b; Scott et al. 2021). Ebony, a married Black mother in the Los Angeles focus group, explained how she leveraged her voice combined with her husband's voice to protect her bodily and decisional autonomy and avert an unnecessary cesarean birth.

> When I had my second baby, they had—we insisted that I'm not going to get a cesarean. I was in the operating room, every—they was prepping me and my baby started to come out. I was like I'm not doing this. You do not have my consent. And they still pushed me in there. Was like she's coming. Her heart is dropping. I was like—she's—I'm not going to get cut. And my husband's like,

> she's not getting cut. They left. The nurse delivered my baby because they were prepping for surgery.

Ebony and her husband united in their collective acts of refusal and resistance against the hospital in the operating room while she was lying on the operating table. In this situation, Ebony and her husband assert their autonomy and agency to decline participation in the medicalization and pathologization of her birth. Both focus groups in Oakland and Los Angeles revealed a pattern of Black mothers and their husbands, independent of the race of the husband, deploying their own will against the control of the hospital system and the demands of involuntariness. The will of Black mothers and Black fathers represents a force dyad in the battle against obstetric racism. As Davis argues, the act of refusal is a response informed by a clear sense of responsibility to recognize and reject the possibility of coercion, medical intervention, abuse, disrespect, and the power of contemporary obstetrics in hospital systems used to dominate the Black reproducing body and her creations (Davis 2018; Davis 2019; Davis 2020; Davis, Varner, and Dill 2021; Davis 2022a; Davis 2022b). The act of refusal extends beyond people's understanding of the implications of not doing something (Davis 2018; Davis 2019; Davis 2020; Davis, Varner, and Dill 2021; Davis 2022a; Davis 2022b); rather, they understand the risks, benefits, and alternatives of medical interventions and remain more concerned about agreeing with medical advice within the context and conditions of their lives and birth plan. The rise of the Black mother-father force dyad also provides a model of resistance as another response to obstetric racism (Davis 2018; Davis 2019; Davis 2020; Davis, Varner, and Dill 2021; Davis 2022a; Davis 2022b). The Black mother-father force dyad utilizes their experiential, spiritual, ancestral, and mainstream knowledge to push back against forced cesarean birth or other forced practices or procedures. The Black mother-father force dyad represents an act of mobilization against the obstetric racism permeating throughout the hospital system. As a response against obstetric racism, resistance is deeply grounded in a vision of how a Black mother, her partner, her parent, and any other member of the Black mother's given or chosen kinship desire, dream, and deserve to be treated by hospital systems, teams, and individual clinicians and staff members (Davis 2018; Davis 2019; Davis 2020; Davis, Varner, and Dill 2021; Davis 2022a; Davis 2022b).

Battling Over Birth: Black Women and the Maternal Health Care Crisis offers a critical report and timely resource that interprets the birthing experiences of Black women as they navigate the horrors of the manufactured Black maternal health crisis in the U.S. (Oparah et al. 2017). Using research justice methodologies (Jolivétte 2015), Black Women Birthing Justice (BWBJ) researchers gathered data directly from Black women instead of relying on existing databases such as birth certificates or large administrative datasets (Oparah et al. 2017; BWBJ n.d.). The overreliance on administrative datasets in measurement design, selection, and monitoring strategies in quality improvement and implementation science creates and exacerbates the hypervisibility of Black women as victims (Scott 2018; Scott 2019a; Scott 2019b; Scott 2021), and not as victors in the battle over Black bodily and decisional autonomy. The other problem with existing structural, institutional, and disciplinary efforts toward innovation and transformation in quality improvement is the structural exclusion and erasure of Black women as patients, community, and content experts (Scott 2018; Scott 2019a; Scott 2019b; Scott 2021; Scott and Davis 2021; White VanGompel et al. 2022). Racism denial leads to inaction in the face of need, which Jones identified in 2020 as institutionalized racism (Jones 2020). More importantly, racism denial across multiple disciplines, including the public health literature (Hardeman et al. 2018), and the perinatal QI literature continues to absolve obstetric quality and patient safety leaders, hospitals, and health plans from taking responsibility for the actions that create and worsen the deplorable services and conditions of birthing while Black in U.S. hospitals (Scott 2018; Scott 2019a; Scott 2019b; Scott 2021; Scott and Davis 2021; White VanGompel et al. 2022; Lett et al. 2023; Scott and Lusero 2023).

Above and beyond holding hospitals accountable for how they "handle," rather than "care for," Black women (Scott 2021) in the battle over who controls the Black reproducing body and Black births (Roberts 1997; Oparah et al. 2017), hospital systems, teams, and individual clinicians and staff lack the appropriate ethical, legal, moral, and epistemological oversight for naming, measuring, monitoring, preventing, and mitigating the violence enacted against the Black reproducing body, baby, and kinship (Scott 2021; Scott and Davis 2021; Scott and Lusero 2023). The prioritization of being safe (as defined by quality and safety systems and structures) over feeling safe (as defined by the experiential, ancestral, and spiritual knowledge of Black patient, community, and content experts) (Lyndon et al. 2023) creates and exacerbates epistemic injustice (Fricker 2007; Scott 2021).

Three excerpts from three different Black mothers in the Los Angeles focus group illuminate the ongoing tensions and struggles Black mothers endure to affirm, actualize, and protect their bodily and decisional autonomy. The imagery of Black mothers preparing for warfare, whereby Black mothers exercise agency in carefully choosing which armor and weaponry to use in the war for their desired birth, based on the threat and conditions for each series of battles, permeates the feelings, thoughts, and spirit in the room.

> *Felicia:* I think I read every article imaginable, especially when it came to, like, what I wanted as for as, like, late cord clamping, or vaccinations, or any

eye ointments, or, like, who I wanted in the room or who was allowed, and—Who I wanted in the room. I think I—I'd have like every baby app, and they have—a list of things that you can go down through to just make sure you—you are aware of what might happen and what you want in different type of things. And just as far as consent, like, nothing happens in that room without my consent—despite what the doctors may say or what the nurses might say. So just going through those things to try and prepare myself for it, because I expected just to have, like, a full-out battle, because I—I understood what I wanted was probably contrary to what a lot of doctors, or nurses, or staff would have wanted.

Tiara: To touch on that battle portion, it was, you know, really interesting going to all of the prenatal visits and everything, because I was very adamant that I didn't want to vaccinate—you know, vaccinate immediately, nor did I want the vitamin K shot. I didn't want anything injected into my baby, you know, and they were really adamant about the vitamin K and the—the eye ointment, like to the point where they did the eye ointment, you know, and I had requested them not to.

Mariah: She said battle, and that resonated with me because throughout all of my prenatal visits—I carried twins—and—not that there's anything wrong with a C-section, but my—my two previous births were vaginal, so it just made logical sense for my twins to be a vaginal birth. And I got opposition the minute I opened my mouth about the—the possibility to have a vaginal delivery. Well, if baby A is head down, then we can try for the vaginal, but if baby B is breech, you know, it might be, you know, we might have to do emergency C-section—emergency surgery and it was a lot of fear being pushed by Hospital 1.

In the battle to secure a SACKRED Birth, Black mothers, like Felicia, Tiara, and Mariah, deployed multiple strategies of resistance, refusal, and racial reconnaissance as responses to obstetric racism. At the opening of this dialogue, a Black mother searched for and read every article about medical interventions such as cord clamping, vaccine administration, and application of the Erythromycin eye ointment for prophylaxis against Chlamydia. She also downloaded multiple pregnancy- and baby-related apps. She also determined who would take up space in her birth. Davis describes the Herculean efforts made by Black women to avoid or mitigate racist encounters including being hypervigilant about procedures and finding providers as racial reconnaissance (Davis 2018; Davis 2019; Davis 2020; Davis, Varner, and Dill 2021; Davis 2022a; Davis 2022b). At the core of childbirth hospitalization in the U.S. is the longstanding battle over a Black woman's or person's right to control what happens to, within, through, and about her reproducing body and the byproducts of her body including her baby, her blood, her urine, and her placenta and the umbilical cord.

Tiara's decisions for her baby regarding newborn vaccinations and administration of vitamin K and the topical eye ointment highlight the ongoing battle over whose authority determines the well-being and development of a newborn baby, the Black mother or the hospital system, acting as an agent of the state (Roberts 1997). Just as Roberts' scholarship explicates how the prison and foster care systems operate together to overpolice and punish Black mothers in service to maintain the hierarchy of human value based on racism, gender oppression, and class exploitation in a neoliberal state (Roberts 2011), this Black feminist hermeneutic phenomenology provides the evidence to argue that modern-day obstetrics and insurance companies, in synergy with quality and safety organizations, weaponize reproduction, pregnancy, and childbirth to maintain hierarchies of motherhood, family planning, and legacy building. By medicalizing, pathologizing, and commodifying pregnancy and birth, hospital, insurance, and quality systems justify the translation of human beings and human experiences into numerical values that require hyper-surveillance, frequent visitations under the supervision of a licensed health care professional, and recurrent monitoring and documentation of visits for the purpose of reimbursement based on risk stratification and resource reimbursement. In chapter 3, Tiara clearly felt the commodification, quantification, and devaluation of her Black reproducing body, birth, and life by the obstetric medical-industrial complex, "I'm just I'm a product. I'm a number. I'm not a person. I'm money." Risk, resources, and reimbursement usurp the rights of Black mothers to authorize actions and govern decisions about their bodies and babies. The presence and permeation of anti-Black racism and misogynoir throughout hospital policies, processes, practices, and procedures threaten any pathway toward obstetric quality, patient safety, and institutional accountability and oversight. Thus, any strategy or solution that requires the acceptance and actualization of Black women's human right to bodily and decisional autonomy feels so monumentally daunting and disingenuous to oppressive systems and structures, and to the people benefiting from the oppression and power inequities. Tiara provided additional insights into her feelings and thoughts about the ways health systems and structures see and treat Black women throughout pregnancy, childbirth, and postpartum.

> I think it's very stereotypical. They—they look at us as we're dumb, we don't know, so therefore, we're going to tell you what you're going to do. Everything is costly now. So automatically, it's like, oh, no, you're high risk because you're black. You have to get a C-section automatically. Surgery and then how long you have to stay in there. That's all money. Versus you're having a vaginal birth. You're out, what, the next day? I was also going to say I feel they should explain or give you that option of having a birthing plan from the beginning. Do I want a cesarean in the beginning, why do I want a cesarean, give me the

> risk of a cesarean? Do I want a vaginal birth? Why do I want a vaginal birth? Give me the risks of a vaginal birth. Run the testing for—for everybody. Like is it—would it be okay for me to have a cesarean because I could actually, you know, I would rather not.

When the selling of enslaved Black women, men, girls, boys, and gender expansive-adults and children can no longer generate profit, then the new slavery is the medicalization, pathologization, commodification, and desanctification of Black reproducing bodies and Black births (Roberts 1997; Sharp 2000; Cooper 2015). The societal circumstances and conditions of Black women's reproduction and reproductive health provide deeper insight into the racialized and pathological oversight that obstetricians and other reproductive health professionals deploy to control, govern, and monetize Black women's reproduction and births throughout U.S. history. Reproductive dominance and governance over Black women's reproduction, birth, and parenting are asserted in many ways. For example, racial capitalism forces, coerces, and constrains Black women's reproduction, birth, and motherhood. A more accurate and precise assertion is that racial capitalism and racialized medical procedures, specifically in the field of gynecology and sexual and reproductive health, such as sterilization, contraceptives, and assisted reproductive technologies, control and stratify Black fecundity (Davis 2018; Weinbaum 2019). By design, the state weaponizes and then mobilizes structures and systems within the law, the courts, prisons, child welfare, and health care to carry out diabolical plans that facilitate the obstruction and eradication of Black life (Roberts 1997; Roberts 2011; Roberts 2012; Roberts 2017; Goodwin 2017; Goodwin 2020; Scott and Davis 2021).

With increasing rates of maternal death (Hoyert 2023), infant death (Hagen 2023), and preterm births (March of Dimes, n.d.) that disproportionately and unfairly impact Black mothers and Black babies, combined with the removal of Black children from the home and the incarceration and criminalization of Black mothers, the state lacks any interest in the liberation and vitality of Black lives. With the emancipation of enslaved Black people, the overpolicing of pregnant women and individuals, particularly Black mothers and gender-expansive parents, becomes increasingly justified and shaped by the coordinated communications and actions of reproductive, perinatal, and infant health workforce, hospital security, law enforcement, and CPS. Goodwin's scholarship also speaks to the weaponization of state statutes in undermining Black mothers' autonomy and privacy, facilitating coerced and forced care to protect the fetus. Fetal safety then justifies the criminalization of pregnancy and motherhood and the concomitant prosecution and incarceration of pregnant and parenting women and individuals, particularly individuals and families navigating poverty and class exploitation (Goodwin 2014, 2017, 2020).

In adding the scholarship of Davis, one sees the patterns of harm manifested as hospital acts of obstetric racism enacted against middle-stratum Black mothers navigating reproductive injustice during the provision of obstetrics, neonatal, and perinatal services across different hospital and health care settings. When reflecting on the Black hospital birth narratives of Felicia, Tiara, and Mariah and the use of birth as a battle metaphor, one reads how the system of obstetric care disregards the ethical and legal principles and practices of autonomy and informed refusal. Tiara is a free-thinking Black mother who weighed her options of various medical interventions affecting her newborn. She repeatedly declined the administration of vitamin K to prevent vitamin K deficiency bleeding (and subsequent brain damage and death) (CDC n.d.) and erythromycin eye ointment as prophylaxis treatment against Chlamydia. She asserted her right to informed refusal, and the hospital system, team, and individual clinicians proceeded to administer the eye ointment. When medical professionals perform procedures without consent and/or intimidate patients to make decisions, Davis identified this behavior of violating a Black mother's autonomy as coercion (Davis 2018; Davis 2019).

For Mariah, she expressed how the battle metaphor resonated with her experience of advocating for a vaginal birth during her third pregnancy, which resulted in twins. She examined the risks of both vaginal birth and cesarean birth with twins. She also examined the facilitators for a vaginal birth, two prior pregnancies that resulted in two prior vaginal births. As soon as she expressed disagreement with a scheduled cesarean birth and her intentional plans to focus on a vaginal birth, especially if the presenting part of the first baby (identified as baby A) is the fetal head, she disturbed the obstetric power dynamic. When Mariah asserted her right to bodily and decisional autonomy, the hospital weaponized fear to assert reproductive control over the Black mother. Davis identified this type of behavior as medical abuse, when medical professionals engage in experimentation and/or (repetitive) behavior that serves to validate the clinicians' self-worth and upholds their domination over the patient. Medical abuse is never motivated by fulfilling the expressed concerns or needs of the patient, but rather to fulfill the desires or plans of the hospital system, team, and individual clinicians and staff (Davis 2020).

One Black mother in Los Angeles, Charlene, shared her decision to watch the 2008 documentary, The Business of Being Born, by executive producer, actress, and television host Ricki Lake, who recruited filmmaker Abby Epstein as the director. The documentary, inspired by Ricki's disappointment with the birth experience of her first child, explored the maternity care system in the United States and chronicled Ricki's home birthing experience and the work of her midwife (IMDb n.d.).

> Yeah, it (the documentary) talks a lot about the mortality rate for African American women --In different hospitals—around—around the world. And the reason why I watched that was because, that was like my fear, you know, of just being—like, having the experience of being pregnant to term and then delivering the baby, and then not being there. Like, I—for whatever reason that, like, resonated with me. That was, like, my ultimate fear was not being able to really be a mom. So I really wanted to watch that, not because I was afraid of, you know, my—my mortality, but just educational. You know, I wanted to know what the hospitals were—were going to do—like, what they were capable of because I, too, wanted to go to a birthing center, or do, like, a homebirth or something, but I ended up being anemic, and I didn't qualify. Like, I had—I was borderline, like, I was almost going to have to get a transfusion. But I worked really, really hard to raise my—my blood count by taking chlorophyll—I don't know if anybody knows about that. Yeah, so that's what I did in order to get where I needed to be in order to deliver, but anyway. That documentary was very, very helpful for me to just—allow me to take control over my birthing process. You know, and I actually—spoke a lot with—I wanted to do, you know, the doula thing and everything. But once I found out about my blood count, you know, they were, like, we're not going to allow, you know, other people to come in the room. So I couldn't go forth with the doula thing. Right, which is just weird. But then at—on the actual day of delivery, like, I had family and everything, like, it was more people, so I'm, like, what? And my doula could've been here. But I think that that was by design, you know—because my doula was going to follow my birth plan, you know, to the T—and make sure that all of these things—and they know that, you know. They know that when you're educated about certain things, you know, they try and lie and manipulate—at least that's my experience—is that I felt very manipulated out of what my desires were, in order, you know—so, like she said, they—they're—Tiara, like you mentioned—the—interest that the hospital staff have is for the hospital.

Once again, the hospital system and team demonstrated their own disdain for and intimidation by a free-thinking, liberated, and well-informed Black mother who desires a doula to be present as a prevention and mitigation strategy against hospital acts of violating her autonomy. Consequently, birthing hospitals exert reproductive control over the reproducing Black body through coerced or forced medical interventions such as labor inductions, cesarean births, or postpartum family planning. Medical coercion, as defined by, for, and with thirty-six Black mothers, means feeling pressured to have a cesarean birth for medically unnecessary reasons as a barrier to optimal and autonomous birthing experiences. Like the focus group dialogue about birth as a battlefield in Los Angeles, one Black mother's oral narrative of medical coercion to endure a cesarean birth sparked a series of admissions by multiple Black mothers in Oakland.

> *Tasha:* I feel like I was made to have a C-section, too. Like, you know how they do emergency C-sections. I was all like it wasn't that much of an emergency to rush it through. And he [the obstetrician] was so you know how you don't feel like the—you're looking at the doctor and you can tell by the vibe like it's not a—it didn't seem like it was really an emergency. But it was like more so against the clock—let's just go and do the C-section. And that's how I felt. They was saying that the umbilical cord was wrapped around him. But when he came out he was perfectly fine, you know what I mean? And I don't know if a fever had anything to do with it. I have like a 103 fever. So, I don't know if that was cause for emergency C-section. But they weren't telling me whether or not it was.
>
> *Dominique:* Yeah, I have one. I felt like when I was giving birth, they were trying to pressure me into having a C-section, too. And I knew I wouldn't [make it] because they said my baby's heart rate was dropping. But I think they were just saying that because it's easier for them to give you a C-section than to go through all like you screaming in pain and stuff and everything. Like I felt like it was just easier for them so they would want to pressure you to doing it. And plus, they get like extra money they have to use essentially.
>
> *LaToya:* I think it was like that too. Because it was like so oh, yeah, we're just going to give you a C-section. And was no—like and when he did it, it was like quick. Like you can't really—you're in pain and you can't really talk to them. They're just rushing you on over there I was like—and me, my family members wasn't like speaking up for me. They would have basically made me get a C-section when I really didn't need it.
>
> *Dr. Scott:* So, ultimately, you did end up having to have one [a cesarean birth]?
>
> *Imani:* Yeah. Uh-huh.

The Oakland focus group dialogue about navigating a coerced or forced cesarean birth revealed commonalities across the different individual patient experiences and hospital systems, cultures, leadership, and workforce. Black mothers felt unsafe due to a lack of belief or trust in the obstetrician performing the cesarean birth or the obstetrician's reason for the cesarean birth. Given the repeated pattern of Black mothers' individual and collective inability to accurately or precisely name the maternal, fetal, or placental indication for the cesarean birth, the practice of coerced or forced cesarean births among Black mothers raised great concern for a deliberate, calculated, organized, and incentivized attack on Black women's autonomy, agency, and self-efficacy during communication, consent, and decision-making.

If one were to obtain and review a copy of the medical records, including the pre-operative, operative, and post-operative documentation, would the medical record reviewer find a medical indication that fulfills the standards of obstetric care and matches the clinician *and* patient account of events? The obstetricians and hospitals would like to defend their behaviors and motivations as being safe for the mother and baby. Yet, Black mothers felt unsafe as the decision to perform a medical intervention occurred within the circumstances and conditions of the Black mothers feeling vulnerable and in pain, stripped of their autonomy and humanity. Moreover, given the power relations, dynamics, and differentials, the Black mothers were unfortunately in a position of least influence in decision-making. Based on Black mothers' understanding and interpretation of the behaviors of the hospital system, team, and individual clinicians and staff, the lack of comfort, clarity, and confidence during care supports the analogy of birthing in hospitals as both a war zone and a horror film. Application of Davis' analytic and phenomenon, obstetric racism, onto the lived experiences of the Oakland Black mothers aligns with at least three of six previously explained dimensions: coercion, medical abuse and neglect, dismissiveness, and disrespect (Davis 2018; Davis 2019; Davis 2020).

In reflecting on the opening chapter narrative, the weaponization of fear by hospital systems, teams, and individual clinicians and staff to coerce or force any medical procedures, particularly cesarean births need to be criminalized at the federal and state level. Throughout Kendra's pregnancy, fear overwhelmed her being and body. Based on technology to predict an estimated fetal weight from images and measurements of specific fetal body parts through the use of obstetric ultrasound, Kendra's prenatal birth team repeatedly warned her of the threat of forming and then birthing a three-pound baby. And as a result, the anticipated smaller-than-expected birth weight, her prenatal team insisted on scheduling a cesarean birth, due to the baby being "*too small to come through the birth canal.*" The implications of constantly navigating coerced or forced care or interventions place Black mothers in a perpetual state of stress and stressful responses such as "fight, flight, freeze or fawn." Violations of psychological patient safety may hinder optimal patient participation in effective and efficient communication, comprehension, consent, and decision-making. Based on the lived experiences of Black mothers, one must interrogate the association between violations of patient psychological safety and the integrity of autonomy, agency, and self-efficacy in consent. In the battle over birth, hospital systems, teams, and individual clinicians and staff maintain control and governance by curating a culture of fear, intimidation, and psychological torture during childbirth hospitalization. By the way, Kendra birthed her baby into the world through her vaginal birth canal. Her baby weighed five pounds and six ounces.

Returning to the Black mother in Los Angeles, Mariah, with two prior healthy pregnancies ending in two prior successful vaginal births, and with a third pregnancy creating two babies, she provided additional details about her experience.

> Their [birthing hospital in Los Angeles] fear tactics was ridiculous. So finally got up to the 39th week and was still, you know, really pushing for—for that [a cesarean birth for a twin pregnancy, no other complications. And it just—it was—it was wow. Amazing, but—I—I got what we desired, but it—I mean, it was a long four-day battle in [birthing hospital in LA] with—I—I spoke to maybe six different doctors, finally had the specialist come in and said we want a vaginal birth after everything I had been through, because if I would have got the C-section, I would have hemorrhaged—long story because of how long I had been in [labor] on the Pitocin. So anyway, the specialist came in, everyone was mad at him, and finally we had the vaginal birth.

Despite repeated psychological pressure and assaults on her bodily and decisional autonomy, Mariah persisted and enjoyed her intended vaginal birth of twin babies. One of the primary drivers in actualizing her autonomy was the presence and participation of a high-risk OB specialist. The recommendation of the specialist aligned with Mariah's birth intention and priority, and provided additional insights that revealed the risks of cesarean birth outweighed the benefits of cesarean birth. Therefore, Mariah experienced a twin vaginal birth. In this instance, the dual opposition of an assertive Black mother and a high-risk OB specialist to a cesarean birth represents a response to obstetric racism as defined by Davis, resistance (Davis, Varner, and Dill 2021; Davis 2022a; Davis 2022b). Mariah uses her experiential knowledge while the high-risk OB physician specialist uses their formal professional knowledge to push back against the primary team's recommendation to pursue a cesarean birth. Resistance serves as an act of mobilization against the system and involves interrogating the terms of intervention and negotiating various forms of involvement in decision-making. Both the Black mother and the high-risk OB physician specialist shared a mutual vision of how the Black mother wanted to be cared for, based on the Black mother's birth plan. Black mothers and their given and chosen kin deserve more obstetricians, high-risk OB physician specialists, and other physicians to respond to obstetric racism in solidarity with Black mothers with acts of resistance.

In chapter 2, Kiara, a Black mother in the Oakland focus group, initially shared her experience of showing up to L&D triage with her mother, who was also a doula, and navigating dismissive and delayed care. She presented with regular painful contractions with her baby in a breech position, and the nurses chose not to trust and believe yet another Black woman about her own bodily experiences. She remembered arriving at triage at 4:00 p.m. and being checked one or two hours later, with a dilated cervix at 3.5 centimeters and 100 percent effaced, or a paper-thin cervix. She noted giving birth by cesarean at 9:50 p.m. However, her mother, a doula, felt her grandchild was not in the breech position when Kiara presented to the hospital in active labor. Kiara also never mentioned any hospital attending physician, resident physician, or radiology technician performing an informal or formal ultrasound to confirm fetal presentation or location of her placenta before the cesarean birth. Between 4:00 p.m. and 9:50 p.m., the hospital team had ample time to locate the nearest ultrasound on the unit and determine whether a cesarean birth, a major abdominal surgery with risks, remained a necessary clinical option.

> Another thing—so, I, unfortunately had to have C-section. My son was breech, so he was butt down. But my mom doesn't feel like he was breech at the time I went into labor. So I—I went in for an ultrasound to see if he was still breech. So they had me—and they—it turns out I was actually in early labor, and I didn't know it. So because I had already went into labor, they said he was still breech, so they had to schedule the C-section. I was really pushing—I wanted to give him that time to flip, because I've heard stories of him—you know, the babies flipping literally at the last week. I gave birth to him at 39 weeks, and it—during the C-section—so I had my mom in the room with me, my—his father, unfortunately, is incarcerated at the moment. So my mom was in the room with me, and they wouldn't allow her to look over the thing [surgical drape]. And usually, I've heard—you know, like some people have the clear curtain (with a window for the patient and support person to view the surgery at time of birth) where you can actually watch. Yeah. So they didn't offer that. They said they couldn't—they don't—they don't have the clear one, and you're not allowed to look over. Which was strange for me, because I'm, like—there are people who literally watch the whole—like, I didn't—I didn't understand why I couldn't watch, or see, or anything, and they wouldn't allow her to look. She really believes that he wasn't breech, and she strongly—like, she feels strongly about that. And then—and I – they [the obstetrician surgeon and surgical assistant] literally argued, like, in front of me while I'm open, paralyzed—I'm—I'm panicking. I can't see anything, and they wouldn't—they wouldn't let her look over until he was out. Once he was out, they let her stand up and she could see.

Multiple factors coalesce in a manner that support the hospital possibly conspiring to hide the fetal presentation from the Black mother and maternal grandmother of the baby. The decision to deny the Black mother or maternal grandmother the opportunity to view the birth of the baby raises suspicions of duplicitous intentions, language, and behaviors by the hospital system. The decision to restrict the maternal grandmother from watching the actual mechanisms for facilitating an abdominal birth, combined with the denial of a surgical drape with a clear anesthesia screen or a clear window, facilitating the observation of the abdominal birth and immediate skin-to-skin contact, increases the concern for system-level deceit and violation of patient autonomy. The argument between the obstetrician surgeon and surgical assistant also increases the Black mother and maternal grandmother's concerns about performing a coerced or forced cesarean birth without any proof of a valid maternal, fetal, or placenta reason.

The presence or participation of learners in nursing, midwifery, or medicine must be included in the continuous process of informed consent, which is upheld by the ethical and legal principles and practices of autonomy. Black mothers shared experiences in which the hospital system prioritized teaching, training, and supervising learners over actualizing patient autonomy and providing patient and family-focused care. Simone, a Black mother in Oakland, questioned the process and rationale for multiple people, unknown to her, standing idly or walking aimlessly during her cesarean birth,

> Since we all had a C-section, I want to add to that. Because they had like three or five people just standing there. It's like a study, or something. They have all those new people [staff, nurses, physicians, trainers, and learners] and you can only bring like in one person. So, why are they standing there? It was a lot of people just standing and walking around.

The structure, procedures, practices, and processes of undergraduate (medical students), graduate (medical and surgical resident physicians), and post-graduate medical education (medical, surgical, and research physician fellows) require exerting control and governance over the reproducing body. At times, medical education feels like experimentation and exploitation to Black mothers and their given and chosen kin (Washington 2006; McClurg et al. 2022; Lin et al. 2023).

In consideration of Black mothers' feelings and the ethical and legal principles and practices of actualizing patient autonomy, hospital systems that also serve as medical training institutions need to practice continuous consent or refusal for learners to participate in care provision, communication, consent, and decision-making. Jada, a Black in the Oakland focus group, shared how she consented to the presence of learners in her care as observers only. She declined allowing learners to practice on her, "I felt it was fine to let somebody who's training come in. I just didn't want them to do the work. They can [shadow]—or they can just look over the person's shoulder. So, they said they were fine with that." Denying Black mothers the right to refuse care provision by a learner, even in the presence of a supervising physician attending, is considered coerced or forced care. A few Black mothers in the Los Angeles focus group, like Patrice, expressed regret for not speaking up and out about their lack of interest or desire in having learners present or involved in their care.

> And I have a seven-month-old now. And for the second time around, I wanted to give myself an excellent way to speak up more about this delivery, because with my—with my son, I felt like I didn't—I didn't—there were things that were happening during my labor that shouldn't have, like, there were students in—in my room when I was pushing. And I was just, like, why are they here? Oh, they—this is a practicing [teaching] hospital—I didn't know about that. You know, so with --I didn't—I wasn't aware of that in the beginning. I would just—it was—it was all—can—you can imagine, I was embarrassed, I was in pain, you know, it was just weird.

Many times, Black mothers felt the hospital system took additional steps to create and take up space in the birthing spaces for learners at the exclusion or erasure of the partners, parents, or loved ones of the Black mother. In the Oakland focus group, Jada expressed experiencing a flood of anxiety-driven emotions and thoughts upon entering the operating and seeing multiple people in the room except the one person she trusted, loved, and valued and loved her in return.

> I had a bad experience though in the operating room. Because when I walked in, I felt like, you know, they had students—probably like eight people in the room. And they asked my husband to wait outside. I'm like I need to have him. And they were all like—first, you know before they laid me down, I'm like I need to have him in the room right now. Because it's all like white and I don't see anything that I'm familiar with and she was in there at that time. So, I was like have him in here. They were like oh, you have to wait a little. I had to scream and start crying like I need to have my husband right here like right now. So, he came in a little earlier.

To Jada, the hospital system provided preferential treatment to the students as opposed to making sure she and her husband felt comfortable and confident in the manner in which the hospital system, team, and individual clinicians and staff treated and cared for them. After the cesarean birth, once Jada and her husband were transferred to her postpartum room, her husband removed his shirt to prepare to participate in skin-to-skin bonding with his newborn baby. In chapter 2, the reader first engages with Jada's narrative by learning about the nurse dismissing the value and benefit of skin-to-skin daddy-baby bonding, disrupting the physical connection between a Black father and his newborn, and removing the Black baby from the arms and chest of the Black father.

Based on the lived experiences of Black mothers, childbirth hospitalization in the U.S. serves to impose surveillance, control, and governance over the Black reproducing body, baby, and kinship ties. The pathologization and racialization of the Black reproducing body, pregnancy, and birth facilitate the translation of human beings and human experiences into numbers that correspond to diagnoses, procedures, and levels of care. The numbers then correlate to risk stratification and resource utilization to justify reimbursement and referrals. The most optimal method to constrain and deny Black mothers' autonomy, agency, and self-efficacy is the imposition of perpetual psychological terror.

Chapter 5

Communication and Information Exchange

He told me—well, I broke down crying. He watched me deal with my crying, so—because I was like I don't want to be pregnant no more and I was just crying. He let a nurse come in and explain to me that you have a higher risk of a C-section if we induce you, we would like for your body to do it on its own so that's what we're going to do. And so, I was doing stress tests and they found out he [the male fetus] didn't have any more liquid [referring to low amniotic fluid in the pregnancy or amionitic sac that holds the fetus]. Like I had a stress test on a Friday, and then that Monday I didn't have any fluid. They were like were you leaking. I'm like I can't tell the difference between regular—you got pregnancy discharge and, you know—but they explained it to me to not get an induction and I appreciated that once I learned more about it. I still ended up being induced because he ran out fluid and wasn't coming. I had a reason. And so, I was really glad that he [the Obstetrician] didn't just go for the money and be like, oh, she's tired of being pregnant, you know, get the baby out and we can get more money, as opposed to this time being told to be induced. But for the health of me and my baby, I felt like I was given enough information. You know, I learned about preeclampsia. I was scared of preeclampsia and for the fact that my blood pressure hit so high the day I got out the hospital. I was [in] ER for two days after I had him because my blood pressure was extremely high. And so, I was thankful that they made that decision and took him out on the 5th as opposed to the 12th. But I also feel like it depends on the moms who ask and educate herself, not just let—you can't let them tell you anything and why—and they try to tell moms, and don't let them tell you anything. If they want an induction, ask why. If they want to do a C-section, ask why.

The opening Black birth narrative about Maya describes the expressions, expectations, and experience of communication and information exchange, the third patient and community-identified quality domain in the SACKRED Birth framework. Four dominant perspectives of communication and information exchange emerged from exploring meanings and measurements of quality as described by thirty-six Black mothers in Oakland and Los Angeles, California, in 2019: (1) seeking help, information, or health care from the hospital/health system; (2) informed consent and informed refusal; (3) need to dispel myths and misconceptions about the possibility of a vaginal birth after cesarean birth (VBAC); and (4) communication, information, and education (absence/presence).

During the Oakland focus groups, Maya recalled the experiences of seeking help, information, or health care information from a certified birth professional within the hospital or health system. When seeking health care information, support, or service from a hospital or health system, Black mothers and birthing people desire and deserve scientifically and culturally robust, rigorous, relevant, and responsive information about different options, opportunities, optics, and experiences during hospital-based births, including but not limited to pain relief, mobility, pushing/birthing positions, support persons, lactation and infant feeding, birth attendants, birth types/methods, and birthing facilities/locations. In the opening Black narrative, Maya expressed relief and delight that the physician avoided moving immediately to a riskier, more invasive and expensive birth process (induction of labor) and modality (cesarean birth, which is a possible consequence of labor inductions). Throughout this Black feminist hermeneutic phenomenology of Black mothers' expectations, expressions, and experiences of communication and information exchange, Black mothers set forth seven demands to protect and uphold their right to communication, consent, and decision-making. Black mothers desire and deserve the right to: (1) Black mother-parent focused language and information that affirm partner, given and chosen family, and community relationships; (2) recognition of power structures and differentials that maintain, reproduce, or disrupt the hierarchy of knowledge evaluators, incubators, accelerators, and disseminators in the medical-industrial complex during communication, counseling, and consent; (3) assertive patient and family inquiry and communication without anticipation of or actual hospital discomfort and retaliation; (4) feeling heard, seen, listened to, believed, believed in, and comforted; (5) inclusive, diverse options, opportunities, resources, and optimal conditions that acknowledge, affirm, activate, and amplify the power, promise, potential, and passion of Black mothers, birthing people (now described as pregnant and postpartum Black gender-expansive individuals), and Black chosen and given kin throughout childbirth hospitalization for vaginal and abdominal births (e.g., cesarean surgical birth); (6)

optimal and equitable communication, information, and education on linkages to services and resources within hospitals and in community settings; and (7) more time, truth-telling, trust, and transparency in communication, consent, and decision-making.

In this chapter, we will examine and explore communication and information exchange, one of seven patient-identified care domains for defining quality of care during childbirth hospitalization. Thirty-six Black mothers define the communication and information domain as verbal and nonverbal gestures (e.g., language and behavior), interactions, and cues utilized for explaining, understanding, and exchanging scientifically and culturally robust, rigorous, relevant, and responsive information. The actors involved in the communication and information exchange include maternity hospitals, maternity health systems and structures, individuals and teams of perinatal health administrators, clinician administrators, clinicians, and support staff. Black mothers desire communication and information exchange to focus on diverse, inclusive, Black woman-person focused, family-affirming, and community-centered expectations, experiences, options, and opportunities that impact hospital-based births (i.e., different options and expectations for birthing, pain relief, mobility, pushing/birthing positions, support persons, lactating/infant feeding, birth attendants, birth types/methods, and birthing facilities/locations).

Across many sectors in society, from the ivory tower to professional sports, Black women encounter varying degrees of disrespect, dismissiveness, mistreatment, neglect, and abuse during verbal and nonverbal communications (Bailey 2016; Bailey and Trudy 2018; Bailey 2021; Davis 2018; Sue and Spanierman 2020). In health systems, sexism, racism, misogynoir, and other forms of domination, degradation, and control structure the quality, function, context, and impact of social and clinical interactions between patients and hospital clinicians, staff, and administrators (Cooper et al. 2003; Koerber et al. 2004). A study published in 2004 examined audiotape and questionnaire data collected in 1998 and 2002 and found that the quality of medical-visit communication differed among African American versus White patients (Johnson et al. 2004). The study sample consisted of 458 Black and white patients who visited sixty-one physicians in the Baltimore, Maryland–Washington, DC–Northern Virginia metropolitan area. The researchers measured three outcomes: communication process, patient-centeredness, and emotional tone (affect) of the medical visit. Study findings revealed that physicians were 23 percent more verbally dominant and engaged in 33 percent less patient-centered communication with Black patients than with white patients. The results also demonstrated that both Black patients and their physicians exhibited lower levels of positive affect than white patients and their physicians did (Johnson et al. 2004).

Nearly two decades later, researchers decided to seek evidence to support reported experiences of Black individuals and women, as two different groups navigating structural marginalization and minoritization, feeling dismissed or doubted by the health care workforce (Beach et al. 2021). The researchers set out to identify the types of linguistic ("language-producing") systems of communication used by physicians to show that they doubt or disbelieve patient narratives of their lived experiences (committing acts of testimonial injustice) and then explore racialized and gendered differences in the use of such linguistic mechanisms. The three primary measures included utilization of three linguistic features that suggested disbelief based on content analysis of 600 clinic notes for patients seen in an academic ambulatory internal medicine practice in 2017: quotes (e.g., has a "reaction to the medication"); specific "judgment words" that suggest doubt (e.g. "claims" or "insists"); and evidentials, sentences made by physicians to label patients' symptoms or experiences as hearsay versus truth. The researchers used natural language processing to evaluate the prevalence of each linguistic feature in the remaining notes and assessed differences in the prevalence of each linguistic feature by race or gender. To account for clustering of notes within patients and providers, the researchers applied mixed-effects regression analysis. Study findings from 9,251 notes written by 165 physicians about 3,374 unique patients showed that 74 percent of patients identified as Black individuals and 58 percent identified as female. In the practice of documentation and dissemination of health care information in the health records, physicians were more likely to write clinical notes about Black patients using at least one quote, at least one judgment, and more evidentials, compared to their written communication about white patients. Study findings demonstrated no difference in notes based on patient sex (female vs. male) for the use of judgment words or evidentials. Physicians were more likely to use at least one quote to show they doubt female patients. The researchers concluded that physicians are more likely to subject Black patients to systematic bias in physicians' perceptions of Black patient credibility, a practice identified by the researchers as testimonial injustice (Beach et al. 2021). Therefore, any health care professional holds the power and potential to weaponize communication and information in the documentation and dissemination of health care information in patient handoffs, patient sign-outs, and paper or electronic health records.

Engaging and then entering the medical-industrial complex places structurally and historically marginalized and minoritized communities at greater risk for violations of patient safety based on differential and dynamic levels of power and varying power relations that shape and bestow certain types of privilege and positionality on a select few structurally protected classes or groups. The power differentials and dynamics within the medical-industrial complex determine the onset, frequency, timing, duration, intensity, and content of communication and information exchange in a manner that reinforces a hierarchy of human value and knowledge based on skin color, genitalia, and attainment of medical training (Cooper et al. 2003; Johnson et al. 2004; Korber et al. 2004; Penner et al. 2010; Beach et al. 2021). The hierarchy of human value and knowledge establishes medical normativity, which is a concept based on four assumptions: (1) medical knowledge, training, and certification are the preferred or normal modes of knowing and understanding health and disease in humans; (2) the patient-physician binary is the standard model of healthcare service provision and utilization; (3) healthcare relationships are best established between patients and physicians wherein the medical-industrial complex asserts and then elevates medical knowledge as superior to cultural, spiritual, and experiential knowledge (Jolivétte 2015); and (4) knowledge acquisition and application follow a hidden algorithm that asserts and reinforces race as a biological construct that defines norms and narratives for healthcare-seeking behaviors, outcomes, and experiences.

The consequences of medical normativity include the development and sustainability of a healthcare hierarchy and economy that facilitates the exclusion, erosion, and erasure of other forms of healthcare relationships and service models beyond medicine, such as midwifery, nursing, doula support, mental health, lactation support, and spiritual advisors. Second, medical normativity justifies the reproduction of biological determinism, which then establishes white people, particularly white cis-gender heterosexual women, as the default and desired patient in sexual, reproductive, and perinatal service provision and training. Third, medical normativity facilitates control and domination of Black women, girls, and gender-expansive people within the patient-physician binary model of care, and willfully adopts and expands upon racist, sexist, and classist archetypes of Black women, girls, and gender-expansive people that originated from slavery. Thus, medical normativity standardizes medical language and behavior that reinforce its four assumptions and sustain differential power relations and dynamics between physicians and patients. In the provision of medical care during childbirth hospitalization, Black women, girls, and gender-expansive people report repeated episodes and experiences of medical mistreatment, neglect, dismissiveness, delays, and denials (Chambers et al. 2018; Davis 2018; Davis 2019; Attanasio and Hardeman 2019; Scott, Britton, and McLemore 2019; Vedam et al. 2019; Davis 2020; Chambers et al. 2020; Chambers et al. 2021; Davis, Varner, and Dill 2021; Scott and Davis 2021; Davis 2022a; Davis 2022b).

The greatest deception created by the medical-industrial complex is convincing the public that medicine, specifically, science, and therefore, science communication is evidence-based, driven, and objective, free of bigotry and bias (Bueter 2022). Additionally, medical normativity assumes a bi-directional flow of information that labels the information obtained from patients as subjective while information obtained from the physician as objective (Larimore and Jordan 1995; Cameron and Turtle-Song 2002). The organization of medical information and its subsequent packaging and dissemination of medical information in oral (patient handoffs and patient sign-outs) and written communication (electronic health records) follows standard format divided into four sections, collectively called the SOAP note: (1) subjective (information about the patient's history elicited by the physician, physician in training, or medical student from the patient); (2) objective (additional information collected about the patient's existing or new medical conditions using a physical exam and technology such as lab tests, imaging studies, monitors, and extraction of samples of saliva, blood, urine, tissues, stool, including amniotic fluid using invasive or non-invasive tests); (3) assessment (physician-centered list of potential causes of the medical condition, sometimes prioritized by most likely to least likely primary causes or contributors to medical symptoms, discomfort, or disease); and (4) plan (physician-centered prioritization of a sequence of steps or events to gather more information to narrow the list of potential causes (differential diagnosis), to offer options to ameliorate any pain or other forms of discomfort, or to lessen the progression of discomfort or disease) (Larimore and Jordan 1995; Cameron and Turtle-Song 2002).

The quality, timing, and sequence of supportive steps described by physicians in the plan are usually dependent on several multi-level independent and intersectional factors, usually organized into five dimensions of institutional capacity accessibility (approachability; acceptability; availability and accommodation; affordability; and appropriateness) and five corresponding patient abilities to access care services and support (1) ability to perceive; (2) ability to seek; (3) ability to reach; (4) ability to pay; and (5) ability to engage) (Levesque, Harris, and Russell 2013). Many times, physicians and patients are unaware of how robust, rigorous, relevant, and/or restrictive the plan of care can be since physicians and patients collectively lack control over options available to them from their institutions and insurance plan. Until grave illness combined with structural and systemic incompetencies impact physicians and hospital administrators, they usually lack nuanced insights into the power relations and dynamics of navigating health care communication during counseling and decision-making.

Throughout pregnancy, labor, childbirth, postpartum, and beyond, Black mothers actively search for answers to questions about their growing bodies, babies, and placentas from multiple informal and formal sources. Black mothers constantly solicit and elicit advice about how to adjust to their growing bodies, babies, and placentas from family, community, and maternal-fetal medicine ("high-risk OB") specialists or other licensed birth professionals such as OBGYN physicians, nurse midwives, or nurses. In the quest for knowledge and understanding of the physiological changes of pregnancy, childbirth, and postpartum, including the possible and subsequent onset of new and/or the exacerbation of existing medical, social, or behavioral conditions and diagnoses, Black mothers desire and deserve to trust the physicians and nurses assigned to care for them and the integrity of the information given to them. Black mothers desire and deserve a perinatal workforce that possesses both interest and capacity to offer information customized to their patient preferences and priorities. Black mothers desire and deserve health care services and health care information that extend beyond textbook pregnancy age (e.g., first trimester) or pathology (e.g., hypertension) specific anticipatory guidance. Black mothers desire and deserve the art and science of medicine and nursing that better aligns with and activates person-focused, humanistic perinatal health care.

Black mothers repeatedly expressed their expectations for physicians and nurses to actively facilitate and participate in a culture of explaining, understanding, and exchanging information in the most optimal and equitable manner for themselves and their given and chosen kin. Earlier in chapter 2, during one of the Oakland focus group discussions, Ayana demonstrated an act of vulnerability by sharing her desire for hospital nurses to provide care with more understanding and to form genuine human attachments with Black mothers. In chapter 3, Ayana reflected upon the actions of a nurse who returned to visit her on her day off and how the nurse's generosity of care and compassion caused her to feel valued, connected, and safe. In considering her expectations and experiences of communication and information, Ayana explained the impact of guidance from her health informed her planning and preparation for childbirth in a hospital setting,

> Then I got some advice from them and also from the doctor that was visiting, and a midwife. There was a lady that she was there every three months, six months, and nine months, and then she would go in and she would give you advice [on] what you need, even in the hospital and what—what do you have to take. She was giving me a list and then I—so I had a plan for what I need[ed] before I bought everything.

While Black mothers also shared their expectations for hospitals and health systems to provide scientifically and culturally robust, rigorous, relevant, and responsive information about different expectations, options, and experiences during hospital-based births (e.g., different birthing attendants, positions, methods, spaces, facilities, and locations), Black mothers asserted their need for their care team to acknowledge, activate, and amplify their autonomy, specifically their bodily autonomy, lived experience, and intuition as the mother preparing for their childbirth. Kiara, one of the Black mothers in the Oakland focus group, previously shared in chapter 2 how the L&D triage nurse dismissed her pain when she showed up in active labor, with prior ultrasound findings of her baby in breech presentation. In chapter 4, Kiara recalled how the hospital never confirmed her baby's position and presentation with an ultrasound prior to the nighttime cesarean birth and prevented her and her mother, a doula, from observing the birth of her baby by denying access to peek over the sterile surgical drape or using the customized surgical drape made with a clear window to view the birth while maintaining the sterile field. As a first-time Black mother whose own mother was a Black woman and doula, Kiara offered meaningful insights about navigating the tensions between seeking help or health information and having the space to think freely and make decisions on one's own. She explained how she managed to receive an abundance of information from multiple sources while also making space to clearly hear her own voice and make her own decisions.

> I think for me I had too much information given. I guess because I felt like it was good and then it was just too many—too much. It was overwhelming. It was just—I felt like everyone had their own opinions. And I'm the type of person where, okay, well, it happened for you but let me see what happens once I finally have her. So, I feel I guess a lot of information was given, even from doctors, but sometimes I feel like doctors don't have the last say so either in hospitals, so they even—Don't have the last say so. So, I felt like it was more so like trusting myself and my own instinct as a mother. I was—being a first-time mom, I was just given too much, you should do this, you should do that, this and that, that and the other, the doctors—it was too much and I was like, you know what, let me just do this. And I want to be able to have that experience as a first-time mom and I don't want it to be taken away and I did that. And it was the best decision I could have ever made by not taking so much information in at once. I took some things, but some things it was just—it was just too much.

Black mothers also demonstrated a knowing of the power differential, dynamics, and relations that influence the role of the physician as the harborer and disseminator of medical information and the role of patients as the recipients of medical information. Yet, in their knowing as consumers of physician-centric medical information, Black mothers continuously expressed their desire and need to feel heard, seen, listened to, believed, believed in, and comforted during communication and information exchange.

At the same time, Black mothers also conveyed a yearning for equitable communication and information exchanges that first recognize and then disrupt power structures and differentials in the medical-industrial complex that maintain a hierarchy of knowledge incubators, accelerators, and disseminators. Without hesitation, Black mothers demanded the right to reclaim their bodily autonomy, lived experience, and intuition as mothers during decision-making. In fact, Black mothers demanded the right to seek and synthesize information in their own way and on their own time. Black mothers eloquently described their own internal information filtration system where they choose the onset, timing, frequency, magnitude, and duration of information to accept, absorb, analyze, arrange, adopt, or abandon. In doing so, Black mothers solidified the role of physicians as facilitators, and not as owners, governors, or managers of health care communication, information, consent, and decision-making. More importantly, Black mothers firmly established their right and role to actively participate in health care as autonomous agents. Rhonda was one of the Black mothers in the Oakland focus group who offered critical feedback on the attributes of nurses that make them safe(r) to care for Black mothers. In the narrative below, one can better appreciate her perceptions and perspectives about the different roles, responsibilities, and impacts of nurses during childbirth hospitalization.

> For me because I was in the hospital for like literally ten days, so I kind of got a feel like for the nurses that were there. And like I said me and my daughter's dad is like on the rocks a little bit, like we was always arguing but not really kind of. And then like I said I had ended up getting to know like a lot of the nurses because I was in the labor and delivery, and then like I said the doctors came in and was like okay, we're going to just deliver you at 37 weeks. And then—so some of the nurses that was there, they just kept giving me all this information and it worked out fine because one of my nurses was one of my friends from elementary school, so—and she was pregnant as well too. So, like she got to help me a lot and then I got to help her too to get ready for her son and it was cool. Like I didn't get as much breastfeeding information as I'd like to. I didn't even think I was going to breastfeed for this long so I'm really proud of myself. And even though it's been a struggle, but I'm still going strong. And like I said, it was—it was stressful, but like I said I got to know a lot of the nurses and then it was cool, too, because like when some of them went home for their two days off and then they come back, is (inaudible) still here, and then they give you more information. And then sometimes they give me diapers or they'll give me like extra chugs or whatever the case may be, so when I go home and I like didn't have a bathtub because I got kind of cool with them and I, you know, let them know I didn't have a lot of stuff yet because I didn't prepare for her to come that early, they just started giving me like, you know, extra stuff so that like when I did get home like I have like a whole bag full of like Enfamil or whatever, like the little small little tubes, or whatever. I haven't used them but she gave me a big supply to go home with just in case my breastfeeding didn't work out. So, I got a lot of information being able to stay there. And they all told me like, you know, if you want to get the epidural, you know, it's good and—it wasn't more—like they—to me my nurses showed me a lot of love compared to what I thought it was going to be, so I'm excited about that.

One positive unintended consequence of the disproportionate obstetric practices of clinician-initiated labor, when the physician or nurse midwife recommends mechanical or medication "induced" cervical ripening or labor contractions to facilitate non-spontaneous childbirth due to maternal, fetal, and/or placental reasons, is the extended time spent with the hospital clinicians and staff, sometimes over a long period of time. Despite changes in the composition of the hospital care team within and across different shifts during the weekday and weekend, increased time with familiar faces can curate both a professional and personal type of bond and attachment, grounded in trust, truth, and transparency. Black mothers named the four Ts—time, trust, transparency, and truth—as the core criteria for fostering an optimal communication and information exchange between Black mothers and individual clinicians and staff, hospital teams, and the hospital system as a whole. In contrast to the possible fractured personal relationships in the Black mothers' lives, hospitals possess a tremendous responsibility, privilege, and opportunity to be a haven, a soft place to land, particularly throughout pregnancy, labor, childbirth, postpartum, and parenting. In the above narrative, Rhonda shared the details of her hospitalization for an unexpected timing in her pregnancy and the duration of time during which she experienced safety and social kinship with the nurses. For her, the labor and delivery nurses offered greater insight into the processes and procedures of her medical care. Nurses provided comfort care that included information and education on linkages to services and resources within the hospital, prior to hospital discharge. When Rhonda recognized one of her assigned nurses as one of her elementary school friends, who also happened to be pregnant, one could feel and hear the joy and relief in her voice and the wave of peace flowing across her body as she recalled the added value and impact of establishing and expanding social ties or kinship bonds across power differentials between the patient and hospital team.

Labor and delivery nurses, particularly Black nurses, carefully navigate a fine line between two different worlds, the personal and professional, and the politics within and between each world. The capacity and willingness of the hospital nurses, in general, and in the case of Rhonda, to choose to participate in building community and parental capacity by fulfilling many unmet material needs (e.g., bathtub, bottles) of a Black mother demonstrates the vital role of nurses in building new and strengthening existing trusting relationships between community members and hospital systems (Dalton et al. 2020). For many mothers, particularly Black mothers in our society with inaccessible, inadequate, or absent social networks and capital, an unplanned physician-initiated hospitalization for labor induction may result in disrupted and/or terminated preparation and planning for parenting. Thus, the hospital acts of generosity led by the hospital nurses demonstrated the nurses' capacity and willingness to curate a spirit and praxis of belonging, acceptance, and collective responsibility for and with a Black mother during a period of uncertainty and stress.

More importantly, a Black mother as a patient encountered her pregnant peer in the role of her nurse and participated in a form of reciprocity with a kinship bond that transcended hierarchies of knowledge, power, and positionality between a patient and a nurse. Yet racial and cultural concordance combined with their shared experiences of childhood, pregnancy, childbirth, and parenting provided a type of inclusive insight and a growing communication and information exchange between the Black mother and hospital nursing staff based on increased time, trust, truth, and transparency. Optimal information and communication exchange between Black mothers and hospital teams requires appreciation, activation, and amplification of the humanity of Black women as Black mothers, beyond meager attempts at awareness and acknowledgment of Black culture and Black maternal health. If love is an action, then language and behavior, including verbal and nonverbal gestures, interactions, and cues, represent the various musical notes, harmonies, rhythms, and lyrics of a song that facilitates optimal patient and public (i.e., patient's partner, loved one) participation in all aspects of communication, counseling, deliberation, and decision-making. For this Black mother, the soundtrack to her childbirth hospitalization featured the incredible, and often untapped, power, promise, and potential of hospital nurses and activated feelings of belonging, safety, and worthiness. In Rhonda's words, "*to me, my nurses showed me a lot of love compared to what I thought it was going to be, so I'm excited about that,*" communication and information exchange manifest love and serve as the foundation for advancing obstetric quality and patient safety.

Independent of the duration of the hospital triage visit and admission for pregnancy-related care, the ethics of the patient-clinician-hospital triad require a continuous exchange of information and communication that explores and prioritizes patient lived experiences and expectations in communication, consent, and decision-making. The continuous engagement within the triad needs to be a standardized, non-negotiable practice and process of explaining and exchanging information to facilitate patient awareness, comprehension, and voluntariness during informed consent or informed refusal, in the most optimal and equitable manner for Black mothers and their given and chosen kin. For Brianna, who likely experienced one of the most SACRKRED Birth experiences in Oakland from admission to discharge, including an all-Black hospital team led by Black midwives with all Black nurses and support staff, she benefitted from virtual support during her prenatal care that curated the 4Ts: time, trust, truth, and transparency (Birthing Cultural Rigor n.d.).

> It was like the best. And then also [a health insurance plan] sent me a lady—like I never met her because she was in another state. But she would just call as a nurse. And I think she was an old White lady. I can't tell from her voice. But she was just like a grandma basically, that would like call me and ask if I had questions and give me suggestions about morning sickness and offer information that I didn't even know I didn't know. She was like a nurse. And I didn't seek her out either. They called me. And she was like I just I just wanted to know if you wanted me to call you. I was like thanks, yeah, you can call me. And like she—I feel like she would call right on time. Like right when I was this is not it. And then she would call and like tell me like oh, well maybe you can try, you know. She was like an old lady. Sometimes her dogs would be barking in the background. So, I think she was like working from home, but she was a nurse. And so, I could trust that her information was like, you know. And that was it but that was enough. That was a lot.

Black mothers expressed they desired and deserved consist, reliable, comprehensive, accurate, and dependable sources of information and guidance, particularly during the use of telehealth prenatal education and support, nearly three years prior to the genesis of the COVID-19 pandemic. The lack of physical proximity within the same facility or state between a pregnant patient and prenatal health professional could complicate both the dyadic communication and relationship. Instead, Brianna's graphic and detailed depiction of her relationship with her telehealth nurse again proves the value and impact of repeated patterns of language and behavior that convey to the Black mother that she is seen, heard, wanted, listened to, believed, believed in, and comforted throughout the entire telehealth encounter.

First, her health insurance identified and then paired her with a white nurse who sought out mothers to offer telehealth prenatal health education, support, and anticipatory guidance. Second, the white telehealth nurse in another state also continuously practiced informed consent, checking in with Brianna to determine whether she wanted the nurse to call her. Such an action by the telehealth nurse communicated to Brianna that within the hierarchy of knowledge, power, and positionality within telehealth visits via a phone call, the white nurse acknowledged, affirmed, and activated the free will of a liberated Black mother and the power of a Black mother to serve as the main actor in her life, at least during these routine and frequent phone calls. The professional conduct of one white nurse who consistently showed up in a timely, attentive, and responsive manner, throughout the series of telehealth calls, without video, embodied the practical knowledge and skills of cultural humility (Murray-García and Tervalon 2014). The spirit and praxis of these particularly designed phone calls honored and amplified a Black mother's autonomy and agency. More importantly, the telehealth communication and information exchange reflected one singular, specific message to a Black mother "you are worthy." By sharing her prenatal telehealth care journey in a room full of nine other Black mothers, she then elevates their current expectations and future experiences in perinatal telehealth care and perinatal care, in general. Imagine the state and conditions of the perinatal health system between 2017 to 2019 in Oakland and the East Bay, California, for a Black mother to express that getting the right amount of trustworthy information felt overwhelming, "*And so, I could trust that her information was like, you know. And that was it but that was enough. That was a lot.*"

The previously described exemplar of affirming and activating the dignity, autonomy, and agency of Black mothers during prenatal telehealth care perfectly aligns with Black mothers' repeatedly expressed desires and demands for person-focused, equitable communication that recognizes how power structures communication and information exchange. Black mothers in Los Angeles also expected perinatal health professionals to possess and apply critical thinking and practical, yet sophisticated, skills to facilitate patient conversations that recognize and thereby avoid reinforcing power differentials within the medical-industrial complex. Mariah vocalized her relief and gratitude for having anemia with a twin pregnancy, which then marked her as high-risk status by the maternity health system. Without the high-risk designation, she felt she would have never encountered the high-risk OB physician specialist who advocated on her behalf to both refuse and resist the hospital team's pressure to birth abdominally via a cesarean birth.

> My specialist—if I had not been high risk and been anemic and needed the specialist to follow me, then he would not have had a voice in me not trying for the vaginal birth. Which means that I could have been another dead African-American woman from bleeding to death. And that is just really concerning. And traumatizing. And t's just—wow. Unbelievable. Unbelievable.

Black mothers in Oakland, like Yolanda, demanded a higher quality of communication and information exchange that disrupts the longstanding hierarchy of knowledge incubators, evaluators, accelerators, and disseminators in perinatal medicine and nursing. However, repeated evidence from the recollections of Black mothers demonstrated that being assertive in seeking information, demonstrating autonomy and agency, and expecting informed consent or informed refusal without hospital retaliatory actions is a privilege only afforded to white women.

> I think for me it was being defiant or asking so many questions. Because they were pushing me and basically forcing me to have a C-section. And I was so against it. And so Dr. XX, she was like my regular doctor was telling me like you've got to go see the person who will do the C-section. So, I went but when

> I got there, I expressed my self and from then on it was like oh, here she comes and, you know. The lady was really honest. Every time I came in there to see her to ask her questions, she would be like you're always questioning me—and, you know, blah—blah—blah. And I was just like I don't feel comfortable getting a C-section. And I don't—why do I have—so I questioned it. I had like three visits with her and I questioned every visit. And they were telling me like it's unsafe to have a vaginal birth because I have fourth degree tears from my son who is 14 years old. And I'm like that was 14 years ago.

Of the Black mothers who endured a cesarean surgical birth, or abdominal birth, the majority shared experiences of hospital acts of coercion, medical abuse, ceremonies of degradation, and force during the process of informed consent. The presence and participation of an assertive and active Black mother, Black parent, and/or Black family member threatens the fabric and foundation of the medical-industrial complex. A Black mother and Black father dyad or a Black mother birthing alone, who knows their worth and chooses to interrogate medical expertise and decision-making, represented the single most formidable threat to the hierarchy of knowledge, power, and authority in maternal and perinatal care. Maternity hospitals and health systems repeatedly fail to uphold and protect the civil and human right to persistently inquire about the medical necessity, timing, risks, benefits, burdens, and alternatives of medical recommendations and intervention (Scott and Lusero 2023). The obstetric medical-industrial complex, particularly OBGYN physicians, view Black women, individually and collectively, as both infantile and subhuman, one who is by nature unfit to make autonomous decisions with agency, including the decision to bring forth a Black baby into the world through her body and be a mother (Wiegman 1995; Roberts 1997; Roberts 2011; Roberts 2012; Roberts 2017; Goodwin 2017; Weinbaum 2019; Goodwin 2020).

The nature of an OBGYN physician trained in the U.S. is to control and regulate the body and autonomy, or bodily autonomy, of Black women, Black girls, and Black gender-expansive individuals. To be more precise and accurate, the professionalization of contemporary twenty-first- century OBGYNs requires successful completion of an initiation grounded in the "violent appropriation of the (m)other and entanglement with colonialism, slavery, bio- and necropolitics, and patriarchal subjectivity" (Da Silva 2007; Mbembe 2006; Van der Waal et al. 2021, 36). Yolanda's repeated acts of resistance and refusal (Davis 2020; Davis 2022a; Davis 2022b), as so boldly and explicitly stated by the OBGYN physician, "you're always questioning me," represent an affront to the established controlling and dominating nature, culture, and praxis of U.S. obstetrics and gynecological care. An OBGYN demonstrating frustration and annoyance at a Black pregnant woman's intuition and instinct to critically examine and then resist and refuse obstetric motivations and intentions to force a cesarean birth is unethical. Imagine the unnecessary risks, barriers, and burdens that many unapologetic authentically assertive Black women must confront and navigate after being labeled in the electronic health record as "angry, non-compliant, combative, disruptive, abusive," as well as a "danger to self, unborn baby, staff, and others around her" (Bailey 2016; Bailey and Trudy 2018; Bailey 2021).

In chapter 2, Destiny, a Black mother in the Oakland focus group, explained the misogynoir endured by Black women when health care professionals, and any individual, system, or structure in society, weaponize words, messaging, and imaging against Black women who speak up and out about their pain and suffering from various forms of violence. Although Destiny did not share experiences of misogynoir or weaponization of the angry Black woman trope during her childbirth, her decision to contribute to the discussion by sharing the harm of others demonstrated both empathy and humanity in making space for different hospital birth experiences within and across Black birthing communities.

> And so, I think we as Black women get labeled for when we do speak up. When we speak up, they feel like well that attitude and anger or, you know, whatever. And it's also it's like the nurse or whoever could say oh, she had an attitude or she could make this up. And, you know, and it may not be what happened or they can, you know, but they'll make it look like that. Oh, she had an attitude, she was just defiant or, you know, she wouldn't let me do anything. So, even though we speak up it's not going to be taken seriously because we have that stereotype of being like attitude or, you know, angry. That's what I'm looking for, yeah.

Based on the data about linguistic bias and testimonial injustice (Beach et al. 2021), I wondered about the presence, frequency, and types of quotes, specific "judgment words" that suggest doubt, and evidentials (a sentence made by physicians to label patients' symptoms or experiences as hearsay versus truth) in health records of Black women who speak their truth, express their feelings, or voice their dissent. Imagine the back and forth between an unapologetic, authentically assertive, and active autonomous Black pregnant woman and a medically abusive and coercive OBGYN physician, their physician peers, their office or clinic staff, and the hospital administrators, clinicians, and staff. In chapter 4, a Black mother in the Los Angeles focus group, Mariah, recalled her clinical interactions, communications, and debates with multiple physicians who asserted their dominance over her bodily and decisional autonomy. For the purposes of this chapter, I included Mariah's full description of her battle against OB physicians to secure and achieve her fourth vaginal birth.

> She said [the word] battle, and that resonated with me because throughout all of my prenatal visits—I carried twins—and—not that there's anything wrong with a C-section, but my—my two previous births were vaginal, so it just made logical sense for my twins to be a vaginal birth. And I got opposition the minute I opened my mouth about the—the possibility to have a vaginal delivery. Well, if baby A is head down, then we can try for the vaginal, but if baby B is breech, you know, it might be, you know, we might have to do emergency C-section—emergency surgery and it was a lot of fear being pushed by Hospital #1, so—So finally got up to the 39th week and was still, you know, really pushing for—for that. And it just—it was—it was wow. Amazing, but—I—I got what we desired, but it—I mean, it was a long four-day battle in Hospital #1 with—I—I spoke to maybe six different doctors, finally had the specialist come in and said we want a vaginal birth after everything I had been through, because if I would have got the C-section, I would have hemorrhaged—long story because of how long I had been in—on the Pitocin. So anyway, the specialist came in, everyone was mad at him, and finally we had the vaginal birth. Thankfully I had the specialist because I was high-risk. So I was really anemic—I had to get iron infusions, so on and so forth. So he had been following me from day one. But my—my doctor—the babies should have been taken way before the 39th week, so that had a lot of other complications that I'm still healing from as a result. But when every—you know, when every other doctor said, we need to do a C-section, we need to do a C-section, his—his medical professional opinion was, because of your uterus has already been on this Pitocin for 24-hours, your uterus is now overworked. So if we cut your uterus and injure it trying to get these babies out, it could fail—tire out basically, and then you die, because you're hemorrhaging. Grateful for my specialist. So when he went [left] all the other doctors were still like, oh—scare tactics. It was ridiculous—it was crazy.

In Mariah's characterization of her prenatal encounters, one observes how multiple OBGYN physicians refuse to honor her decision to experience a vaginal birth for her twin pregnancy. During multiple communication and information exchanges about the optimal timing and type of delivery method, or birth modality (e.g., vaginal birth or abdominal birth by way of a major abdominal surgery called a cesarean surgery), Mariah shared details about physician behaviors that align with Davis' analytic and phenomenon of obstetric racism. Specifically, the narrative highlighted physician acts of coercion, which Davis defines as the moment during the provision of obstetric care to Black pregnant women and people when medical professionals perform procedures without consent and/or intimidate patients to make decisions (Davis 2018; Davis 2019; Davis 2020). Instead of accepting Mariah's patient right to informed refusal, multiple physicians then engaged in a series of repeated behaviors during each encounter, weaponizing the anticipation of a bad event that had yet to present itself, and exploiting the power of fear and the threat of losing the lives of two babies. According to Mariah's own account of her experience and prenatal health status, the physicians had not identified any maternal, fetal, or placental indication to move toward an emergency cesarean birth at 39 weeks pregnancy age, particularly given the implied optimal presenting fetal parts in the uterus: head-down presentation for both babies.

The cogent narrative offered by Mariah also illuminated the different utilities of communication and information as either a dimension of or a response to hospital acts of obstetric racism. From the perspective and positionality of the OBGYN physicians, they deployed military-style defensive strategies as acts of retaliation to undermine the confidence, authority, and agency of an assertive and vocal Black women patient. OBGYN physicians heavily depended on the collective practice of fearmongering through communication and information exchange as an attempt to reestablish control and dominance, not only over the entire situation and condition, but more importantly, over the bodily autonomy and decision-making power of a strong-willed Black woman.

In the re-reading and revising of this text, particularly this chapter, combined with images Mariah's words conjure in my mind, I was reminded of the practice of slave breaking, the process of violently abusing and beating an enslaved person to shatter their resolve and sense of dignity, humanity, and hope. Senseless and endless brutality to achieve docility, control, and domination. Specifically, my thoughts returned to past readings of how slave owners and plantation owners designed and utilized different strategies to abuse and whip enslaved Black women. If the enslaved Black woman was pregnant, then the slave owner sometimes would force enslaved Black pregnant women to dig a hole in the ground, and then lie face down with the belly (and unborn baby) in the ground. This practice facilitated the beating of enslaved Black pregnant women to establish and maintain fear, control, and domination while also protecting future property and wealth (Lowcountry Digital History Initiative n.d.). Adding historical context of abuse, brutality, control, and dominance during chattel slavery provides deeper meaning to contemporary acts of mobbing, gaslighting, bullying, and coercion utilized by OBGN physicians under the guise of standards of care and medical expertise. Davis describes these specific and repeated acts of physician retaliation against a patient as medical abuse, repeated language and/or behaviors that can occur when medical professionals engage in experimentation and/or (repetitive) behavior that is motivated not by concern for the patient but serves to validate the clinician's self-worth and upholds physician domination over the patient (Davis 2020).

In re-focusing the attention on Mariah, one observes that her persistent and heightened situational and conditional awareness throughout each outpatient medical encounter during her pregnancy and inpatient labor, birth, and postpartum interaction with the hospital demonstrated all three responses to obstetric racism (Davis 2020; Davis, Varner, and Dill 2021; Davis 2022a; Davis 2022b). Racial reconnaissance describes the Herculean effort made by Black women to avoid or mitigate racist encounters, including being hypervigilant about procedures and finding providers. In Mariah's efforts to practice racial reconnaissance in avoiding a coerced, near-forced cesarean birth, Mariah also responded to hospital acts of obstetric racism (e.g., medical abuse, coercion) through resistance and refusal. Davis defined resistance as a strategy whereby a person applies knowledge they possess to push back against medical mandates or requirements to intervene. Resistance to obstetric racism is an act of mobilization against systems and structures within the medical-industrial complex. According to Davis, resistance to obstetric racism manifests as actions that involve questioning the terms of intervention and negotiating various forms of involvement in decision-making. A foundational prerequisite of resistance to obstetric racism is the possession of a vision of how one wants to be treated based on one's own terms (Davis 2020; Davis, Varner, and Dill 2021; Davis 2022a; Davis 2022b).

Resistance to obstetric racism also suggests a core attitude or belief in one's own autonomy (e.g., free will) and agency (e.g., power to act on one's free will). Upon further critical analysis and reflections, all three responses to obstetric obstetric infer that many Black mothers and birthing people possess, and then act upon, a fundamental core attitude about and/or belief in their own worth as a human being desiring and deserving of the human right to autonomy, agency, and dignity during service provision. When positioning both race and gender as modes of knowledge production and application in medical communication, consent, and decision-making during childbirth hospitalization, particularly among Black women and gender-expansive people, I noticed four common themes among Black women's responses to hospital acts of obstetric racism that mapped onto the four tenets of Black feminist theory (Collins 1990; Collins 1996; Collins 2004):

1. Innate power and worth—Black women acknowledge and activate their own power and worth by creating self-definitions and self-valuations that enable them to establish positive, multiple images and repel negative, controlling representations of Black womanhood.
2. Disruption of systems & structures: Black women confront and dismantle the "overarching" and "interlocking" structures and systems of domination in terms of race, class, and gender oppression.

3. Thoughts & activism: Black women intertwine intellectual thoughts and political activism in their individual or collective recognition, reporting, responses, and reconciliation with various harms and oppressions.
4. Resistance & transformation: Black women recognize a distinct, shared cultural heritage that gives them the energy and skills to resist and transform daily discrimination.

As modeled by Black feminist scholars (Collins 1990; Collins 1996; Collins 2004; Collins and Blige 2000; Davis 2018; Davis 2019; Davis 2020; Davis, Verner, and Dill 2021; Davis 2022a; Davis 2022), the stories of Black mother's expectations, experiences, and expressions of their pregnancy, labor, birth, and postpartum generate knowledge about the particular ways that hospitals reproduce obstetric racism and how Black mothers respond to hospital acts of obstetric racism. As Davis beautifully wrote, "Black feminist theory situates Black women's stories as both the evidence and source of theory" because of the interlocking, reciprocating ways in which racism, sexism, gender oppression, and classism wax, wane, collide, and explode in the daily expectations, lived experiences, and routine expressions of Black women (Davis 2018, 5). Furthermore, I noticed how Black mothers and birthing people, and sometimes their chosen and given kin, acting as their proxy, promoter, or protector, embody the core tenets of Black feminist theory as a praxis for preventing or mitigating obstetric racism.

Simply, each of the three responses to obstetric racism (e.g., racial reconnaissance, resistance, and refusal) (Davis 2020; Davis, Varner, and Dill 2021; Davis 2022a; Davis 2022b) serves as a mechanism of action by which Black mothers and birthing people, including their given and chosen kin, achieve alignment between Black obstetric care expectation and Black patient care experience throughout care encounters. Responses to obstetric racism by Black mothers when seeking guidance, help, or care through communication and information exchange demonstrate a Black feminist praxis as the source and driver of their knowing (e.g., theory), doing (e.g., praxis), and being (e.g., reflection). Yet, none of the thirty-six Black mothers in Oakland and Los Angeles spontaneously identified as Black feminists, nor did they name Black feminist theory or praxis as the organizing force behind their responses to obstetric racism.

Although not named by Black mothers in 2019 during the sharing of perinatal stories, one of the most powerful manifestations of Black feminist praxis through a Black mother's response to obstetric racism is refusal. As defined by Davis, refusal occurs during care provision, specifically during communication, consent, and decision-making whereby one does not consent to participate in the medicalization of birthing (Davis 2022a; Davis 2022b). As an act of informed refusal, a Black mother or pregnant person asserts their own free will against a system of control and the demands of consent. According to Davis, refusal, as a response to obstetric racism, is informed by a clear sense that one rejects the possibility of coercion, medical intervention, abuse, disrespect, and the power that is used to dominate Black obstetric patients and their Black babies, their partners, their given and chosen kin, and their team of community support persons without hospital affiliation or alignment. Refusal goes beyond people understanding the implications of NOT doing something, but rather they understand the implications of acting against medical advice. According to Davis, Black mothers and birthing people, including their given and chosen kin who choose the pathway of informed refusal, may be more concerned about agreeing to do something recommended by obstetricians and other hospital clinicians, and the social, political, reproductive, and other medical implications of medical compliance (Davis 2022a; Davis 2022b).

Complementary to seeking help, information, or health care information from the hospital or health system as part of the communication and information exchange quality domain, Black mothers and birthing people identified a second criterion for quality communication: informed consent and informed refusal. The American Medical Association (AMA) first published the Code of Medical Ethics in 1847, which includes opinions on Consent, Communication, and Decision Making (AMA 1847). Ironically, the AMA asserts that the opinions in the chapter are to be viewed as guidance for physicians to shape their ethical approaches to care provision, and not as established standards of clinical practice or rules of law. While the AMA did not mandate a standardization of clinical practice or state or federal laws in the implementation of consent, communication, and decision, the AMA did assert that the practice and process of informed consent to medical treatment is both legally and ethically fundamental (AMA 1847).

According to the AMA, patients possess the right to receive information and to pose questions to physicians about recommended treatments. The reader must consider the AMA's deliberate decision to use the word recommended, and not required, treatments. The implication of this word choice of recommended both establishes and strengthens the following expectations for a physician's role and responsibility as well as environmental conditions for facilitating consent, communication, and decision-making through explicit language and behavior: (1) physician recognition, acceptance, and actualization of a patient's right to bodily autonomy; (2) physician provision of scientifically and culturally accurate, rigorous, relevant, and responsive information about various treatment therapies and modalities, including indications, risks, benefits, and alternatives; and (3) physicians elicit participation by a patient or a patient's surrogate (a person who provides informed consent in the event that the patient lacks or loses decision-making capacity or the patient declines to participate in consent) in the practice of informed consent. The AMA ethical guidance excludes a mandate that a patient or a patient's surrogate accept and/or consider physician recommendations as medical requirements in the provision of care. According to the AMA, a surrogate is a person who provides consent on behalf of the patient if the patient lacks decision-making capacity or refuses to participate in making decisions about medical care (AMA 1847).

The AMA Code of Medical Ethics, specifically chapter 2 titled Consent, Communication, & Decision-Making, asserts that the communication and information exchange process between a patient and physician includes the patient's right to receive information and make inquiries directed to the physician about recommended treatment therapies. The AMA goes on to justify this type of communication and information exchange process as an accountability mechanism for ensuring patients possess and practice the capacity to consciously choose and then act on decisions about care. Then the AMA asserts that successful communication in the patient-physician relationship fosters trust and supports shared decision-making. The AMA also defines the temporality of the informed consent process as beginning when communication between a patient and physician leads to a patient's agreement or authorization to participate in a specific medical intervention. Prior to the patient's agreement or authorization, the physician is required to implement the informed consent process which consists of three core practices: (1) sharing of medically accurate, relevant, and comprehensive information in a sensitive manner that acknowledges, affirms, aligns with, and activates patient preferences and needs for engaging and receiving medical or health care information; (2a) assessing comprehension or a patient's actual skill or ability to understand information and learn new things shared by the physician, including the possible things that might happen if the patient chooses a particular treatment plan or pathway; (2b) assessing a patient's ability to make an independent, voluntary decision, free of coercion or force; and (3) documenting the conversation, the communication and information exchange, and the patient's (or surrogate's) decision in the medical record (AMA 1847).

The AMA provides additional guidelines for performing a sharing of information procedure in the informed consent process. Specifically, the AMA expects the physician to communicate information about three components of the recommended medical care: (1) the diagnosis of the condition that warrants a medical intervention, when the diagnosis is known; (2) the purpose, process, and components of the recommended medical intervention; and (3) the risks, benefits, and burdens of all options, including the consequences of declining treatment (e.g., informed refusal) (AMA 1847).

In the event of a medical emergency, during which a decision to accept medical care must be made expeditiously, and the patient lacks the capacity to participate in decision-making, in the context of an absent or unavailable patient surrogate, the AMA states physicians may initiate medical treatment without prior informed consent. The AMA goes on to stipulate that physicians are obligated to inform the patient or surrogate at the earliest opportunity and obtain consent for ongoing care, in alignment with AMA ethics for communication, consent, and decision-making. In such situations, the physician should inform the patient/surrogate at the earliest opportunity and obtain consent for ongoing treatment in keeping with these guidelines (AMA 1847).

A process is a series of well-defined, repeatable steps that are implemented to achieve a predictable result. Based on the AMA's Chapter 2 titled, "Consent, Communication, and Decision Making," one could argue the informed consent process, when both governed and performed correctly and ethically, yields a predictable result that includes two outcomes: (1) an exchange of information and communication between the physician and patient, and (2) a well-thought-out and thoroughly researched decision about care made by the patient.

One necessary yet rarely discussed critique of the AMA expectation of informed consent is an explicit set of standards for physicians to provide high-quality, medically and culturally accurate, precise, relevant, responsive, and robust information and communication, as well as high-quality and equitably accessible information dissemination designs and approaches. The AMA description of informed consent with respect to medical ethics and the law is predicated on a series of hidden, perhaps rarely tested, assumptions: (1) physicians are innately excellent and impactful data collectors and disseminators of patient-reported information about their health, wellness, discomfort, and disease; (2) physicians possess the capacity and will to define, recognize, and uphold informed consent, informed refusal, autonomy, and medical consent surrogacy; (3) physicians participate in optimal initial and ongoing education, training, and evaluation in the performance of communication about and during informed consent, informed refusal, autonomy, and medical consent surrogacy; and (4) patient and community representatives participate in the optimal initial and ongoing education, training, and evaluation in the performance of physician communication about and during informed consent, informed refusal, autonomy, and medical consent surrogacy (AMA 1847).

At the time of writing this chapter, I was unaware of any previous or current Black feminist hermeneutic phenomenology of Black women's expressions, expectations, and experiences of informed consent and informed refusal, the second theme that emerged from the focus group interviews of thirty-six Black mothers in Oakland in February 2019 and Los Angeles in March 2019. Black mothers defined informed consent and informed refusal as an exchange of high-quality communication and information between physicians and Black mothers, with optimal timing and delivery of both scientifically and culturally rigorous, relevant, and responsive information about the indications and conditions for all interactions, exams, tests, and procedures, including cesarean birth, throughout the entire birth experience. Black mothers also expressed an expectation that communication and information exchange between them and hospital clinicians acknowledges, affirms, upholds, and protects patient autonomy ("free will") and patient agency ("power to act one's free will") throughout the entire duration of all three components of consent: information, comprehension, and voluntariness.

> He told me—well, I broke down crying. He watched me deal with my crying, so—because I was like I don't want to be pregnant no more and I was just crying. He let a nurse come in and explain to me that you have a higher risk of a C-section if we induce you, we would like for your body to do it on its own so that's what we're going to do. And so, I was doing stress tests and they found out he [the male fetus] didn't have any more liquid [referring to low amniotic fluid in the pregnancy or amionitic sac that holds the fetus]. Like I had a stress test on a Friday, and then that Monday I didn't have any fluid. They were like were you leaking. I'm like I can't tell the difference between regular—you got pregnancy discharge and, you know—but they explained it to me to not get an induction and I appreciated that once I learned more about it. I still ended up being induced because he ran out fluid and wasn't coming. I had a reason. And so, I was really glad that he [the Obstetrician] didn't just go for the money and be like, oh, she's tired of being pregnant, you know, get the baby out and we can get more money, as opposed to this time being told to be induced. But for the health of me and my baby, I felt like I wasn given enough information. You know, I learned about preeclampsia. I was scared of preeclampsia and for the fact that my blood pressure hit so high the day I got out the hospital. I was [in] ER for two days after I had him because my blood pressure was extremely high. And so, I was thankful that they made that decision and took him out on the 5th as opposed to the 12th But I also feel like it depends on the moms who ask and educate herself, not just let—you can't let them tell you anything and why—and they try to tell moms, and don't let them tell you anything. If they want an induction, ask why. If they want to do a C-section, ask why.

The above narrative served as an opening to this chapter, highlighting Maya's experience in receiving lots of information about the myriad of medical challenges she and her baby endured. With the additional knowledge and understanding of the AMA's ethical guidance on consent, communication, and decision-making, Maya's narrative demonstrated all components of consent from the patient's perspective of her own experience: information, comprehension, and voluntariness. Maya applied the information component of informed consent to ensuring the safety and health of her and her baby.

She also explicitly identified the reason for the induction (low amniotic fluid produced by the fetus during fetal urination) and easily provided the evidence (low fluid found on her obstetric ultrasound) to support the reason for medical interruption of pregnancy duration. She also explicitly explained the mechanism of action for medical interruption of pregnancy continuation as an induction of labor. Labor induction is a form of medical treatment or a series of medical treatments that prompt the uterus to contract during a time in pregnancy before the onset of spontaneous labor, usually done for maternal, fetal, and/or placental reasons when the continuation of the pregnancy is no longer safe(r) or optimal for the pregnancy, fetus, and/or placenta. Despite experiencing an unexpected phenomenon such as an induction of labor, Maya expressed joy and relief in knowing the why and how: an interruption of pregnancy via labor induction.

Her physician's response to the Black mother's crying culminated in a decision that facilitated optimal communication and information exchange between the Black mother and the hospital team. One possible interpretation of the physician's decision and subsequent action to leverage the role of the nurse as a reliable mediator between hospitals and patients is that the OBGYN physician recognized their limitation, in that singular moment, in creating a safer, non-hierarchical space for uphold patient autonomy and agency during communication, consent, and decision-making. Including the nurse in the consent process disrupted medical normativity and redistributed power from the physician to the patient and centered the patient during the information exchange and comprehension components in medical decision-making.

An underappreciated consequence of the hospital practice of optimal communication and consent is gaining new knowledge about different pregnancy-related conditions. In the above narrative of a hospital seeking consent to interrupt pregnancy by inducing labor for fetal reasons (e.g., low amniotic fluid), Maya described the unexpected yet desired benefit of learning about preeclampsia during communication and consent. The additional knowledge she gained during the communication and information exchange with the hospital teams prepared her for the subsequent unexpected postpartum return to the hospital emergency room (ER) and possible hospital re-admission for postpartum preeclampsia.

Black mothers repeatedly expressed concerns about the misalignment between their expectations and experiences of having hospitals uphold, protect, and secure their autonomy ("free will") and agency ("power to act on their own free will") during childbirth hospitalization. Violations of autonomy and agency frequently occurred during the hospital process of informed consent for procedures including, but not limited to, labor inductions, epidural preparation and placement, pain relief beyond epidurals, cesarean births, newborn immunizations, infant feeding, and immediate postpartum family planning, including contraception and sterilization. The power relations, particularly the power dynamics and differentials, between hospital teams and Black mothers play out in a very predictable, meticulous, and insidious manner during the necessary communication and information exchange for consent and decision-making. Black mothers raised concerns about their capacity to choose the most optimal clinical course of care based on the quality of options and opportunities made explicitly accessible to them by hospital physicians and nurses.

> I would say choice. Choice and option. So, there's power in choice. And so, if you lay out the options, then the person is willing—the person is informed and they can either make a choice. And when a person gets to make a choice, they get the opportunity to own their choice and be empowered by their choice. And they'll take accountability for their choice if they had too; right? I think there needs to be more compassion towards Black women in their—in any birth setting, and particularly the hospitals because statistically Black women and—well, let me say African-American women, even some Latino Brown women, don't necessarily get the option to have access to a birthing center or a home birth with a midwife and a doula because these things are associated with more affluent communities. It's more associated with people of Caucasian or White descent. And so, it's not even like shared, communicated, like, oh, this is an option, I think give birth like this if you want to, or you can refrain from having a birth like that if you want to; right? So definitely having options and choice. And then I feel like there should be more patience and individuality, like more individual care and compassion, not just like, oh, this is what we do.

The accuracy and precision of a Black mother's mind to distinguish between a choice and an option strengthens the argument that the communities most proximal to the crisis are most capable of designing the solutions. Based on Chantelle's keen awareness and understanding of power and the power to choose, hospitals are responsible for presenting patients with a menu of diverse and inclusive options of birth setting, attendant, position, and conditions. In contrast, choice is an opportunity to make a selection from a list of options. Power is then the capacity to choose based on access to both options and resources to make the most optimal choice or informed decision. Chantelle's unsolicited yet necessary and relevant analysis of choice, option, and power is supported by a similar analysis published in a 2017 blog (The Boring Bug 2017). Both the blog author and Chantelle asserted that options precede choice. Likewise, both suggested that structures and systems of power influence the delivery of information and the quality of information about options, which then subsequently affect choice and decision making.

In the case of Chantelle, she suggested that the delivery and quality of information about options from hospital clinicians and staff to patients varied based on racism, classism, and elitism. Thus, thirty-six Black mothers in Oakland and Los Angeles shared a dominant perspective that a primary determinant and driver of informed consent and decision-making included power in patient-provider communication and information exchange. Similarly, twenty-two self-identified women of color (eight of whom identified as non-Hispanic Black or African American) in San Francisco shared a dominant perspective that power and privilege shaped patient-provider communication and information exchange (Altman et al. 2019). Specifically, women of color in San Francisco (who likely navigated similar cross-pollinated health systems with similar clinicians and staff in San Francisco and Oakland) expressed a desire for "complete, truthful, and comprehensive information about their care and options available to them" (Altman et al. 2019, 3).

Like Oakland Black mothers, San Francisco mothers of color felt providers determined the quality and quantity of information to share with them based on how providers saw them as individuals. Furthermore, San Francisco mothers of color perceived providers packaged information in a manner by which to either facilitate or block their ability to make autonomous decisions about their own care during pregnancy and birth. The study investigators deliberately coined the phrase "packaging" to describe a process by which patients perceive providers to be intentionally or inadvertently using information sharing as a mechanism for controlling interactions with and influencing patient decision-making agency (power to act in the world) and autonomy (freedom from external control or influence) (Altman et al. 2019).

Another point of symmetry between the experiences of Oakland Black mothers and San Francisco mothers of color is the role of structural marginalization in shaping provider perceptions of mother "worthiness and fit" which then translated into the differential "packaging" of information by providers, not based on individual needs, but instead based on racism, classism, and elitism. Given Chantelle's breadth and depth of birthing experiences in hospital and community (e.g., midwifery-led birthing center) settings and with physician-facilitated versus midwifery-facilitated births, she consistently offered critical analyses about the uneven determinants and distributions impacting access to and utilization of options, opportunities, choices, and conditions for achieving optimal birth care. During one of the Oakland focus group discussions, Chantelle raised concerns about the uneven access to birthing centers, home births, midwives, and doulas for Black and Latino women compared to white women,

> well, let me say African American women, even some Latino Brown women, don't necessarily get the option to have access to a birthing center or a home birth with a midwife and a doula because these things are associated with more affluent communities. It's more associated with people of Caucasian or White

descent. And so, it's not even like shared, communicated, like, oh, this is an option.

Based on the analysis of experiences shared by the San Francisco mothers of color, three subtypes of packaging reflected the provider's assumptions about the patient's ability to make good *and* autonomous decisions: withholding information, providing partial information, or providing misleading information (Altman et al. 2019). Based on the experiences of Oakland Black mothers, I would argue for the expansion of packaging to be defined as a patient or community-reported experience of harm that consists of a series of flexible and adaptable practices utilized by hospital administrators, clinicians, and staff to silence patient voice or sabotage patient agency and autonomy during clinical interactions, communication, counseling, decision-making, and documentation and dissemination of information in patient handouts, patient sign-offs, and electronic health records.

Based on the initial definition of packaging (Altman et al. 2019) and my expanded definition, packaging directly violates the guidance clearly articulated in the AMA Code of Medical Ethics on Consent, Communication, and Decision Making (AMA 1847). Specifically, packaging violates all three components of informed consent: information, comprehension, and voluntariness. Packaging hinders patients and community support persons from optimal participation in the inquiry process to gather a higher quality or quantity of information to make an informed decision—either informed consent or informed refusal. In fact, packaging erodes and erases trust and accountability in the communication and information exchange process, particularly among historically and structurally marginalized and minoritized communities.

Consider the deliberate practice of de-packaging as a structural act of prevention and mitigation against quality and patient safety violations. Based on the application and integration of health equity, as defined by Dr. Camara Jones, MD, PhD, MPH (Jones 2014), into communication and information exchange, I define de-packaging as a patient, community, or hospital-reported experience or observation of a healthcare professional who provides all patients and their given or chosen kin with opportunities, options, and resources to achieve the highest level of communication, consent, refusal, and decision-making, based on individual and community-level needs, independent of social, economic, demographic, or geographic circumstances *and* with the assurance of optimal conditions for accessing and utilizing communication and information exchange for all people. In accordance with Jones' 2014 definition of health equity, de-packaging, unlike packaging, is a perpetual process whereby systems and structures are required to "value everyone equally, rectify historic inequities, and distribute resources according to need" (Jones 2014, S72). Thus, I argue that de-packaging is a "360 structural or systems measure of progress and performance" that serves as an accountability metric and mechanism by which to operationalize equity and justice in communication, consent, refusal, and decision-making.

De-packaging activates the provider's responsibility to offer an array of options and the patient's power of choice based on options, opportunities, and optimal conditions made accessible to them. De-packaging shifts decision-making power from hospital and health systems and structures to patients, caregivers, and communities. A Black mother in the Oakland focus group, Brianna, expressed excitement and enthusiasm when she chose a birthing tool to facilitate being both actor and witness in her birth based on information shared during a hospital tour of the L&D unit,

> Like when I went in to go like to my visit of where I was going to be at for—like a tour of the labor surroundings they had gave me a paper with all those options about it. It was presented to me, and I chose to pick the mirror so I could watch her come out.

The simple act of offering all options facilitates access to opportunities that can optimize an experience. In the above example, options precede the choice, and the power to choose an option that affirms and aligns with one's expectations or desires radicalizes the care experience and outcome.

The power to choose how one participates in one's own birth, as both the actor and audience, is priceless and indescribable. Based on the lived experiences of Black mothers in Oakland and mothers of color in San Francisco, packaging perpetuates inequity and injustice in choice and option by favoring historically and structurally centered and over-represented individuals and communities. Subsequently, packaging violates communication, consent, refusal, and decision-making as explained by the AMA Code of Medical Ethics (AMA 1847). I argue then that de-packaging advances processes and practices of equity and justice by the activation of power of all through the redistribution of resources to facilitate optimal communication and information exchange, by first prioritizing those in greatest need, thereby rectifying historic and contemporary inequities and injustices.

De-packaging will require more flexibility and adaptation from both patients and hospital clinicians and staff. A major determinant and driver of trust, equity, justice, and accountability in communication, consent, refusal, and decision-making is nurse participation, partnership, and leadership. Optimal de-packaging will lead to the de-centering of physicians as the architects, incubators, accelerators, and beneficiaries of power and privilege in communication and information exchange in the patient-physician relationship and the physician-nurse relationship. Nurses, when contexts and conditions favor nurse intervention free of anticipated or actual physician, administrator, or peer retaliation, can serve as mediators between physicians and patients to facilitate optimal communication, consent, refusal, and decision-making. For Destiny, a Black mother of four children who participated in the Oakland focus group, she brought up the memory of being advised to consider an induction of labor for elevated blood pressures to prevent, not treat, preeclampsia. And during the process of discussing risks, benefits, and alternatives, the nurses expanded the conversation to explore the severity and a sense of urgency versus emergency in the timing of the induction of labor. Destiny expressed both relief and shock in the nuanced communication approach that prioritized her concerns, conditions, and choices.

> Again, because I could—this was like one of my best experience out of all four births. This was the first time they actually were just like on me about what I needed and wanted. And with me being induced at 38, too, to prevent preeclampsia, the nurses were like, well, your blood pressure has been fine, do you want to be induced, you don't have to be induced, I can talk to the doctor. Everything was fine for me, like you could go home, do you know you have a choice, like she was you don't have to, you can wait. And I was shocked.

De-packaging as prevention and mitigation against violations of autonomy and trust in communication and information exchange shapes the naming and meaning of the third dominant perspective within the Black mother-identified quality domain: informed consent and informed refusal. Black mothers in Oakland and Los Angeles describe informed decision-making as a process by which any health care professional must elicit ongoing informed consent or informed refusal. The perpetual process of informed decision-making requires quality and quantity of communication dependent on the assurance of information, comprehension, and voluntariness about the indications and conditions for all interactions, procedures, policies, exams, and tests, including cervical exams and cesarean birth, throughout the entire birth experience.

De-packaging in hospital policies, particularly visitation policies, requires contextualizing visitors in the birth space beyond family members. For example, the inclusion and involvement of medical learners (e.g., physician residents and physician post-doctoral fellows) in the provision of services to obstetric patients during childbirth hospitalization is not mandatory, independent of the teaching or academic status of the maternity—birthing hospital. Any policy or practice that mandates participation of medical learners without optimal communication, consent, and decision-making is a violation of patient autonomy and trust in the patient-provider relationship. As demonstrated in the experiences of San Francisco postpartum mothers of color, the impact of hospital violations of quality in communication and information manifested in three different ways: inadequate information, biased or incomplete information, and packaging of information in a manner that shaped the interactions, communication, counseling, and decision-making to benefit the individual clinician or the larger hospital system (Altman et al. 2019).

Black mothers in Oakland and Los Angeles frequently shared violations of bodily autonomy and experience autonomy when the medical-industrial complex exploited and favored birth and bodies, particularly Black births and Black bodies, as sites for observation, surveillance, experimentation, extraction, exploitation, teaching, and supervision. De-packaging during communication and information exchange about the participation of visitors during the experience of birth in spaces and bodies must include communication, consent, refusal, and decision-making about the inclusion and involvement of medical learners, partners, and other community support persons in biological or social relationship with the obstetric patient. One of the many reasons Destiny enjoyed her fourth hospital birth experience included the option and choice of having her three existing children bear witness to the birth of their baby sister. Destiny's hospital birth also aligned with the SACKRED Birth framework, "This was at Hospital XX, they actually let me have—I had like eight people in my room while I gave birth, and my kids were included. My kids were like right there in it like watching their sister be born. And they didn't kick out my kids out or nothing. My kids were like right there in it watching their sister be born. And they didn't kick my kids out or nothing. My doctor said you are okay with everyone in the room. I said I don't even care."

The process and practice of informed consent must also make space for informed refusal as part of authentic decision-making that more accurately and precisely aligns with the AMA Code of Medical Ethics on Consent, Communication, and Decision Making (AMA 1847). When a physician seeks and then obtains enthusiastic consent for the inclusion and involvement of hospital staff, medical learners, and family members, the patient feels like a valued participant and partner in determining the care process, outcome, and experience. Curating a spirit and practice of inclusion (participation) and belonging (psychological safety and connectedness) in communication and information exchange also applies to informed decision-making about procedures performed during childbirth hospitalization, including but not limited to, labor induction, pain management options, and cesarean births. One Black mother in Oakland, LaToya, who previously talked about not having access to a midwife for her prenatal care, birth, and postpartum care or a doula for support, also reflected on the quality and quantity of information shared about epidurals. Her experiences with hospital communication, consent, and decision-making resulted in the packaging of information and subsequent coerced or forced epidural placement.

> So, with the epidural situation, I really feel like the hospital should really just be clear with the women about what is taking place and how serious and dangerous an epidural can be. And like for me, I had the epidural that one time and that was going to be my last time because I was stuck twice. So, she inserted it wrong or some kind of mishap and it was very painful and I still have pain there on certain days from that experience, so—more information about epidurals, the side effects—risk and benefits, not just like, oh, well, people get them all the time. I don't care that people get them all the time.

LaToya's experience offers both a critique and analysis of communication, consent, and decision-making about the process and procedure of epidural placement. In her critique, she highlighted a key flaw in the process: lack of transparency to women about the actual procedure and potential serious short- and long-term complications to their body. Her expression of her care experience reveals greater insights into the suboptimal communication performance of the anesthesiologist or nurse anesthetist who placed the epidural. Beyond the acute and long-term pain, LaToya expressed greater concern with the quality, quantity, and intention of the hospital clinician's communication. Her analysis as an Oakland Black mother about the clinician's poor communication aligns with the expressed care experiences of failures in communication among the twenty-two San Francisco mothers of color (Altman et al. 2019). According to Altman et al. 2019, failures in information exchange between clinicians and the San Francisco mothers frequently involved three key indicators of unsafe and low-quality communication and information exchange: lack of information, biased or incomplete information, and "packaging" of information to coerce or force interactions, consent, and decisions to favor or protect the clinician (Altman et al. 2019). The clinician's unsafe and poor-quality communication and information exchange with LaToya resulted in the subsequent denial of her right to bodily autonomy and overall care, autonomy, and agency in communication, consent, refusal, and decision-making. The expectation for an anesthesiologist to provide scientifically and culturally accurate, rigorous, relevant, and responsive information about various treatment therapies and modalities, including indications, risks, benefits, and alternatives is the bare minimum behavior as outlined in the AMA Code of Medical Ethics (AMA 1847).

The conversation in the Oakland focus group then shifted to deeper explorations of clinician use of packaging to coerce or force Black mothers to accept other procedures such as an induction of labor, or a cesarean surgery, or abdominal birth. An induction of labor is a procedure that involves a medicinal (e.g., administered by way of mouth, intravenous line, vagina) or mechanical (e.g., laminaria sticks, foley bulb catheter) agent to modify the cervical vertical or horizontal length and consistency and/or initiate uterine contractions prior to spontaneous labor for a maternal, fetal, or placental reason (American College of Obstetricians and Gynecologists (ACOG) n.d.). Chantelle continued to share her knowledge and wisdom about the disproportionate rate of labor inductions among Black women and the increased likelihood of a labor induction ending in a cesarean birth, especially within the context of unfavorable clinical conditions (e.g., a closed, thick, long, hard cervix located high in the female pelvis).

> I feel like they push a lot for—what is it when they try to bring the baby earlier? An induction. Yeah. And inductions—if I'm just getting my own little percentage of what I know. Eighty percent of inductions—it probably is not correct—ends in a cesarean, at least from every single person that I've seen have inductions end in a cesarean, because they're rushing the baby instead of letting the baby come naturally. I understand like if it gets past the 42-week mark and you're like listen, we have to do this, but for the most part, I've seen women get induced at 38 weeks when they have no medical issues, baby is fine, the baby isn't even in the canal yet ready to come, and that's why at least those inductions end in cesareans.

For the purposes of my Black feminist phenomenology of expressions, expectations, and experiences of pregnancy, birth, and postpartum as a Black mother, I focus on race and gender as modes of knowledge production to make sense of structural and systemic oppressions, incompetencies, and inequities in the provision of obstetrics care. Likewise, I assert that knowledge production manifests through the interpretation of shared individual and collective experiences. What happens during this part of the conversation is a collective desire to acknowledge and pursue an analysis of shared experiences of intimidation, control, and domination imposed on Black mothers by U.S. hospitals and health systems to subject them to the ongoing medicalization and pathologization of birth and Black reproducing bodies.

> *Dr. Scott:* But outside of that [medically unnecessary inductions] do you think that in your peers and your communities [of Black women] there are a lot of women being induced.
>
> Black mothers in Oakland: Yes. (In unison)

What I repeatedly witnessed throughout the series of focus group interviews in Oakland and Los Angeles was the evidence that obstetrics as a profession weaponizes the status of "high risk pregnancy" as a tool to reinforce the biological inferiority of Blackness, to sustain and control a pregnancy, and justify forced labor onto an entire group of women based on race. The pervasive culture to force womb evictions (separation of babies from the bodies of Black mothers) to better care for and protect Black babies (through an entanglement of tubes and lines within a transparent box, a new womb owned and overseen by agents of the state) is felt and therefore experienced differently as a Black mother in community with other Black mothers navigating a similar unspeakable hell. In the Oakland focus group, Dominique extended the conversation on the phenomenon of increased inductions to her sister-in-law, who was not a participant in the Oakland or Los Angeles focus groups. Unfortunately, Dominique shared her feelings that the unnecessary induction might have contributed to the impaired development of her sister-in-law's child. But Dominique never voiced her opinion to avoid shaming or blaming her sister-in-law (McLemore 2018; Scott, Britton, and McLemore 2019).

> And I feel like—my sister-and-law and me were pregnant at the same time, and—well, she was supposed to be 3-1/2 weeks behind me. They induced her before it was even my delivery date and she was already 3-1/2 weeks behind me. And I was sitting there—I kept telling her, like, you know, your first baby, you want them out, so she was like—well, the doctor kept saying, oh, well, we can induce you. She's like oh, yeah. And I kept telling her don't do it. And she didn't listen, and I don't want to say that her son is delayed, he does a lot of stuff slower and there's certain things that he doesn't do, and I don't want to put it on that, but I—part of me feels that if they would have let him develop longer and get everything he needed from his mom, he would be better off.

Packaging then becomes the mechanism of subordination by which obstetricians, maternal fetal medicine specialists (high-risk obstetricians), and neonatologists impose forced inductions and labors onto the bodies and beings of pregnant Black women and their families. Packaging resembles a medical mob mentality by which a team of hospital clinicians and staff act as a large group, usually forsaking their own internal sense of morality, fairness, and science, and adopting the dominant actions and behaviors that reinforce the obstetric attitude that Black pregnancies are best ended through cesarean births. Based on my integration of Davis' dimensions of obstetric racism (Davis 2018; Davis 2019; Davis 2020) and packaging as defined by Altman and their co-authors (Altman et al. 2019), packaging then facilitates coercion when medical professionals perform procedures without consent and/or intimidate patients to make decisions, such as forced inductions and forced labors. Furthermore, packaging is an insidious yet impactful act of medical abuse, another dimension of obstetric racism that occurs when medical professionals engage in experimentation and/or (repetitive) behavior that is motivated primarily by seeking validation of their own self-worth as health care professionals and not by concern for the patient. Davis asserts that medical abuse upholds the domination of hospital clinicians and staff over Black obstetric patients (Davis 2020).

Packaging, when contextualized through histories of anti-Black racism, eugenics, plantation colonialism, chattel slavery, and reproductive control and dominance, emerges as an immensely powerful lever in the cascade of events leading to predictable, preventable, and unfair forced cesarean births among Black mothers and birthing people. Packaging is then the catalyst that expedites forced transfers of Black babies from Black wombs to hospital tombs through forced cesarean births, reincarnating admissions in the neonatal intensive care unit (NICU) as shackling, the modern form of chattel slavery of Black communities, starting with our Black babies.

Chantelle: Can we add onto that about how hospitals now push you more for a cesarean instead?

Simone: Right.

Dominique: They push for it because it gives the hospital more—

Latoya: Money.

Dominique:—money.

Dr. Scott: Do you think that's the reason why?

Chantelle: I—that's the reason I feel they do it, because a lot of times I've known—okay, my brother and his —

Angie: Especially if you've got government-funded health care.

Chantelle: My brother and sister literally just had a baby a week ago and they're military. And in turn, they didn't have—they're right now in North Carolina. So, the military hospital didn't in general have a facility for births. They sent them to sources outside of the military hospital. And the doctor kept trying to push my sister-in-law for a C-section and this is her first baby. It was—he kept trying to plan for a C-section and she was like I want to try and give natural. And he's like, oh, well, he's not coming so maybe the best is cesarean. And I told her don't—if that's not what you want, don't go for that, tell him no. And even my brother was becoming very PO'd because this isn't his first baby but it's her first baby. And he's like she doesn't need a cesarean, like he's going to come when he comes. And they kept pushing for the arrival, if he's not here by the weekend, we're going to do the cesarean on Monday.

Over and over again, Black mothers shared the horrors of packaging as mechanisms by which hospital clinicians and staff violate patient safety, avoid accountability, undermine autonomy, exploit communication and information, dismiss given and chosen kinship, reinforce anti-Black racism and misogynoir, discard empathy for and humanity of Black people, and dismantle the dignity in Blackness and holistic care. Based on the expressions and lived experiences of Black mothers in our phenomenological study, packaging manifests as harms that engage all seven theorized patient-identified quality care domains of the SACKRED Birth framework. In this example, hospital clinicians and staff use packaging to coerce Chantelle's brother and sister-in-law, who were expecting their first baby together while enlisted in the military, into a forced cesarean birth. The expecting Black military couple had to seek labor support at a civilian hospital as the military hospital did not offer maternity services. At the civilian hospital, the hospital clinicians and staff repeatedly made attempts to coerce the Black military family into a coerced cesarean birth. The supportive sister, Chantelle, and the expecting brother created a shield to affirm, activate, and protect the autonomy of the pregnant patient. In this situation, specifically, kinship is weaponized in a defensive strategy to fortify a shield of resistance and refusal, two of three responses to obstetric racism.

According to Davis, resistance is a strategy of mobilization against the medical industrial complex whereby a person uses their knowledge to push back against the mandates or requirements to intervene during the provision of care (Davis 2022a; Davis 2022b). Resistance by the Black obstetric patient or their given and chosen kin can manifest as questioning the terms of intervention and negotiating various forms of involvement in decision-making. As Davis explains, resistance comes from having a vision for how one wants to be treated based on one's own terms (Davis 2022a; Davis 2022b). Therefore, one could argue that a prerequisite for resistance is some dose of self-efficacy or the belief in one's own ability to accomplish tasks and achieve goals (or affect change). Or if one lacks the belief, at a minimum, one possesses vision.

In comparison, Davis describes refusal as the act of declining consent to participate in the medicalization of birth during circumstances in which the Black obstetric patient and/or their given or chosen kin deploy their own will against the system of control and the demands of consent particularly during the decision-making process for the possibility, necessity, and timing of a cesarean birth. The act of refusal is shaped by a very clear understanding of the consequences or impacts, which include but are not limited to rejecting the possibility of coercion, medical intervention, medical abuse, disrespect, and the associated power that is used to exert dominance over the Black obstetric patient, their body, their decisions, their care, their baby, their partner, or any other chosen or given kin (Davis 2022a; Davis 2022b). Davis goes on to assert that refusal goes beyond people understanding the implications of not doing something advised by medical professionals. Moreover, Davis explains refusal as an act committed by the Black obstetric patient and/or her given or chosen kin with intentionality and an understanding of the intended and unintended consequences of agreeing to do something recommended by any health care professional (Davis 2022a; Davis 2022b). Through the perspective of an Oakland Black mother, Chantelle, sharing her sister's and brother's pregnancy experiences, one sees and feels the clarity and confidence of kinship wielding shields of resistance and refusal to thwart the medical plans for a forced cesarean birth over the weekend if the baby did not arrive by Monday.

Before moving forward about the power of family shielding, I decided to provide some additional context about the phenomenon of coerced or forced cesarean births within military hospitals. Among popular opinions in medicine, nursing, public health, policy, philanthropy, and health care financing, two primary drivers contributing to maternal health inequities include access to care and socioeconomic status. Consider the rates of maternal health outcomes within a closed system where access and socioeconomic status can be eliminated or significantly reduced. For military service members and their dependents, one can test the hypothesis that equal access to healthcare and similar socioeconomic statuses among diverse communities lead to no or minimal differences in maternal health outcomes (Hamilton et al. 2021).

A study published in the *American Journal of Obstetrics and Gynecology* tested a hypothesis that universal access to healthcare, as provided in the U.S. military healthcare system, would produce similar rates of maternal morbidity independent of race or ethnic background. The sample included 1000 births from April 1, 2018, to March 31, 2019. The Inaugural National Perinatal Information Center provided these data from participating military treatment facilities in the Department of Defense during the study period. The primary outcomes included indicators of severe maternal morbidity by race. After comparing the percentages of cesarean births, adult intensive care unit (ICU) admissions, and severe maternal morbidity between Black and white patients, study findings demonstrated that racism, not race, matters significantly (Hamilton et al. 2021).

Military hospitals were 1.5x more likely to perform cesarean births on Black reproducing bodies and were ~3x more likely to admit Black reproducing bodies to the adult ICU compared to white reproducing bodies. Black reproducing bodies were also ~2x more likely to experience severe maternal morbidity, even when excluding blood transfusion, compared to white reproducing bodies in military hospitals (Hamilton et al. 2021). The researchers concluded that "equal access to healthcare and similar socioeconomic statuses in the military healthcare system do not explain the healthcare disparities seen regarding maternal morbidity encountered by Black women having children in the United States" (Hamilton et al. 2021, 512e1). The implications of the study are monumental as the findings indicated that equality, or one size shoe fits all strategies and solutions, will not eliminate or close the death and dying gap between Black reproducing bodies and all other reproducing bodies. Health inequities in severe maternal health complications persisted despite equal access and similar socioeconomic statuses among Black pregnant and postpartum mothers and individuals. Unmeasured structural and systemic factors including, but not limited to, variations in hospital, L&D unit, and individual clinician/staff practices, behaviors, language, communication, continuity, and coordination of care were not measured (Hamilton et al. 2021).

More importantly, patient-reported experience measures and patient-reported outcome measures of quality, patient safety, packaging, de-packaging, or obstetric racism were not included in the analysis of outcomes based on race. Thus, the work of Black women-led, Black feminist ethnographic, phenomenological, applied epidemiological, and mixed methods participatory action research studies and implementation science research studies, grounded in reproductive justice, cultural humility, research justice, anti-racism, cultural rigor, gender justice, and birth justice, are necessary for identifying and contextualizing levers that drive and end the manufactured Black maternal health crisis.

Returning to the sharing of the above story of a family shielding a pregnant Black mother from a forced disruption of pregnancy via a forced cesarean birth without any medical indication prompted another Black mother to further elaborate on the integrity of medical advice. Chantelle then expanded upon her critique by offering a brief analysis of the various levers that illuminate power differentials and dynamics in communication and information exchange around consent.

> Yeah, I wanted to speak on that too because if technically you're supposed to—or you can be pregnant for 40 weeks, right, or up to 42 weeks. I just feel like this, you get pregnant in a natural—for most people, you get pregnant in a natural way. You carry this baby in a natural way. And your onset—and the onset of your pregnancy is all—it's like—it's something you don't control. So why should you try to control when a baby comes out. Now, for health risks or issues like that, yes, we got to take certain precautions, but a lot of times a young mom or a foreign mom or somebody that is not from this country, that don't speak the right languages or there's language barriers, there's culture barriers, there's financial barriers, there's all these things in play, you hear this doctor who is a professional who you're entrusting, and so you feel like, oh, well, they're a doctor, they know best, but they're just a person that went to school maybe longer than you or they went to school to study something you didn't study and so they're considered an expert so you trust them, but they are human—they're human so they can make human error and human mistakes and I just feel like there should be—oh, man, it's—me and my women, we'd like to have kids. We like to have kids. I just got a little real passionate about that, but I just really feel that you should not try to control something that is natural supposed to happen unless there is something—and what that trust thing is if he

> says like, oh, you got preeclampsia or you got high blood pressure or you got this or got that, you're like, oh, I do, oh, shoot, and so you just trust the doctor. And the doctor say, oh—the doctor said you got to do this or do this or do that, you go with it. But that's maybe not what you needed to do.

In her own way, Chantelle explicitly named and then explained how physicians weaponize various intersecting levers in the mechanisms of subordination to exert reproductive dominance in interactions, consent, and decision-making. Chantelle's characterization of how physicians exert dominance illustrates a longstanding hierarchy of knowing and knowledge based on age, nativity, language, class, financial capital, education, professionalization, and prioritization of medical knowledge. The societal pressures or assumptions that physicians are worthy of innate, unearned patient and community trust make all patients, particularly structurally marginalized and minoritized obstetric patients, susceptible to violations of bodily autonomy, care autonomy, and decisional autonomy. Chantelle also spoke to the need for physicians to integrate humanity and humility in their approach to leveraging their medical knowledge and expertise to support patients. At the same time, the Black mother insisted physicians support her and women like herself to practice the freedom to have kids, which is the manifestation of reproductive justice in birth justice,

> well, they're a doctor, they know best, but they're just a person that went to school maybe longer than you or they went to school to study something you didn't study and so they're considered an expert so you trust them, but they are human—they're human so they can \make human error and human mistakes and I just feel like there should be—oh, man, it's—me and my women, we'd like to have kids. We like to have kids.

The expressions of Black mothers' expectations and experiences of navigating power, options, and choices during their perinatal health care encounters prompted me to ask a critical question: "How do Black mothers and people ensure that what's being offered to them is appropriate?" At that moment during the interview, I crossed the boundary of objectivity as a researcher and intentionally stepped into reflexivity as a Black feminist and dissident obstetrician gynecologist. I leveraged my own positionality to ask Black mothers, traditionally excluded from knowledge production that evaluates the quality of communication, consent, and decision-making in perinatal service provision, about how they go about checking system accountability to and alignment with ethical and equitable standards of care. That singular question sparked a dialogue, not just for data extraction to meet a grant deliverable, but for transforming beliefs and practices through influential interaction as explained by Zorn and colleagues (Zorn et al. 2006).

Like many other moments during these 2019 focus groups, I began to reimagine the value and impact of focus group participation and interaction as participatory peer-to-peer interventions to influence participant beliefs about controversial topics such as the principles, processes, and practices of informed consent and informed refusal, particularly in the context of obstetric racism and Black women and gender-expansive individuals seeking and utilizing any pregnancy-related health care services in the U.S. As Zorn explains, the dialogue between participants reveals a peculiar yet powerful series of social dynamics and the implications of these dynamics to the participant, the interviewer, the research team and possibly the general public (Zorn et al. 2006).

> *Dr. Scott:* How do Black mothers and people ensure that what's being offered to them is appropriate?
>
> *Gabrielle:* A lot of times you've been offered that when there isn't no other choices, like this is—or if you're going to do it this way or —
>
> *Maya:* They don't give you second opinions, and it's either what they say or you're screwed, like it's either you go with what I say or nothing.
>
> *Dominique:* Like we have to do this—we have to do this induction now because of da-da-da, and if you don't have the induction—and then the alternative that they tell you sounds farfetched like some people are like, oh, well, if this is the alternative, then I'm going to go ahead and get this induction.
>
> *Tasha:* And it always sounds easier for the doctor, always.
>
> *Chantelle:* Induction just seem like it became more popular recently than before, like I don't remember hearing about inductions as much when I was—when I had my first child, but this millennial stuff, it's like induction left and right and almost giving women the option to induce as though like, oh, you're tired of being pregnant, oh, I'm feeling pressure, oh, I'm feeling that I got some cramping. You're going to have some cramps, you're going to have some pressure, you're going to have some pain, you're going to have a lot of different stuff, but that don't mean it's time for you to give birth.
>
> *Maya:* That don't mean bring the baby here. And those last few weeks are essential weeks, like there's a lot of natural stuff that happens
>
> *Angie:* The critical stuff.

In that moment, I asked a singular follow-up question as I was curious about Black mothers' awareness of the insidious yet impactful ways obstetricians, high-risk OB specialists, neonatologists, and obstetric and neonatal nurses exploit power differentials in clinical knowledge and weaponize fear of death in communications, consent, and decision-making. The dialogue among six Black mothers during the Oakland 2019 focus group shows how group participation and interactions catalyzed a convergence of thought on a substantiative issue, blatant and repeated violations of patient autonomy by hospital obstetricians and other physicians. First, the dialogue highlights in detail the role and performance of packaging in constraining Black mothers' access to comprehensive, relevant medical information and discussion of an array of medical options and opinions, including risks, benefits, and all alternatives. Second, the dialogue illuminates group thought about the motivations behind the use of packaging in violating patient decisional, bodily, and care autonomy, serving the needs, priorities, and interests of the physician (as a representative of larger structural and systemic violations, incompetencies, and inequities in communication, consent, and decision-making). Thus, the focus group, whether in person or online, facilitates a process of influence whereby participants go beyond reporting their pre-existing beliefs and move toward challenging, questioning, and persuading participants. Likewise, the focus group presents an opportunity for one or more participants to either change or build up their own and another participant's pre-existing beliefs. I conducted a literature review on the inclusion of focus group dialogue in the reporting of results in qualitative research to resist the denial of interpersonal influence and acceptance of the utilization of single quotes from focus groups as data exemplars in traditional or positivist approaches to interpreting and reporting of focus group data. Therefore, I applied a more critical or interpretive approach to focus group use, interpretation, and reporting using a Black feminist hermeneutic phenomenological methodology so that the context of the phenomenon itself dictates how the data are analyzed (Crowther and Thomson 2023). In real-time, I both observed, recorded, and experienced the power of focus group influence and interaction in meaning-making construction and negotiation (Zorn et al. 2006) of being a Black woman navigating quality and patient safety violations while simultaneously seeking and utilizing pregnancy-related health services, with a focus on childbirth hospitalization.

When describing how one orients to the expressed lived experiences of Black mothers (phenomenology) and how one interprets the texts of single excerpts or focus group dialogue describing Black mothers' lived experiences (hermeneutics), Black feminist praxis requires me to apply reflexivity in my examination of Black mothers' lived experiences of packaging within the dimension of obstetric racism. As a dissident OBGYN physician-scientist and OB Hospitalist since 2006 and obstetric quality improvement and implementation scientist since 2018, with insider (board-certified in obstetrics and gynecology, with more than twenty years in serving and supporting "high risk" pregnant and postpartum communities throughout the Midwest, West Coast, and South) and outsider (birthed in Black feminism in 1992, reproductive justice in 2010, public health in 2013, cultural humility in 2014, applied epidemiology in 2015, and birth justice and research justice in 2018) ways of being and knowing, I must continuously critique and interrogate the language, actions, and behaviors of any health care professional serving Black pregnant and postpartum (including many Black individuals and families surviving (in)fertility, surrogacy, adoption, or legal abandonment) through the phenomenon and analytic of Davis' obstetric racism.

Earlier interpretations of packaging (Altman et al. 2019) within the six dimensions of Davis' obstetric racism (Davis 2018; Davis 2019; Davis 2020; Davis, Varner, and Dill 2021; Davis 2022a; Davis 2022b) clearly show how coercion and medical abuse are commonly deployed and easily recognized mechanisms of action in the subjugation of Black mothers in obstetrics. Further analysis of the focus group dialogue reveals a more insidious form of quality and human rights violations as captured by the dimension, intentionally causing pain. The second part of Davis' definition articulates a form of pain that typically goes unmentioned in traditional quality and patient safety meanings and measures, the absence of empathy for Black people's physical suffering, leading to a lack of internal motivation to alleviate or reduce Black suffering (Davis 2018; Davis 2019). Packaging, as defined through interpretations of women of color in San Francisco (Altman et al. 2019), results in withholding of relevant medical information necessary for the actualization of the full process of informed consent (e.g., information, comprehension, and voluntariness), even if motivated by beneficence, and is thereby an act of therapeutic privilege (Claude, Lajeunesse, and Lussier 2010; AMA 1847).

According to the AMA's Council on Ethics and Judiciary Affairs (CEJA) report examining informed consent, the onus of responsibility in communicating "all requested medical information sensitively and respectfully, while seeking to minimize any negative effects upon the patient," falls on the physician. The CEJA report concluded by asserting that the act of listening by physicians to patients' concerns and responding to their individual needs can promote the patient-physician relationship and protect against the iatrogenic suffering of patients (Bostick et al. 2006). Triangulation of data from San Francisco women of color (Altman et al. 2006), my Black feminist hermeneutic phenomenological research on Oakland Black mothers, and Davis' Black feminist ethnographic research that informs obstetric racism (Davis 2018; Davis 2019; Davis 2020; Davis, Verber, and Dill 2021; Davis 2022a; Davis 2022b) with the AMA's CEJA report on informed consent (Bostick et al. 2006) situate packaging by physicians as a praxis of therapeutic privilege that facilitates acts of coercion, medical abuse, and intentionally causing pain based on demonstrating an absence of empathy during communication, consent, and decision-making.

The inclusion of the focus group dialogue among six Black mothers clearly shows the architecture of disparate, predictable, preventable, and unjust Black suffering (beyond the act of physical injury) during decision-making, leading to a lack of internal motivation to alleviate or reduce Black suffering. As expressed by Tasha, "And it always sounds easier for the doctor, always," the motivation for initiating and perpetuating Black suffering through mechanisms of packaging favors the physician, a representative of the medical-industrial complex. Oakland Black mothers also speak to the withholding of information, specifically risks, during the praxis of packaging in communication and information exchanges around inductions, cesarean births, and informed consent.

> *LaToya:* They're just like, okay, well, you want to have an induction, all right, that's cool, you want to have a C-section, okay, that's cool, and you tell them instead of mentioning a risk factor, same as with epidurals. Okay, this is the risk that comes with it, are you sure this is what you want to do. More like when you're in pain is when they get to have you sign all these papers—
>
> *Dominique:* Oh, yeah, and you agree when you're like in pain.
>
> *LaToya:* Exactly. You're not reading all the risks that comes with an epidural, when they're putting fentanyl and the baby is going to come out drowsy, all this extra stuff. You don't know because you're signing off your rights at that point. You got to listen. And I don't care what you got to give me, give it to me. Like they should automatically be going over stuff with you, not waiting until your contractions are hitting the charts coming back to back like—I mean I know when you go in there, you're supposed to be five minutes apart and everything, but when you go in there, you're still somewhat okay compared to when the baby starts dropping more and that hurts.

Black mothers offered both a critique and analysis of information, communication, consent, and decision-making about multiple processes, practices, policies, and procedures involved in childbirth hospitalization. Throughout their critique of hospital performance in communication and information exchange, Black mothers highlighted multiple flaws in hospital performance at the level of the system, team, and individual clinician and staff member. The lack of transparency and weaponization of information and communication facilitated the reproduction of five of the six dimensions of obstetric racism throughout childbirth hospitalization: neglect, dismissiveness, and disrespect; diagnostic lapses; intentionally causing pain; coercion; and medical abuse.

Chapter 6

Given and Chosen Kinship

> And then after the baby was born, actually, they had to take her away because they had me on a diet for so long that she didn't have any sugar. So, she was shaking when she came out. So, I was mad about that so I started crying. Because I asked him, I want to follow her. I don't want them to mix up my baby or anything. Just go, as soon as she came out. So, I started crying because why was I on a diet this whole time. So, the first night I didn't sleep with her. I gave birth at 10:30 [am] and I didn't see my baby until like 6 p.m. Yes. And I started crying because I had to breast feed her. And then there was no bond, or anything. So, I was like I'm going to get up and walk to her room. And they came and they drive me there and everything. The whole time I was crying. Because she was all hooked up and everything and she had to spend the night there. And the first thing that they tried to give her was formula. Oh, she needs this sugar right now. And then I said why did you guys have me on a diet for so long if she needed that sugar.

Take a moment to feel the psychological and physical suffering of a Black mother separated from her newborn baby at birth, not by family policing systems or law enforcement (Roberts 1997; Roberts 2011; Roberts 2012; Roberts 2017; Goodwin 2017; Goodwin 2020; Roberts 2022) but by hospital nurses and physicians from the L&D unit, Neonatal Intensive Care Unit (NICU), or Special Care Nursery (SCN) without the involvement of family policing systems. Imagine your obstetricians medicalizing and pathologizing your reproducing body, pregnancy, and fetal development and then assigning a classification of high(er) risk to your pregnancy experience. As a result, the obstetric team mobilizes to compel you to modify your diet throughout your entire pregnancy as a preventive measure to mitigate this high(er) risk and curtail any adverse maternal, fetal, and placental sequelae. Thus, you submit to the medicalization and pathologization of your reproducing body, pregnancy, and birth. Unfortunately, you find out at the birth of the baby you vowed to love, nurture, nourish, and protect that your restrictive diet resulted in inappropriately lowering the blood sugars in the baby's blood below normal after physiological separation of you and your newborn baby (through the clamping of the umbilical cord). Your decision to comply with medical advice led to an actual pathological response and condition in your newborn baby, leading to the admission of your newborn baby into the NICU. In this situation, the medical advice and care provided to you by your obstetrician and prenatal health team resulted in an unexpected subsequent diagnosis and adverse response in your newborn that then required higher-resourced care and a NICU admission.

The phenomenon under interrogation can be classified as one of three types of iatrogenesis, as explained in greater detail in chapter 2. In this specific circumstance, iatrogenesis was previously described as any noxious, unintended, and undesired effect of the actual treating physician. Illich described three types of iatrogenesis: (1) clinical, the direct harm done by various medical treatments; (2) social, the medicalization of ordinary life; and (3) cultural, the loss of traditional ways of dealing with and making sense of suffering, death, pain, and sickness (Peer and Shabir 2018; O'Mahony 2016; Smith 2003). The opening Black narrative describes Dominique's response when she found out that her restricted diet led to clinical iatrogenesis, impacting her newborn's health and requiring parent-child separation to stabilize her newborn's blood sugar levels. Dominique's narrative is shared repeatedly throughout the various chapters as manifestations of hospital acts that actualize or violate different Black mother-identified and defined obstetric quality care domains in the SACKRED Birth framework. Given the evidence in her experiential knowledge shared during the 2019 focus groups, she never revealed the exact diagnosis given to her by the obstetrician that required her to restrict her dietary intake. Thus, the obstetrician's undetermined diagnosis and subsequent specific therapeutic intervention of diet and caloric restrictions resulted in newborn hypoglycemia at birth (inappropriately lower-than-normal blood sugars for a newborn baby).

Based on the interpretation of her experiential knowledge, the hospital then facilitated the clinical, social, and cultural iatrogenesis. Then the iatrogenesis, independent of type, ultimately led to unplanned Black mother-child separation, which then catalyzed a series of quality violations when quality is defined for, by, and with Black mothers in equitable and dignified partnerships with Black women community and content experts. For this chapter's purpose, unplanned or undesired Black parent-child separation at birth is one of six themes or manifestations of how hospitals recognize and respond to given or chosen kinship. Unplanned or undesired Black parent-child separation is an event that can occur as a consequence of decisions made by the hospital system, team, or individual clinician or staff that leads to the removal of the baby from the birthing parent, supportive parent, or both for prolonged periods of time, with no regard to the impact on parent, child, or parent-child bonding. When kinship is defined and discussed within the constructs of the seven patient-identified domains of the SACKRED Birth framework, the focus of analysis is the role of an individual hospital administrator, nurse, or physician, hospital teams, or the hospital system (e.g., policy, practice) in facilitating the denial, exclusion, or disruption of given or chosen relationships or relationship-affirming activities that involve the Black mother or birthing person and their new child, existing child or children, partner(s), parent(s), siblings, other family members, friends, community doula, community midwife, and other birth workers in the community (birth educator, lactation educator). When kinship disruptions or violations involve parent-child separation after childbirth, the focus and analysis will be based on the evidence presented in the narratives of thirty-six Black mothers in Oakland and Los Angeles, which does not involve CPS or other family policing systems such as social workers, case managers, mental health/behavioral health specialists, law enforcement, or hospital security.

In returning to the opening Black birth narrative detailing Dominique's experience of kinship disruption, specifically unanticipated and undesired parent-child separation due to neonatal hypoglycemia, imagine the scene not in a birthing hospital in Oakland, but on a plantation in the Deep South during the antebellum period. Now re-read the opening narrative from the perspective of an enslaved Black woman who had just given birth in the slaves' quarters. Imagine giving birth and the plantation owner or overseer immediately snatching your newborn Black baby from your arms, disrupting your capacity to hold, body feed, bond, know, love, and see your own baby. Now your newborn baby is chained and constrained by various tubes in a box that prohibits you from touching and tending to your baby's needs as their biological, birth, and social mother. You can no longer exercise your right to independently nurture and nourish your own baby. The situation and the experience cause you unplanned, undesired, and unnecessary psychological torture that also includes an element of physical suffering as your mind, heart, spirit, and body yearn to establish physical, emotional, and spiritual attachments to your baby that are now forbidden. And the actions and policies of the individual obstetrician, prenatal health team, hospital L&D team, and hospital neonatology/pediatric team go unaddressed. To date, the obstetric quality and patient safety paradigms in the U.S. lack any shared meaning, measurement, monitoring, reporting, or mitigation standards, structures, or strategies for the role of recognizing, affirming, protecting, including, and maintaining kinship in establishing or facilitating obstetric quality or patient safety. Moreover, hospital performance and reimbursement for maternity care in the U.S. exclude a measure of affirming or disrupting kinship ties between the mother—birthing parent and the newborn baby, partners, and other individuals or communities recognized by the mother or birthing parent. Given the historical and contemporary acts of violence in the U.S. enacted against Black mothers and birthing people and their Black reproducing bodies to destabilize, disrupt, and dismantle Black families, the absence of a kinship measure in the evaluation of obstetric quality in existing improvement and implementation initiative feels ahistorical, atheoretical, unethical, irresponsible, and unscientific (Scott 2018; Scott 2019a; Scott 2019b; Scott 2021; Scott and Davis 2021; White VanGompel et al. 2022).

To date, the obstetric quality and patient safety literature lacks a shared meaning and measurement of kinship in the provision of hospital-based obstetrics care. Based on the lived experiences of thirty-six Black mothers, the shared meaning of kinship includes the following elements:

- acknowledgment, affirmation, activation, and amplification of Black mother-identified given (biological) and chosen (social) family relationships and roles by making space for kinship in the form of a live person at the bedside or by technology such as a partner, parent, chosen or given family, friend, or birth professional such as a doula, community midwife, birth educator, or lactation educator.
- inclusion and integration of partners, especially Black men or masculine presenting partners, in care provision, including communication, information sharing, interactions, decision-making, and documentation and dissemination of health care information during patient hand-offs, patient sign-outs, and in electronic or paper health records.
- having support, protection, and advocacy that is specific and loyal exclusively to the Black mother and birthing person, with no association or affiliation to the hospital or health care team (Lett et al. 2023).

Black mothers and birthing people believe kinship shows up in clinical & social interactions (measures) as:

- increased perception and experience of belonging (psychological safety and connectedness), cultural, social, and physical safety, and trust for Black mothers and birthing people, their given and chosen kinship, and additional community support persons;
- having mechanisms or strategies of resistance and resilience in place to communicate and reinforce the rights, priorities, needs, and wishes of the Black mother and birthing person;

- having accountability and oversight meanings, measurements, and mechanisms of action (e.g., reporting, response, and reconciliation) established in writing within hospitals and health systems for practicing informed consent and informed refusal with Black mothers and birthing people, and their given and chosen kinship with oral or written authorization by Black mothers and birthing people; and
- having accountability and oversight meanings, measurements, and mechanisms of action (e.g., reporting, response, and reconciliation) established in writing within hospitals and health systems on acknowledging, supporting, and incorporating the capacity and capability of Black mothers and birthing people to optimally heal and recover in community with kin from life challenges (external and internal) that impact pregnancy, birth, postpartum, and beyond.

The synthesis of the shared meanings and measures for kinship in the provision of hospital-based obstetrics care established four overarching themes or manifestations of activating or violating Black mothers' kinship:

1. Clinician or hospital facilitated parent-child separation at birth with subsequent disruption, destabilization, and dismantling of Black parental and family caretaking roles and responsibilities for the Black newborn baby with or without involvement of family policing systems;
2. Inclusion or exclusion of a Black mother's partner, parent (grandparent to the baby), or any given or chosen family intervenes in the provision of care and support;
3. Learners in the health care profession affect the optimal presence and participation of any given or chosen kin (e.g., Black mother's partner, parent, sibling, friend) or additional community support person; and
4. Social networks (non-peers)—interveners and advocates.

Like the unintended yet impactful physician-facilitated parent-separation at birth, due to clinical iatrogenesis and without the involvement of family policing services in the chapter opening, another Black mother shared her experience of preventing undesired parent-child separation in the middle of the night. For context, as the focus group interviewer and facilitator, I asked Black mothers if anyone felt they had received too much or too little care during the immediate postpartum period of their childbirth hospitalization. A Black mother in Oakland who experienced a hospital water birth, Gabrielle, expressed she felt like the postpartum care and attention was inadequate. After the hospital postpartum nurses discovered she knew how to breastfeed and confirmed optimal breastfeeding, the nurses no longer seemed interested in providing any additional care or attention. However, during the middle of the night, the postpartum nurse discovered co-sleeping, specifically, bed-sharing between Gabrielle and her newborn baby girl. At that point, the hospital postpartum nursing team regained interest in Gabrielle and her baby.

> I felt like I had too little [care]. Because [the nurses thought] she knows how to breast feed. They came in and asked if I was breastfeeding okay. I'm like yeah, it's okay. Then after that it was like they checked on me when they wanted to. They left me alone, they came in the middle of the night and tried to take her one time. Because I was sleeping in the bed with her and they stressed that you can't sleep in the bed with the baby. Which I was totally against. So, we argued about that. And then afterwards they never came in there. I felt like once they saw me breast feeding cool and I was so defiant against her to be put in the little thing, they just left me alone.

Without providing a discourse on the science and safety of different co-sleeping behaviors (e.g., bed-sharing or surface-sharing, room-sharing, rooming in) and focusing on critiquing and judging the Black mother's behavior and choices, this chapter applies a Black feminist hermeneutic phenomenological analysis of the lived experience of childbirth hospitalization and meaning-making of quality as measured by affirming or violating kinship through the written birth narratives of Black mothers. The object of critique then becomes the impact of the hospital postpartum nurse's initial reaction to the discovery of co-sleeping and the subsequent series of harmful responses in which the postpartum nurse's goal was to facilitate kinship disruption as felt and experienced by Gabrielle. The discovery of a successful breastfeeding Black mother by a team of hospital postpartum nurses first resulted in neglect, dismissiveness, and disrespect during the immediate postpartum period, which Davis describes as ignoring or dismissing a Black mother's expressed need for reproductive help or care and/or treating them with disdain (Davis 2018; Davis 2019). During one of the most powerful times to promote Black mother-child vitality as systematic acts of refusal and resistance against system drivers of the 53 percent of pregnancy-related deaths occurring between postpartum day 7 and 365 (CDC 2022), the hospital system and postpartum team abandoned the Black mother and her baby, "*Then after that it was like they checked on me when they wanted to. They left me alone,*" according to Gabrielle.

A more meaningful use of the immediate postpartum period would be to apply and integrate the Scott and Davis 2022 "Building and Bridging Black Futures Beyond Birth Model of Postpartum Care, a 12-Step Black Woman-Person First Approach," which offers a more humane and holistic model of culturally affirming and clinically responsive postpartum care (Scott and Davis 2022). Integration of this Black feminist model of care during the immediate postpartum nurse evaluation and provision would provide enhanced insights into how the Black mother views herself, her reproducing and life-sustaining body, and her kinship roles, including being a Black mother, in relationship to her postpartum healing and recovery. The postpartum nurse had the opportunity to explore the desires and intentions of rest and sleeping for Gabrielle and her baby, as determined and understood by Gabrielle, in a non-threatening, non-confrontational, and non-judgmental manner. Instead, the postpartum nurse's response and impact to discovering co-sleeping conjures ancestral and contemporary memories of the forced removal of Black children from their Black mothers, fathers, and families and the forced disruption and destabilization of Black family lives and relations.

"They came in the middle of the night and tried to take her one time" reads like an excerpt from a Black slave narrative or a sci-fi film that mixes the genre of war and horror. As previously described in chapter 2, "they" would be defined as plantation owners, overseers, or slave catchers during the antebellum period. In modern times, "they" means nurses, physicians, social workers, case managers, or CPS. In the case of Dominique and Gabrielle, kinship disruption manifested as the actual or threat of system/clinician facilitated parent-child separation without involvement of family policing systems. Instead of involving the state, the medical-industrial complex exerts control and dominance over the placement of Black babies during the immediate postpartum triggered by a clinical finding or a clinician's concern for the welfare of the baby, as defined for, by, and with clinicians and the health system. The medical-industrial complex continues to exclusively define, value, and shape newborn safety and well-being before, during, and after pregnancy and childbirth without ethical and equitable participation by or partnership with patients, particularly Black mothers and birthing people, and their given and chosen kin. Therefore, the development and validation of new quality and patient safety theories, domains, and measures defined for, by, and with Black patient, community, and content experts are vital to disrupting epistemic injustice, testimonial injustice, and hermeneutical injustice (Scott 2018; Scott 2019a; Scott 2019b; Scott 2021; Scott and Davis 2021; Lyndon et al. 2023; Scott and Lusero 2023). Designing and implementing system or clinician-centric metrics or protocols without interrogation of patient-caregiver-community identified and defined unintended or hidden negative consequences can potentially generate new and/or exacerbate existing quality, patient safety, and human rights violations (Scott 2021; Lyndon et al. 2023; Scott and Lusero 2023).

In response to the postpartum nurse's threat to forcibly remove the newborn from Gabrielle's arms (and bed) and facilitate forced Black mother-child separation within the confines of the postpartum room and without an exploratory conversation or involvement of family policing systems, Gabrielle resisted and refused. Gabrielle stood her ground and defied the nurse's authority to facilitate "iatrogenic" parent-child separation.

> And then afterwards they never came in there. I felt like once they saw me breast feeding cool and I was so defiant against her [baby girl] to be put in the little thing [small crib next to Gabrielle's bed], they just left me alone.

And yet again, the unexpected behavior of optimal breastfeeding and asserting one's autonomy repelled any future supportive or care-based interactions, evaluations, or communication. The postpartum nurses' behaviors in the day and night may reflect hidden institutional policies that determine standards of care. However, the standardization of obstetric care in the U.S. is deeply embedded in anti-Black racism and anti-Black misogyny (e.g., misogynoir) as explained in detail in chapter 2.

Moving from system or clinician-facilitated or iatrogenic kinship disruption to iatrogenic delayed kinship reunification, a Black mother in the Los Angeles focus group shared her experience of another unexplained and hidden policy whereby postpartum and NICU nurses required Aaliyah to demonstrate competency in walking independently after cesarean birth prior to being able to hold her baby. One must interrogate the evidence requiring a Black mother who endured a major abdominal surgery to demonstrate walking proficiency to gain the privilege to sit down and hold her newborn baby. The Black mother's own mother, the maternal grandmother, was present with her. If the unsubstantiated hospital policy was that at least one person must demonstrate proficiency in independent ambulation, then the presence of the maternal grandmother was sufficient. Therefore, the system or clinician-facilitated decision to sustain parent-child separation in this situation served no higher purpose than to reinforce a hierarchy of power that resulted in social control and dominance over a Black mother's right to parent, visit, nurture, bond, attach, and hold her existing child. Such social control, dominance, and disruption of kinship reunification violate one of the core tenets of reproductive justice (Ross et al. 2017; Ross and Solinger 2017). Clearly, the communication and information exchange between the nursing team across two differed yet inter-related departments lacked humanity, empathy, and optimal explanation and justification.

> *Aaliyah:* When you talked about the walking around. My thing was, they wouldn't let me hold her if I couldn't walk and then they're yeah, you only could sit with her. I was sitting. My mom wheeled me in there.
>
> *Dr. Scott:* If you couldn't walk in the NICU, they didn't want you to hold her?
>
> *Aaliyah:* Yeah. And I'm like why do I need to [walk to] hold her? I'm sitting down.
>
> *Dr Scott:* Why do you have to walk with her in the NICU unit?
> *Aaliyah:* So, my mom pushed me in the wheelchair after me not seeing her for over a day. Because I was [hanging] off the bed—they put me back on bedrest

after it happened. So, then they were like, okay, you can feed her but you can't hold her. I'm like, why? And they were like, because you have to be able to walk. And I'm like well, when they give people their baby and they just had them, aren't they laying in the bed?

Dr. Scott: Exactly. And I've seen them roll people in their wheelchair into the NICU.

Shante: Yeah.

Toni: Yeah.

Aaliyah: Yeah, I was rolled on in there. They would not let me hold her. So, then the next time I went back, which was like that night and it was a different nurse. That nurse, yeah, she closed the curtain and handed me my baby. And was like, are you fine? And I'm just like, I don't understand like who makes these rules.

Dr. Scott: Rules. Yep.

Aaliyah: And having just changed them, why is not everyone on the same page?

Shante: They're not.

Toni: You guys all work the same [job].

Aaliyah: They have their own beliefs and then you put them all on me and it's like the nurses, some are more informed, some don't care. You know, they don't.

Without focusing on the reasons why Aaliyah needed additional support to ambulate and immediately judging Aaliyah, the more appropriate response is an ethical, legal, and scientific interrogation of hospital systems weaponizing the NICU as the new chattel slavery. An online dictionary definition of chattel slavery reads as follows: "the enslaving and owning of human beings and their offspring as property, able to be bought, sold, and forced to work without wages, as distinguished from other systems of forced, unpaid, or low-wage labor also considered to be slavery" (Dictionary n.d.). The hospital system's pattern of forced removals of Black newborn babies to occupy empty SCN or NICU beds, without the need to involve family policing systems, combined with the system's delay, denial, or disruption of Black mother-child reunification, bonding, and attachment, seems oddly reminiscent of the ideologies, practices, and impacts of chattel slavery.

What about demonstrating ambulation competency signifies caretaking competency? Even if the hospital documented a valid concern with evidential material to question the Black mother's capacity to independently care for her newborn in the immediate postpartum period, where was the corresponding psychiatric or social worker evaluation or hospital-initiated adult supervision? Where was the more humanistic and empathetic approach to ask Aaliyah's mother, the maternal grandmother to the Black baby, to supervise the Black mother-child reunification and attachment? Meaning-making of Black women's lived experiences of childbirth hospitalization during the provision of contemporary hospital-based obstetrics feels more and more like the new chattel slavery. Iatrogenic parent-child separation, independent of intention, is a valid harm as expressed and experienced differently by a people forced to endure disproportionate rates of kidnapping, human trafficking, chattel slavery, mass incarceration, and CPS involvement. Ahistorical and atheoretical approaches to obstetric care in medicine, nursing, social services, and mental health, that are also void of empathy and humanity, justify and perpetuate iatrogenic Black parent-child separation and isolation throughout multiple components in the continuum of hospital-based maternity and perinatal services. Iatrogenic parent-child separation within the boundaries of hospitals, even without involvement of family policing systems leads to disrupted kinship and other forms of emotional harms, including distress, anxiety, and fear.

When asked about the quality of care after childbirth hospitalization, during the first twenty-four to seventy hours postpartum, Black mothers shared a feeling of being abandoned and dismissed. Black mothers also shared additional testimonies of iatrogenic parent-child separation without parental notification or consent. When interrogating the NICU as the new chattel slavery, I am interrogating the institutionalized policies that define and shape physician and nursing practices and behaviors that endow physicians and nurses with unfettered authority to enter the room of a sleeping adult Black mother and Black father, remove the Black child, relocate the Black child to another room in another department/unit, and then proceed to initiate extraction of bodily fluids or injection of various substances via insertion of other various needles and IV lines without the expressed and enthusiastic consent of one or both Black parents. When does consent to childbirth hospitalization automatically revoke parental rights to make decisions about the health, safety, and well-being of one's own child? These birth narratives of Black families navigating system- or clinician-facilitated parent-child separation or delayed reunification, without the involvement of family policing systems, are violations of the right to parent existing children in safe, healthy, and sustainable environments (Ross et al. 2017; Ross 2017), free of the threat and/or real acts of violence or retaliation from the government and other systems and structures of power. Kinship disruption as a consequence of reinforcing power inequities between the medical-industrial complex and Black mothers, Black fathers, Black grandmothers, and Black families will never be sustainable or supported, and therefore remains a major violation of quality, safety, and human rights.

Jasmine, a Black mother in Los Angeles, recalled the memory of birthing her second child, holding her child, and then awakening in the middle of the night to her baby missing from her postpartum room, with her husband sleeping in the room with her and the baby girls.

> So with my son, that was great. With my daughter, though, I can remember having her, holding onto her, and then she was gone. And I was, like, well, where is my baby. Like, what time is it? What's happening. Oh, well, she's downstairs in the nursery. She was five-seven [five pounds seven ounces]. They said she needs to be downstairs because—because of your high blood pressure and because of the medicine that you're on. I was having the ear infection, so they gave me the medicine. So I kept going back and forth to sleep. I was, like, but her dad is right here. Like, why does she have to be in another area. I don't know how long that was, but I felt like it was forever. I had my baby at 12:26 in the afternoon. I have a feeling like I didn't really have her until like 7 o'clock at night. Like, on a full-on, like, I'm holding my baby. She's here with me. This is what's happening. And I didn't—I don't even think I really had her until they moved me to the other room. So I didn't—that communication was off to me. Granted, I was in and out of sleep because I was so exhausted, but I'm, like, her father's right here. Like, there's no reason for her to be in a whole nother [*sic*] area with other people when I'm here, you know, when he's here. So—and then even when I got to the second room, they didn't really check on me as much. It was kind of just, like, oh, you're here. Okay. And then when it was time for me to go, they were, like, all right, it's time to go. Like, hurry up and get your stuff. Like, I felt rushed the second time around. And I just didn't like that.

In the above scenario, Jasmine awakened to find her newborn Black baby girl missing. Once again, the opening line of a Black mother's postpartum narrative starts off like a scene in a Hollywood movie adaptation of a kidnapping or a day in the life of an enslaved Black mother on a plantation, "*I can remember having her, holding onto her, and then she was gone. And I was, like, well, where is my baby. Like, what time is it? What's happening.*" Jasmine included her baby girl's birthweight in her narrative as a clue to point the listener or reader to interrogate the weight criteria for a newborn to be admitted into the NICU, 5.5 pounds or 5 pounds and 8 ounces. What about the Black baby girl's condition, with a birthweight that was one ounce below weight criteria, warranted a NICU admission? Assuming the Black baby girl is a term infant birthed to a Black mother navigating preeclampsia, I wondered about the additional neonatal indications for the iatrogenic parent-child separation. As Jasmine explained in exquisite detail, the reasons provided by the hospital team focused exclusively on the Black mother's condition. If there was no other reason to take this Black baby girl from her Black mother and Black father, then one must interrogate the motivation for what feels like a forced Black parent-child separation, motivated to reinforce the clinician's self-worth or hospital policies and to uphold hospital domination over the Black mother and Black father and their Black baby, hence the framing of the NICU as the new chattel slavery. Forced Black parent-child separation and the motivations are the exact definition of Davis' dimension of obstetric racism, medical abuse (Davis 2020). The overall quality of care also violates other patient-community driven quality domains such as safety and accountability, autonomy, communication and information exchange, kinship, and empathy and humanity (discussed in greater detail in chapter 7). Likewise, forced parent-child separation reinforces anti-Black racism and anti-Black misogynistic notions that threaten the humanity and dignity of Black men and Black women. Uninterrogated acts of forced parent-child separation means hospital policies and practices and the people making and enforcing such policies and practices support the portrayal of Black men and Black women as "unfit and indecent" human beings, incapable of raising their own family and parenting their own children in safe and healthy environments, within their hospital postpartum rooms.

Ultimately, iatrogenic parent-child separation violates reproductive justice. Again, one must interrogate the motivation of the obstetric and NICU teams to forcibly remove a Black newborn baby from the presence and protection of her two physically and emotionally available and capable Black parents. Based on a prior analysis, the annual costs of NICU admissions were estimated at 26.2 billion US dollars per in the U.S. Additionally, the average cost of a NICU admission per term infant was calculated in the range of $2,500 to $2,900, with the average NICU stay being 2.2 days, compared to the cost of a NICU admission for a newborn with no complications at $800 (Cheah 2019). Cost analyses by the Health Care Cost Institute (HCCI) revealed that from 2017 to 2021, the number of newborns admitted to the NICU and the spending per NICU admission increased to higher levels (Valencia, Sen, and Martin 2023). Additional study findings revealed that increases in per-day spending contributed more to the escalating admission-level spending than actual increases in the number of days in an average NICU admission. The authors also provided insights into the drivers of increased daily spending, such as changes in service provision from low to high/more complex/resource-intensive services and/or increases in unit prices. The trends of NICU admissions, durations, and spending raised concerns about the possible overuse or misuse of these services, especially in situations where the high level of care may not be medically unnecessary, and sometimes incurring more medical risks than benefits. Likewise, the authors raised concerns for underutilization in situations where a NICU admission could be more valuable. In returning to the impacted families with a newborn in the NICU, the authors expressed concerns that activate empathy and humanity, the sixth and seventh patient-identified quality domains in the SACKRED Birth framework, discussed in greater detail in chapter 7. The data suggested that the additional costs of a NICU admission, in combination with potentially high out-of-pocket expenses for a recent childbirth hospitalization, possibly complicated by a medical co-morbidity requiring higher/more complex/resource-intensive staffing, services, and procedures, could leave families facing significantly higher than expected bills for both maternity care and newborn care (Valencia, Sen, and Martin 2023).

Turning our attention back to Jasmine's postpartum narrative, a forced iatrogenic parent-child separation for the purposes of a NICU admission of a term infant at five pounds seven ounces, with no other neonatal indications, seemed very suspicious. An empty NICU bed makes no money. As briefly mentioned in chapter 2, one must begin to interrogate NICU admissions as the new chattel slavery of Black newborn babies, with incubators and multiple IV lines serving as the new forms of incarceration and shackling of Black babies, funding a multibillion-dollar industry. With increasing rates of maternal death (Hoyert 2023), infant death (Hagen 2023), and preterm births (March of Dimes, n.d.) that disproportionately and unfairly impact Black mothers and Black babies, combined with the March of Dimes giving the U.S. a D+ for the second consecutive year in the context of forced inductions, forced cesarean births, and disproportionate rates of severe maternal health complications among Black reproducing bodies in military hospitals, including the performance of cesarean births and adult ICU admissions, compared to white reproducing bodies (Hamilton et al. 2021), the manufactured U.S. maternal health crisis is clearly profitable to powers that benefit from divestment, disruption, destabilization, dysregulation, and denial of Black kinship, liberation, and vitality. Again, examining the culture and practice of hospital-based obstetrics and neonatology outside of historical contexts, contemporary implications, and theoretical concepts such as empathy, humanity, health equity, obstetric racism, and reproductive justice leads to a very myopic, inaccurate, and imprecise evaluation of the root causes of the manufactured Black maternal and perinatal health crisis in the U.S.

Re-reading the narratives on kinship, particularly iatrogenic parent-child separation without involvement of family policing systems, reminds me of a Black mother in Los Angeles who shared her reflections on birthing in a hospital during the March 2019 focus groups, "You push out the baby, and then you go back to the fields, and you keep picking the cotton." Nearly two years after writing my initial draft of this chapter on kinship, I realize the Black mother, Tamara, never mentioned her role as a mother or the whereabouts of the Black baby she birthed. She never spoke of any of her kinship roles or relationships or the location of any other given or chosen family members. Her oral narrative focused exclusively on performing the reproductive labor of birthing another enslaved Black person and increasing her master's property and the productive labor of maintaining her master's land to sustain and advance her master's profit. The synthesis of both lived experiences of childbirth hospitalization while Black, Black forced parent-child separation or delayed and denied kinship reunification, and the system's need to keep NICU beds occupied with Black babies reinforces the analysis of Black hospital births as the new strategy for maintaining system profit. Thus, the system lacks any motivation to curtail the rising rates of Black maternal deaths, Black near deaths, Black infant deaths, and Black preterm births. One could then argue that the paucity of social capital at the level of individual Black mothers and Black families, as well as at the local community, county, state, regional, and, perhaps, national level, fuels the unnamed and unmitigated weaponizing of childbirth hospitalization as tools for disrupting, destabilizing, and dismantling Black kinship.

Putnam defined social capital as "features of social organization, such as networks, norms, and social trust that facilitate coordination and cooperation for mutual benefit" (Putnam 1995, 67). When asked to define social networks and social capital during childbirth hospitalization, Black mothers described the meaning and value of a live person at the bedside who exists outside of the medical-industrial complex, such as a partner, parent, chosen or given family, or a community birth professional such as a doula, community professional midwife, birth educator, or lactation educator. Black mothers often identified and described complex, dynamic, and nuanced social relations and strategies to activate and assert their autonomy during childbirth hospitalization. Black mothers also utilized existing or created novel social identities and relationships to curate experiences, conditions, and boundaries as acts of resilience and resistance when navigating power relations and inequities between them and hospital clinicians and staff both within and across phases of care (labor, birth, and immediate postpartum). Black mothers reimagined their worth within their self-defined social capital and then interpreted and responded to anticipated or actual experiences of hospital neglect, mistreatment, and abuse through given or chosen social relationships, which I renamed as kinship in 2019 during the initial development and validation of the patient-reported experience measure of obstetric racism©, also known as the PREM-OB Scale® suite (introduced in chapter 1 and discussed in greater detail in chapter 8) (Scott 2018; Scott 2019a; Scott 2019b; White VanGompel et al. 2022; Lett et al. 2023). Given the value and power of kinship in affirming the worth of Black mothers, Black mothers demand that hospitals acknowledge, affirm, and make space for kinship in its varied forms and modalities. Black mothers demand trust in birth workers and teams who will continuously prioritize and amplify their value, voice, wisdom, and lived experience even if the protection and advocacy serve as an indictment of hospital-based perinatal services.

The second manifestation of kinship, as defined for, by, and with Black mothers, is the inclusion (affirmation) or exclusion (denial or disruption) of a Black mother's partner, parent (grandparent to the baby), or any given or chosen family included in the provision of care and support. Black mothers also felt that they deserved support, protection, and advocacy that is specific and loyal exclusively to the Black mother, with no association or affiliation to the hospital system, health care team, or individual clinician or staff. Black mothers expressed the desire to have and harness the power to determine the number and types of support persons to be included or excluded during childbirth hospitalization, independent of birth attendant, setting, or modality (e.g., vaginal birth or cesarean birth). They expressed the desire for hospitals and health systems to include support persons and partners in clinical interactions, care, counseling, support, and decision-making. Black mothers voiced their need for capacity-building and support to align their birth expectation with their birth experience, especially with support persons during their labor, birth, and immediate postpartum. According to Black mothers, the imposition of control or constraint by hospital policies and practices that dictate who gets to be in the room where birth happens violates Black mothers' sense of belonging (their psychological safety and connectedness). Thus, Black mothers clarified how they utilized their social networks as conduits to achieving, protecting, and sustaining safety and accountability. Specifically, Black mothers leveraged the presence and participation of their support persons, particularly their husbands or mothers, as a shield, forcefield, overseer of their birth plan, or as an advocate to prevent or mitigate harm. A disruption of kinship as defined for, by, and with Black mothers occurs in hospital birth with the overlooking, exclusion, silencing, or diminishing of the presence or participation of support persons and partners in the provision of care and support, regardless of birth setting, space, attendant, position, or modality in the hospital. Previously, in chapter 4, Jada, a Black mother in Oakland, disclosed how the L&D team prevented her husband from being with her in the operating room, where she noticed a prioritization of other hospital workers.

> I had a bad experience though in the operating room. Because when I walked in, I felt like, you know, they had student[s]—probably like eight people in the room. And they asked my husband to wait out[side]. I'm like I need to have him. And they were all like—first, you know before they laid me down, I'm like I need to have him in the room right now. Because it's all like white and I don't see anything that I'm familiar with. They were like oh, you have to wait a little. I had to scream and start crying like I need to have my husband right here like right now.

In this example, the participant describes the literal and figurative feeling of unbelonging, psychological terror, separation, and loneliness as a Black reproducing body in a white sterile operating room, preparing to birth. Without knowing the deeper meaning of the phrase "it's all like white," one wonders if Jada meant white walls, bright white surgical lights, being surrounded by white people, or all three. The absence of familiarity tethered to the presence of whiteness illuminates the feelings of abandonment and isolation, especially within the context of desperately wanting and seeking out the comfort and familiarity of your support person, specifically a Black man in the chosen kinship role of husband and father. One can also see in this example the prioritization of other people in birth spaces, such as additional staff and learners in nursing, medicine, and other health care-related fields, especially during an abdominal birth (i.e., cesarean birth), which requires a different set of techniques, expertise, tools, conditions, and settings in comparison to a vaginal birth. The absence of dignity, empathy, and humanity in the operating room etiquette and protocol combined with a near kinship dismissal, disruption, and denial further demonstrates violations of quality as defined by, for, and with Black mothers.

Another Black mother in Oakland, LaToya, contributed to the ongoing discourse of hospital erasure and exclusion of Black husbands as part of the Black parent-child triad and larger given and chosen family. The emphasis on the parent-child dyad fails to recognize and then include the social and emotional needs, as well as the "surgical and sterile" readiness, of support persons unfamiliar with operating room standards of sterile practices. While "performing and managing" a cesarean birth, whether emergent, urgent, or routine, could be considered customary practice in a busy labor and delivery unit, hospital clinicians and staff must be mindful of varied levels of knowledge, comfort, confidence, and exposure to operating room etiquette. Establishing kinship as a valid quality measure linked to reimbursement and value-based incentive models of maternity care could facilitate widespread acceptance, endorsement, and adoption as a key performance and eliminate ongoing erasure or exclusion of given or chosen family in care. In the narrative below, LaToya shared how she wished her best friend could have served as a daddy doula to her husband because the hospital team lacked a combination of compassion, competency, clarity, comfort, and confidence in supporting men, particularly Black men.

> My husband was there but, you know, he was almost about to faint. Like it was crazy. He never seen anything like it, his first baby, he was already scared. He's asking the people and I felt like they should have been talking to him too as well. Because then he's asking them well forget the baby, is she going to be okay. He was nervous about them cutting me open. And they were like yeah, I know, pushing him off. And I felt like if it was my best friend, which my best friend knows him very well she would have been able to, you know—comfort

> him in ways like, she's going to be okay, it'll be okay. But he was a nervous wreck. I mean I feel like they should teach the men also. It was just stressing me out after like.

Establishing kinship as a valid quality measure linked to reimbursement and value-based incentive models of maternity care could facilitate widespread acceptance, endorsement, and adoption as a key performance and eliminate ongoing erasure or exclusion of given or chosen family in care. Incentivizing the design and implementation of clinical policies, protocols, or practices that prioritize the participation of given and chosen kin in patient care, along with the concurrent adoption of regular communication and consent of learners by patients to be involved in care would likely curate a more equitable and ethical participatory experience for all.

In chapter 4, Simone's narrative initially demonstrated how involving clinical learners in patient care without communication and informed consent violated the bodily, decisional, and care autonomy of Black mothers and Black babies. Simone announced to the Oakland focus group,

> Since we all had a C-section, I want to add to that. Because they had like three or five people just standing there. It's like a study, or something. They have all those new people and you can only bring like in one person. So, why are they standing there?

Making space for Black mothers' voices to be heard and felt, and then being held accountable for translating Black voices into victories means one recognizes the power and potential of supporting pathways that facilitate a stronger, more reliable, consistent, and intact Black parent-child bond and attachment prior to, during, and after birth.

At the same time, Black mothers, particularly those whose kinship includes the presence of Black men as husbands, fathers, uncles, brothers, and more, demanded hospital practices and policies recognize and support the presence and participation of Black men as trusted caregivers and protectors of Black mothers and babies. The importance of meaning-making of Jada's narrative in chapter 3 demonstrated how Black mothers' definition of safety and accountability is grounded in feeling love or loved. One pathway explicitly identified by Black mothers to curating love in childbirth hospitalization was the inclusion and integration of Black men, identified by Black mothers as of value to them, into care interactions, communications, and decision-making. Facilitating participation of Black men in care provision creates a culture of belonging (psychological safety and connectedness) and trust.

On the other hand, interrupting or disrupting kinship attachments or kinship-affirming activities ignites a series of harms with potentially very deep psychological wounds based on histories of anti-Black racism, anti-Black misogyny, eugenics, plantation colonialism, and chattel slavery dating back to the antebellum error. Contemporary manifestations of psychological, social, and cultural harms in obstetrics culture include repeatedly asking Black mothers with more than one child if they have one "baby daddy" or if the "baby daddy" is involved. The cognitive dissonance observed and felt by the obstetric medical-industrial complex in fixating on a non-existent problem, absentee Black fathers, in the midst of ignoring an actual problem, intentional exclusion and erasure of Black fathers in childbirth hospitalization, speaks volumes.

Inaction in the face of need is institutionalized racism (Jones 2000). Researchers debunked the notion of the absentee Black father based on science, with the evidence reported in the 2013 publication of a study titled, The Fathers' Involvement With Their Children: United States, 2006–2010, (Jones and Mosher 2013), as discussed in detail in chapter 2. The data revealed that Black fathers (70 percent), in comparison to white (60 percent) and Hispanic fathers (45 percent), who live with their children were most likely to have bathed, dressed, changed, or helped their child with the toilet every day. Black fathers (78 percent), in comparison to white (74 percent) and Hispanic fathers (64 percent), were also more likely to eat daily meals with their children. Black fathers (27 percent), in comparison to white (20 percent) fathers, were more likely to take their children to or from daily activities every day. Black fathers (41 percent), in comparison to white (28 percent) and Hispanic fathers (29 percent), overwhelmingly were also more likely to help their children with homework every day (Jones and Mosher 2013).

Given the data, the act of asking about Black fathers' involvement, in terms of their presence, participation, and persistence in one paternal lineage, outside of inquiries about genetic disorders, is fundamentally racist. Asking questions to Black mothers who show up to the hospital alone while actively excluding Black fathers standing up in the hospital room from participating in skin-to-skin bonding or keeping Black fathers from sitting at the head of the operating room table with anesthesiology with their loved one about to undergo a cesarean birth with eight other clinical learners in the room is egregiously racist. Once again, I shared the narrative of a nurse removing a Black baby from her Black father, in the presence of her Black mother, Jada.

> I want them to be more supportive of the dads. I didn't like . . . .when I had her and did bonding for like five minutes. And then my son's dad was like really excited about this baby, you know. So, he wanted her, and I gave her to him. And he took off his shirt. You know, he was so ready. It was just like we [the hospital clinicians and staff] need her to be with the mom right now and just like wrenched [removed] her out of his hands to give her back to me. And I was

> offended because I wanted him to, you know, [bond]. Yes, you know, he is just as much part of this baby as me. So, give him his time, you know.

Dismissing the value and benefit of skin-to-skin daddy-baby bonding and then physically removing a Black baby from the arms and chest of a Black father without hesitations reveals so much about the nurse, nursing culture, and the ethics, knowledge, and leadership of senior nursing clinical and administrative leaders. The behavior of the hospital nursing staff to physically remove a Black baby from chest and arms of their Black father's embrace demonstrates a form of entitlement and ownership over Black bodies and Black kinship bonds. The words of the Black mothers conjure up images of the antebellum slave period where plantation owners and slave-owners exerted their legal right to control and constrain the formation and separation of physical and social bonds between enslaved Black newborns and their enslaved Black mothers and Black fathers. Additionally, the behavior of the hospital nursing staff demonstrates unintended consequences of promoting a mother-child dyad at the exclusion and erasure of Black men as present, supportive, nurturing, and nourishing partners and parents. Likewise, the mother-child dyad prioritization also negates the possibility of different types of partnering, parenting, and family formation as demonstrated within our Black lesbian, queer, trans, non-binary, surrogacy, and adoption families and communities (Kerppola et al. 2019; Park 2019; Dankwa 2023).

For the first time in sharing the story of Jada, her partner, and their baby, the reader gains greater insight into the depth of the emotional wound made by the nurse's language and behavior, independent of her intention, pure heart, prior performance, years of nursing experience, or duration of employment.

> My boyfriend felt like he was not included. He just felt like well am I not as important as the mother in this situation. Does she [the newborn baby girl] not need to do that skin to skin bonding with me as well? But he prepared for this the whole time he was saying if he comes from work and I'm in labor he wants me to—when I packed my bag, he made me pack him some clothes so he could get in the shower just to make him smell good for his daughter. So, he was highly offended when they just wanted to take her from him and give her back. You know, especially after I gave her to him to give him that [experience]. He thought well what's wrong with him. You know, why are they treating me like this. I'm not a stranger, I'm her dad. And I felt the same way.

One of the most compelling arguments for developing, validating, and endorsing patient and community-identified and defined meanings, manifestations, and measures of "feeling safe" is the story of Jada, her partner, and her baby. The degradation, dehumanization, and devastation by the nurse's language and behavior can never be undone or unfelt. Among Black mothers and birthing people in kinship with Black men, they unapologetically deserve and demand the inclusion and integration of Black men in care, communication, interactions, and decision-making. Inclusion and integration of Black men in hospital-based births lead to increased perception and experience of safety and trust for Black mothers and birthing people. Among Black mothers with Black men as partners and parents, they see affirmations, activations, and actualizations of kinship in birthing while Black in hospital settings between Black mothers, Black fathers, Black gender-expansive parents, Black grandparents, Black babies, and surrounding given and chosen kin as a form of resistance against both the existence and conflation of several archetypes of Black socialization and life: Mammy, Jezebel, Sapphire, Superwoman, single mother, absent father, and dysfunctional attachments between Black mothers and fathers (Childs 2005; Collins 2004; Wyatt 1997; Abdullah 1998; Greene 1995; Greene 1994; Mitchell and Herring 1998; Thomas, Witherspoon, and Speight 2004; West 2012).

Lifting up another narrative from chapter 2, Chantelle expounded on manifestations of anti-Black medical abuse in clinical practice that reinforce anti-Black racism and misogynoir by deploying kinship-negating norms and narratives about Blackness, Black partnering, Black parenting, Black masculinity, Black fatherhood, Black femininity, and Black motherhood.

> They [Black men as parents, partners, family and friends] shouldn't have to force themselves into being included. But they [hospital clinicians and staff] should insure that he—any time they asked a question—something, something, something—he was speaking up. She came out looking like him. So, they didn't even know I was the mom. You know, they're like oh, your baby's so cute. They look at me like who's this dark woman. I think it's because they feel like it's not that common that you see Black women—Black couples because even then you're there they're just like, you know, they don't believe that I don't have more than one baby daddy. Or just that I've got to be a single mom so she needs to put her ring on, you know. And I have to let you know [to] include him. He was included in making this child. It's like they count on he's not going to be here.

Black mothers described and understood kinship as having mechanisms or strategies of resistance and resilience in place to communicate and reinforce their rights, priorities, needs, and wishes.

One act of resistance against degrading and dismissive care is holding hospitals and health systems accountable for continuously practicing (or seeking) informed consent and informed refusal with Black mothers and their given and chosen kin. Black mothers rely on kinship ties to hold hospitals and health systems accountable for acknowledging, supporting, and incorporating the capacity and capability of Black mothers and birthing people to heal and recover quickly from life challenges (external and internal resilience) in service provision. Returning to the kinship with Black men as partners, Black mothers described the strategy of explicitly calling out to their husbands, male partners, or other men in the room to obtain the attention and action needed in response to their implicit or explicit needs. Utilization of kinship in this manner demonstrated two truths: (1) Black mothers and birthing people recognize the patriarchal hierarchy of power in medicine, nursing, and health service provision; and (2) Black mothers and birthing people perceive and expect Black men in kinship to protect their dignity and humanity and to secure their safety.

In the narrative below, first introduced in chapter 2, Mariah spoke about her desire for her mother to be with her during birth based on shared histories of Black womanhood and Black motherhood. In the telling of her story during the Los Angeles focus group, Mariah realized the added yet different value of birthing with her husband, a Black man, as an act of refusal, resistance, and racial reconnaissance in preventing and mitigating hospital acts of obstetric racism and other unanticipated quality and safety violations.

> My husband. Let me tell you all, if that man was not there—I probably would be in tiny little pieces. Like, he was like my number one cheer—like, you can do it, babe. You're almost there. I was like you're right. I can do it. But he was like everything. And I just I was scared because I only had him. You know, that moment to me, I feel like I needed my mom. Like she's the only one who truly understands. But because I couldn't have her there and, you know, I didn't know how he was going to react. But he—I'm telling you all, he put people in their place. And he was like, this is what you're all going to do. He was in there praying. Like this is what's going to happen. And he's egging me on the entire time, and he made me feel like I wasn't alone. Like and that was so important to me. Because I did feel alone because I was going through everything physical. But he was just—it's like he just go in tune with me and I wanted him in that space, and he was there.

Contrary to societal archetypes of Black men in society, birth, particularly in hospital settings, revealed Black men as nurturers, advocates, and protectors based on the meaning-making and knowledge production of thirty-six Black mothers' narratives of childbirth hospitalization in Oakland and Los Angeles. Black mothers in relationships with Black men leveraged patriarchy by activating and exerting a type of kinship force with a male partner to demand respect and ensure recognition and fulfillment of the Black mother's desires and needs. Shanice explained how her husband is the reason she maintained decisional autonomy over her baby's feeding method.

> The only reason he didn't get formula was because of my husband. If I was alone or, you know, and I even think my mother wouldn't have been as forceful.

> As that male, you know, as my husband don't—do not give my baby this. So, I know if it wasn't for my husband, that he would have got formula.

Shanice also recognized the potential limitation in wielding the power of an elder maternal grandmother, given the system's predilection for male-centered and responsive authority in maternity spaces.

Black fathers continued to show up as protectors and enforcers of Black mothers' plans for nourishing and nurturing their Black newborn baby. In the context of the parent-child dyad, Black mothers described experiences of disrupted kinship when hospital clinicians and staff dismissed their expressed wishes around infant feeding and care. Subsequently, Black mothers exerted acts of resistance to obstetric racism in the forms of hospital neglect and disrupted kinship by calling upon their Black male partners, the Black baby's father, to communicate and reinforce their rights, priorities, needs, and wishes of Black women as patient, partner, and parent. Ebony recalled how her nurse repeatedly dismissed her expressed plan of care, demonstrated by the nurse never placing the order for what Ebony requested. Thus, she never received the item, prompting her to transition to a more assertive and persistent mode of communication until her husband intervened and communicated directly with the nurse on behalf of his wife.

> For me, it was my husband. I don't think that I was heard because like when I was—I [spoke] with my nurse over and over and I told her that that was my plan. And it was like she disregarded what I said and never put the order in. And so, I never received it. So, now I have to go get it after. And it was like, but when my husband went after and like so, it was long. Like when he went to go speak to someone, it was, you know, they were aggressive about getting whatever he said—that needed to be done. But when I spoke to the nurse that was directly helping me, it was like I [was't there]. Unless I told him and he was like we'll see.

Based on the prior narratives, kinship serves as a shielding mechanism by which Black mothers reclaim their autonomy, agency, and emotional, cultural, social, and clinical safety. Black mothers activate kinship that situates Black men in birthing spaces in the roles of protector and compliance officer, a type of enforcer who holds systems accountable to and in alignment with optimally recognizing and responding to the needs and desires of Black mothers and birthing people when Black mothers and infants can no longer trust and rely on hospital nurses and physicians to do the bare minimum of their jobs.

As previously described, Black mothers and birthing people utilize existing social identities and relationships to curate experiences, conditions, and boundaries as acts of resistance against obstetric racism in the form of diagnostic lapses, neglect, medical abuses, coercion, ceremonies of degradation, and intentionally causing pain (Davis 2018; Davis 2019; Davis 2020; Davis, Varner, and Dill 2021; Davis 2022a; Davis 2022b). At times, Black mothers benefited from a force dyad, first described in chapter 4, as the combined efforts of a Black mother and Black father in mitigating obstetric racism to preserve, protect, actualize, and amplify a Black mother's autonomy. In this chapter, I explore a second force dyad, the combined wills of the Black mother's husband and mother, the maternal grandmother. During the Oakland focus group, Tasha revealed a series of very harmful events throughout her childbirth hospitalization and extending beyond the hospital. Tasha endured a cesarean birth for unknown reasons that the hospital team failed to adequately communicate to her, her husband, a Black man, and her mother, a Black nurse. Tasha's husband and mother served as advocates and shields, creating a cocoon of love in defense of multiple hospital acts of obstetric racism.

> Okay. I think—well, things I wanted were heard but my husband spoke up for me rather than me saying it myself. When I said something , [hospital response] was kind of nonchalant, but when he said it, they're like, oh, okay, well, let's try that or let's try this, and that was pretty irritating, but it helped that he was there. And my mom, my mom spoke up about a lot. Like I was having convulsions after I gave birth and I couldn't even hold her. Like I was shaking so bad that I couldn't do anything. And they were trying to play it off as if it was okay and that it was my body getting rid of the medicine. But my mom was like—my mom has nursing in her background. She's like no, that's not normal. And they're like, well, her temperature is high and—but the baby doesn't have an infection. So, I guess to them if the baby doesn't have an infection, then my body should be okay since she didn't get it. So that just gave me—they had me doing Tylenol and Motrin back to back to try and drop my fever, but it was kind of—but I think the experience wasn't hard because my mom spoke up for me.

Tasha benefited from the combined yet unique powers in the force dyad of her husband and her mother. With her husband, she recognized and leveraged the power of patriarchy in catalyzing the hospital nurses to respond to her needs through the expressed will of her husband on her behalf. Through her irritation and disappointment in being initially ignored and dismissed, she resisted by utilizing her knowledge and understanding of patriarchy and mobilized her husband to execute her vision of how she desired and deserved to be treated. With her mother, Tasha utilized her knowledge of her mother's experiential, ancestral, spiritual, mainstream, and professional knowledge as a nurse to push back against any diagnostic lapses, neglect, medical abuse, or intentional causes with no motivation to end her suffering as a Black mother. The kinship force dyad of a Black mother's husband and mother demonstrated the importance of exploiting patriarchy and professionalization in favor of mitigating obstetric racism through resistance.

Black women activated kinship with their mothers and sisters (grandmothers and aunties to the Black baby) when they needed to challenge the power differential between patients and the medical-industrial complex within and across phases of care (labor, birth, and immediate postpartum). Black mothers described the use of non-peer social networks, the kinship between Black women as mothers, daughters, and sisters, as strategies to address social and clinical isolation, neglect, and abandonment during the provision of care in hospital settings. Black mothers provided further elaboration about this selective form of kinship with their mothers and sisters, as well as with Black women family substitutes such as hospital nurses and staff who act as advocates, cheerleaders, and other various forms of social, emotional, mental, physical, and clinical supports. In chapter 2, Tiffany's narrative demonstrated one of many ways nurses extend the reach and impact of their tenderness and care beyond their assigned patients. The nurse played a critical role by being with Tiffany in the physical absence of her mother who could not miss work for a second consecutive day. With technology, desire, capacity, and creativity, Tiffany's mother remained virtually present, engaged, and supportive.

> On the day of my induction it felt really, really well and really good for me because like my family wasn't there. My mom had came because she took off work but the baby didn't come. And I didn't want my mom to take off the second day and then she didn't come again. So, my mom was on the phone the whole time while I was giving birth, but just having that—having her there and like those two nurses for the—for the most part was like everything.

Black mothers tapped into a form of sisterhood-kinship as a mechanism by which biological sisters serve as protectors and enforcers of a Black mother's needs as determined in oral or written communication within the family structure. A Black mother's sister also managed the room, serving as the family team lead to oversee the hospital team by re-centering the focus on the Black mother. In the hours leading up to her birth, Ayana discovered that her assigned prenatal health provider, whom she had seen weekly, would not be available to attend or support her hospital birth. Having her trusted sister present and managing the room and the hospital team reassured Ayana, giving her the continuity of care, psychological safety, and connectedness that was missing due to the unexpected and undesired absence of the prenatal health provider with whom she had built a near ten month repoire.

> And I wasn't nervous. Well, I—well, she was coming, but—I was nervous but I wasn't nervous more so as far as like the care that I was in. And I had my sister and her dad there. Oh, and my sister is very outspoken, so she wasn't going to

> let nothing happen. My sister also felt like they were kind of lagging because like I had the ball, the bag [foley bulb] that was inside your vagina. And when it was time to take it out, I started feeling it because they ended up popping my water bag. And that in particular day there were so many moms coming in to like have their babies. And I honestly felt like there wasn't that many nurses there, but like I didn't see all of them so I don't know how many exactly was there, but—at one point, my sister was like, okay, you all need to come on, my sister is in pain, this baby is coming, but they ended up coming, right. So, like as far as all of that, it was good. I had—like I said, I went in knowing that the lady that I see every week wasn't going to deliver my baby.

One Black mother in the Oakland focus group prepared for a battle of wills with the hospital system, team, and individual clinician staff. In Kendra's preparation to resist and refuse acts of obstetric racism, she assembled an army of protectors and enforces to maintain her right to decisional and bodily autonomy. Kendra formed her very own Birth Justice League or the Birthtastic Four to fight and defend herself and her family from quality and patient safety violations.

> Not only that, it was just like the topic of discussion throughout the whole day. Like everybody already knew—Me, my husband, my mother-in-law, my sister-in-law. Like everybody that was in the room, you know, we already knew what I wanted. So, we just made sure that was circulating in the room, yes, to the staff.

Kendra created a human forcefield of belonging and love in the form of her given and chosen kin to ensure she remained safe, seen, heard, supported, comforted, and cared for during her childbirth hospitalization. Assembling one's own Black Futures Birth Justice League and activating their powers to form a kinship forcefield describes the Herculean effort made by Black women to avoid or mitigate racist encounters, which Davis calls racial reconnaissance (Davis 2020; Davis, Varner, and Dill 2021; Davis 2022a; Davis 2022b).

In another birthing narrative from the Oakland focus group, Kiara described a series of quality violations that aligned with the dimensions of obstetric racism: diagnostic lapses; clinical neglect, dismissiveness, and disrespect; ceremonies of degradation; and medical abuse. She presented to labor with regular and frequent contractions occurring every five minutes. Although she did not experience severe discomfort, "it wasn't painful," she realized she could not talk through a contraction. The significance of Kiara's birth narrative for the purposes of this chapter is to highlight the benefit of having the wisdom and strength of one's Black mother, who also happens to be a community doula.

> I just was short of breath. And the lady [the nurse]—they took forever. The nurse. The nurse took forever because she felt like—Took forever to come into the room to check me. She felt like, oh, well, the chart says you're only—you're seven minutes apart so it's not bad, it's not bad, she's still—oh, it's not bad, you're good. Being that I'm—I have a breech baby and I'm telling you that I'm in labor and my mom is a doula. She'd been counting like at the time and everything. I was five minutes apart, even shot to three sometimes. And so finally she came like I want to say an hour or two hours later and checked me and was like, oh, because you would send me home being, I had a breech baby. And she was like, oh, wow, you're 3, 3-1/2 centimeters and completely [effaced], so yeah, we're going to see what we're going to do. My mom said, oh, she's not going home to become complete, she's going to dilate every hour—and which I did by—I went in at 4:00—I went in at 4:00 p.m. and I had her at 9:50 that night. So, if I would have went back home, I would have delivered a breech baby and anything could have happened, you know. And it's just the fact that she didn't trust me.

In Kiara's birthing narrative, her mother was present, listening, watching, and assessing the clinical situation at the bedside during the triage evaluation. Unbeknownst to the L&D triage nurse, the Black maternal grandmother possessed dual lived experience and expertise as a birthing person and birth worker, a doula. Kiara activated a kinship situated at the intersection of parenting and professionalism, a particular type of advocacy and protection driven by the forces of nature and nurture. The utilization of a transitional kinship with hospital nurses to curate experiences of safety, empathy, and humanity repeats throughout the Oakland and Los Angeles Black hospital birthing narratives. Navigating a major abdominal surgery where one is awake, to birth one's child, without anyone familiar or familial at your side can be terrifying. For Simone, forming transitional kinship with the anesthesiologist and the nurses mitigated fear, loneliness, and disconnection. Kinship in this formation, although temporary, sent Simone external cues to her internal sensors that she was worthy of support and love on the day she would bring forth life in the form of a Black baby.

> So, my—is it an anesthesiologist? He was a Black male. He definitely—he assured me everything was going to be fine. He would touch me, say can you feel here, can you feel there, can you breathe, and I'm like I can breathe. He asked me—you know, they were like do you need blankets, are you cold, feel warm.
>
> When they did the spinal, they held me because my mom couldn't be in there with me and her father wasn't there, so I was already really scared—being that my mom couldn't be in the room with me. So, the nurses hugged me as they did the spinal. So, I just—in that way I guess I felt cared for, loved, and safe in that way. They surrounded me with love and care. And they asked me

> if I wanted to—because now H1 offers an option to where the drape can drop clear—so you can see your baby get pulled out. So, they offered that to me, if I wanted to see her getting pulled out and—sorry if I get a little emotional too. But yeah, and—yeah, they like offered that to me, so—it like—it definitely made my experience a little better. [in tears]….t's like always emotional. But yeah, like them being able to just give me that option because I already was just sad that—I would say naturally, but I was sad that I couldn't have her vaginally.

A recurring theme throughout the Oakland and Los Angeles Black birthing narratives in hospital settings is the value of having the Black mother's mother, the maternal grandmother of the Black baby, at the bedside throughout the entire labor, birth, and immediate postpartum experience. Black mothers rely heavily on transgenerational maternal kinship to activate, sustain, and protect their autonomy and safety. Another benefit of transgenerational maternal kinship is the assurance of comprehensive, responsive, and relevant communication and information exchange between Black mothers and hospital staff. In Oakland, Imani shared the transformative and therapeutic power of birthing with one's own birth mother as Black women and Black mothers.

> My mom was there by my side the whole time. She brought me—I don't even remember what I had, but I just know she went somewhere and got me something when I had my first—when I had my son because she knew the hospital food was not going to cut it. But she was my ears, you know, when I was there and not really understanding quite everything. But she was just there for me. I didn't actually find out until, I think, after I had my son that my mom had an abortion when she was younger. So for her to even, you know, be supportive of me being a single mom twice, you know. So this—very supportive 100 percent.

In the same way that Black hospital birthing narratives disrupted societal tropes of Black husbands and fathers as absent or negligent, birth created a pathway for redefining trust and transparency in transgenerational maternal kinship. Birth facilitated a greater understanding, acceptance, and appreciation of norms and narratives around Black womanhood, motherhood, and lactation between Black mothers and daughters. In Los Angeles, Shante reminisced about having her mother be present and show up for her, her birth, and her breastfeeding dreams, although her mother did not breastfeed her. She leveraged transgenerational maternal kinship as a strategy to extend her surveillance and force field beyond her L&D room through the body of her mother. Through the presence, participation, and power of a Black maternal grandmother, a Black mother expands her parental autonomy, agency, and self-efficacy.

> My mom was the same. She didn't breastfeed or anything, but she knew what I wanted with him [male newborn]. So even when I was getting stitched back up, I had her go to the baby and make sure nothing changed. You know, she stayed with us. I said go with him. I don't want—I don't want anything. I don't want them sticking him with nothing. I don't want, like, I need to make sure I'm there to control everything. Like, if I'm not there, you be there.

Based on Black hospital birthing narratives, kinship serves as a form of racial reconnaissance (Davis 2020; Davis, Varner, and Dill 2021; Davis 2022a; Davis 2022b) to avoid or mitigate anti-Black racist or anti-Black misogynistic experiences during social and clinical interactions, communications, counseling, decision-making, and documentation and dissemination of health care information in patient handoffs, patient sign-outs, and electronic health records. Hospital practices and policies that undermine access to and utilization of kinship undermine our dignity, humanity, and justice.

Alternatively, hospital practices and policies can protect and preserve Black kinship, and thereby shift the assumption or narrative that the Black people present for the Black birthing person are not considered social or biological kin. The initial denial of intact, active, and reliable Black kinship ties and practices by hospital clinicians and staff is demonstrated by the immediate and persistent inquiry about the whereabouts of the biological father, as explained by Simone, who contributed to the 2020 revision of the 2019 domain names, meanings, and measures,

> I think the only thing I would change is the assumption that we are not families in the birthing experience because, like I said when I had my daughter, the first thing all the doctors kept saying is "Oh, oh, does she have a different dad than the dad that was actually at the birthing experience?" Multiple doctors asked me that question like it was unbelievable that my daughter could have the same dad as her brother. I'm like, "Yeah, why do you guys keep asking me that?" But it's just the assumption of us just having multiple fathers and that we can't be a united family, you know?

Hospital practices and policies reflect societal tropes of the "dysfunctional, fractured, unstable, disadvantaged, and unreliable" Black family as described in the 1965 Moynihan report (Office of Policy Planning and Research, United States, Department of Labor 1965). The beginning of Chapter 2 on The Negro Family asserts that "at the heart of the deterioration of the fabric of Negro society is the deterioration of the Negro family. It is the fundamental source of the weakness of the Negro community at the present time" (Office of Policy Planning and Research, United States, Department of Labor 1965, 5). When hospital standards of obstetrics and perinatal care reflect the biased, racist, and heteropatriarchal notions and norms of white supremacy found in the Moynihan report, then one better understands and appreciates the origins and perpetuators of separate but equal visitation policies for Black families and other non-Black families.

> Originally, when I—I had my baby at Hospital 8 in Lynwood. And that's my daughter. Originally, they told me I could only have two people in there. And I was, like, kind of want three. Is that possible? Because I definitely wanted my mom and my daughter's father in there. And then I had to have my auntie because she's the nurse. So I got to have somebody that understands all this information. But come to find out I was able to actually have four in there. So my—my daughter's father—my daughter's aunt was in there, as well. So that was nice in addition to her grandmother. So—but when I went there—you know, when you first look at hospital rooms, like, ain't nobody fit in here. Like, you just have that feeling ain't nobody going to be able to be in here with you. But I ended up having the people that I wanted in the room. So I was very blessed in that.

Zaria, one of the Black mothers in the Los Angeles focus group, who activated kinship forces in the form of her mother, maternal grandmother, her daughter's father, Black male co-parent, her auntie, maternal aunt and nurse, and a third Black woman, her daughter's paternal aunt. Hospital practices and policies that preserve, activate, or amplify Black kinship counter the societal narratives of Black family and Black love dating back from chattel slavery to the 1965 Moynihan report to the 2013 study titled "Fathers' Involvement With Their Children: United States, 2006–2010." Based on these data, Black fathers are the best, and, well, other fathers could benefit from a national call to action (Jones and Mosher 2013).

The benefits of kinship recognition, preservation, actualization, and activation positively impact the health care experiences of the Black mother and her family. Likewise, honoring the humanity and dignity of affirming Black kinship extends beyond the patient. Imagine the power of creating a ripple effect within the medical-industrial complex that has the potential to disrupt existing stereotypes, scripts, and stories held by hospital clinicians, staff, and administrators about the existence, structure, function, and impact of Black biological and social kinship. Unfortunately, the medical-industrial complex creates medically unnecessary and ethically inappropriate decisions when Black kinship is denied the right to exist and flourish, especially during hospital births. The denial of transgenerational maternal kinship during a non-emergent cesarean birth for fetal breech presentation, especially given the value and necessity as previously explained through the emotions and experiences of Black mothers, points to the perceived threat of kinship by the medical-industrial complex.

Kiara's entire hospital experience contained invaluable lessons on how hospitals reproduce acts of obstetric racism and violate multiple quality and patient safety violations.

> So they had me—and they—it turns out I was actually in early labor, and I didn't know it. So because I had already went into labor, they said he was still breech, so they had to schedule the C-section. I was really pushing—I wanted to give him that time to flip, because I've heard stories of him—you know, the babies flipping literally at the last week. I gave birth to him at 39 weeks, and it—during the C-section—so I had my mom in the room with me, my—his father, unfortunately, is incarcerated at the moment. So my mom was in the room with me, and they wouldn't allow her to look over the thing. And usually, I've heard—you know, like some people have the clear curtain where you can actually watch. Yeah. So they didn't offer that. They said they couldn't—they don't—they don't have the clear one, and you're not allowed to look over. Which was strange for me, because I'm, like—there are people who literally watch the whole—like, I didn't—I didn't understand why I couldn't watch, or see, or anything, and they wouldn't allow her to look. She really believes that he wasn't breech, and she strongly—like, she feels strongly about that. And then—and I—they literally argued, like, in front of me while I'm open, paralyzed—I'm—I'm panicking. I can't see anything, and they wouldn't—they wouldn't let her look over until he was out. Once he was out, they let her stand up and she could see.

For the first time, kinship was characterized as an organizing strategy for clarifying truth, promoting transparency, and holding systems accountable for achieving a SACKRED birth in hospital settings by preventing and mitigating obstetric racism. The maternal grandmother bearing witness to the birth of her grandchild served two purposes, safeguarding the safe arrival of the passenger and verifying the indication of a low-risk term primary cesarean birth based on a prior diagnosis of fetal malpresentation. Never did the participant share that hospital staff performed an ultrasound prior to the transfer to or during her entry into the operating room to confirm fetal presentation. Birth is both a personal and political act given the degree to which Black mothers exert kinship to protect their autonomy and secure their safety, especially if the kinship extends to professional birth workers such as doulas and nurses.

In the Los Angeles focus group, Aaliyah recalled how the hospital attempted to limit the number of people who could support her and participate in her hospital birth in the community. As time progressed in her labor, she began to push and prepare to welcome her baby. Then she realized how the hospital staff manipulated the visitation policy to exert control and dominance over the quality and quantity of support persons at her birth.

> They limited the amount of people that, you know, could come in. But then at—on the actual day of delivery, like, I had family and everything, like, it was more people, so I'm, like, what? And my doula could've been here. But I think that that was by design, you know—because my doula was going to follow my birth plan, you know, to the T—and make sure that all of these things—and

> they know that, you know. They know that when you're educated about certain things, you know, they try and lie and manipulate—at least that's my experience—is that I felt very manipulated out of what my desires were, in order, you know—so, like she said,—the—the interest that the hospital staff have is for the hospital.

Based on Black hospital birthing narratives, hospital policies and practices sometimes prioritized the presence and participation of learners from different health care professions, such as medical and nursing students and medical residents and fellows. Based on the perspectives and experiences of Black mothers, hospitals were more likely to assign clinical learners to Black mothers or other folks with marginalized voices, sometimes without informed consent. The displacement of Black biological and social kin in favor of clinical learners can be viewed as socially negligent, clinically dismissive, and ethically inappropriate. Patrice, from the Los Angeles focus group, chose vulnerability in the presence of a transitional yet chosen Black kinship to voice her regret for not having the knowledge, courage, or wherewithal to decline the participation of learners in her birth. And in the company of Black women, Patrice felt psychologically safe and connected to speak her truth, nearly seven months after the violation. This is the power of Black femme kinship. PERIODT!

> And I have a seven-month-old now. And for the second time around, I wanted to give myself an excellent way to speak up more about this delivery, because with my—with my son, I felt like I didn't—I didn't—there were things that were happening during my labor that shouldn't have, like, there were students in—in my room when I was pushing. And I was just, like, why are they here? Oh, they—this is a practicing hospital—I didn't know about that. You know, so with—Yeah, [a] teaching hospital, you know. I didn't—I wasn't aware of that in the beginning. I would just—it was—it was all—can—you can imagine, I was embarrassed, I was in pain, you know, it was just weird.

The prioritization of the visibility and involvement of clinical learners at the exclusion or erasure of Black kinship in hospital births, particularly in teaching hospitals, underscores the need for a re-examination of the actors and factors defining and shaping health services provision and interprofessional education and training. At the intersection of health services provision, training, and evaluation is patient-centered access to care, driven by five dimensions of systems accessibility and five corresponding population abilities (Levesque et al. 2013). Thus, medical education requires continuous consensual inclusion and involvement of patients, caregivers, and given and chosen communities.

This chapter identified and characterized a multitude of strategies and solutions that Black mothers leverage through kinship to address quality violations and hospital acts of obstetric racism in clinical practices, decision-making, and care delivery within and across the five other patient-identified quality domains in the SACKRED Birth framework: safety and accountability; autonomy; communication and information; anti-Black racism and medical misogynoir; empathy and humanity; and dignity in Blackness and holistic care. An ethical pathway toward a Black feminist-centered access to SACKRED birth care in hospital settings requires practices, processes, and policies grounded in equity and empathy. The manifestation of a Black feminist birth in a hospital system acknowledges, affirms, activates, actualizes, and amplifies Black kinship as a form of resistance to obstetric racism in health services provision and training. The denial of Black kinship reproduces despair, degradation, disconnections, and dehumanization during labor, birth, and immediate postpartum. At the same time, the celebration and expansion of Black kinship during childbirth hospitalization protects the power, sanctity, and humanity of Black births and Black legacies. Actualizing and amplifying Black kinship during childbirth hospitalization for Black mothers and birthing individuals is an act of political warfare against disproportionate, preventable, predictable, and unfair pregnancy-related deaths and near deaths among Black families and communities.

Chapter 7

Holistic Care

Empathy, Humanity, and Dignity in Blackness

> I think what was missing for me was the afterbirth checkup. So, like I said, they left me pretty much on my own. They didn't do nothing. So, they came in the room, you know. They did the morning shift change and asked me questions. And, specifically, they asked, you know, are you bleeding, how much are you bleeding. And I told them I wasn't bleeding. For two days, I didn't bleed after. It was like oh, that's a miracle, everybody bleeds. And I kept telling them I wasn't bleeding. And on the second—or that night on the second day I went to go use the bathroom and blood came out of me. The whole room was covered in blood. And it scared me so bad because it was something that dropped. It was like it was a drop. And there was blood all, I mean all over the room. And I called my—I was just calling the nurse. Like what's going on? She's bleeding, she's bleeding. And that's how the one lady came in and was like that's where the blood was. She kind of joked, you know. And I'm scared to death. Like I don't know (overlapping). I'm like oh, my God, like I need to go back to, you know, to surgery or what's going on? And she's just like oh, it's fine. This is what we were looking for all these three days. But I'm like if I'm telling you at least that one day that I haven't bled wouldn't somebody go up there and check? You know, something ain't quite [right]. And they cleaned—they had to move the bed out, the towels out. We had to sit outside in the hallway for them to clean up. They had towels everywhere. And then they just was like okay, go take a shower if you can. Do you need help? Okay, and then put a pad on and that was it.

In chapter 2, Dominique, a Black mother in the Oakland focus group, recalled feeling coerced and ultimately forced to undergo a cesarean birth. The obstetric medical-industrial complex included making threats to involve CPS and packaging information as part of their communication, consent, and decision-making process. By chapter 3, Dominique opened up about the regret, guilt, and worry of restricting her diet and caloric intake due to medical advice, and then having her baby born with neonatal hypoglycemia, lower than normal blood glucose levels for a newborn. Dominique never questioned her physician's dietary advice, and he never gave her a medical diagnosis to restrict her diet. Furthermore, her physician never took responsibility for the adverse impact of his unsubstantiated medical advice and therapy. The quality of care provided to Dominique did not align with the six quality domains as established and defined by the AHRQ and NAM (AHRQ 2022), first introduced in chapter 1: safe, effective, patient-centered, timely, efficient, and equitable.

Based on Dominique's detailed and graphic description of her afterbirth, she experienced postpartum hemorrhage. She and her newborn survived a birth complicated by a postpartum hemorrhage without the need for the administration of blood products (e.g., blood transfusion), transfer into the adult intensive care unit, or surgical or other invasive interventions to control the bleeding or save Dominique's life. From a pure clinical perspective, traditional standards of quality care would prioritize and even celebrate the fact that a Black mother and her baby survived childbirth hospitalization complicated by a postpartum hemorrhage without blood transfusion or any other life-saving measures. The absence of a holistic Black woman-person focused approach to obstetrics care, especially for responding to severe maternal morbidity including postpartum hemorrhage, creates a culture of harm (Scott and Davis 2022). The last memory of Dominique's nurse in this very scary situation included an image of a nurse giving orders, "*okay, go take a shower if you can. Do you need help? Okay, and then put a pad on.*" The nurse's bedside manner is methodical and robotic and void of empathy, dignity, and humanity. The nurse and the entire hospital team missed an opportunity to acknowledge and affirm a Black mother's dignity and humanity by emotionally connecting with a Black mother and making space to hold her feelings of living through an obstetric emergency.

Although the mechanics of an obstetric emergency may appear routine and common to the bedside postpartum nurse, the phenomenon may be new and unusual to the Black mother. Therefore, one may interpret the nurse's performance as standard, clinically appropriate, and harmful. All three can be true at the same time. In that moment, Dominique was searching for empathy from her postpartum nurse. And the nurse, like many nurses and physicians, failed to meet a Black mother's expectations for empathy after surviving a postpartum hemorrhage that left her own blood covering the entire room.

> The whole room was covered in blood. And it scared me so bad because it was something that dropped. It was like it was a drop. And there was blood all, I mean all over the room. . .. And they cleaned—they had to move the bed out, the towels out. We had to sit outside in the hallway for them to clean up. They had towels everywhere.

Reading Dominique's deliberate choice of words evoked images of a violent act or series of violent acts culminating in death, like the scenes from a horror movie or a documentary on war. Instead, Dominique granted us direct access to the story behind the statistic. Survival is merely the floor in the battle (more like war) for a SACKRED Birth.

The remainder of the conversation between me and Dominique included my inquiry about the additional support and communication offered to Dominique while living through such a terrifying experience, during which time her hospital room looked like a murder scene.

> *Dr. Scott:* Was there an explanation shared with you as to why for two days you didn't see blood and then at the second day there was all this blood. Did anyone provide any insight?
>
> *Dominique:* They told me they never saw that before and that, you know, they said after that, they're going to check the pad and if you soak up more than two pads in an hour or less than three hours, let them know. That was the only follow up after that.
>
> *Kiara:* I've got a question. So, when you were bleeding, they didn't change your [pad]—because after I had my C-section you're supposed to bleed. Oh, you didn't bleed at all?
>
> *Dr. Scott:* So, for two days there was no bleeding. And no one said anything to her.
>
> *Dominique:* I mean they asked me that night.
>
> *Dr. Scott:* But they didn't respond with like that it's actually unusual to not bleed when you've had a birth.
>
> *Dominique:* They should have checked.
>
> *Kiara:* I know it's hard for you, Participant #3.
>
> *Dominique:* Thank you, Kiara.

The absence of a follow-up explanation from the postpartum combined with the callous, yet clinically appropriate, care provides an accurate snapshot of the impact of obstetric quality in U.S. birthing hospitals. One of many pivotal moments during these transformative healing sessions was the authentic connections being formed in real-time between the focus group participants (peer sharing and bonding) and between me and the focus group participants. The demonstration of empathy from a peer participant about the Black mother's experience reveals the profound scarcity of empathy and humanity in the provision of health and human services in U.S. birthing hospitals. In the field of medicine, medical educators and professional organizations recognize the value of empathy in the provision of care as expressed or modeled in behavior by physicians. However, empathy in medical care differs from empathy in everyday life. Outside of medicine, empathy is defined as an affective mode of understanding that involves being moved by another's experiences. In contrast, the medical field defines and expects a form of empathy that maintains fidelity to the medical norms and narratives of objectivity and detachment.

One medical professional organization defined clinical empathy as an act of properly acknowledging the emotional state of the mother without experiencing that state itself (Halpern 2003; Markakis et al. 1999). An unintended negative structural consequence of the 1999 definition of clinical empathy is the development of a physician workforce that values and prioritizes intellectual or institutional (mainstream) forms of knowing and knowledge over experiential, emotional, spiritual, and cultural forms of knowing and knowledge. The uptake of "intellectual" empathy by medical students, resident physicians, medical fellows, and attending physicians requires dismissing what a patient feels, knows, and thinks as substantial forms of knowledge, data, or information. Intellectual empathy then becomes a primary lever that defines and shapes the ethics, leadership, knowledge, science, measurement selection and monitoring strategies, quality and accessibility, and levels of community participation and partnership that reproduce and reinforce epistemic injustice, testimonial injustice, and hermeneutical injustice (Fricker 2007; Scott 2021; Lyndon et al. 2023).

The 1999 definition of empathy mirrors the definition from the 1950s to 1960s in which "professional" or "clinical empathy" is viewed as cognitive, detached reasoning that avoids over-identifying with patients (e.g., sympathy) (Blumgart 1964; Aring 1958). Neutral empathy allows for predicting a patient's response to their illness through careful observation without feeling grief, regret, or other challenging emotions (Blumgart 1964). Neutral empathy stems from the writings of Sir William Osler, who argued in 1889 that physicians who successfully neutralized their emotions to a point where they feel nothing or numb in response to patient suffering facilitates the numb physician's capacity to "see into" and subsequently "study" the patient's "inner life" (Osler 1910; Sokol 2007). In 2003, a physician scientist synthesized the various empathy definitions to provide greater insight into the meaning of neutral empathy. They described a visual metaphor of detachment that involves projecting the patient's inner life before the physician's third eye.

By taking on the positionality of a viewer who stands separate from what they observe in the patient differs from society's meaning of empathy. In the traditional sense, empathy facilitates "feeling into" or being emotionally moved by another's suffering, which requires emotional attachment (Halpern 2003). A physician who can correctly view a patient's emotions with detached concern begins as a medical student capable of succeeding in anatomy class during the dissection of a cadaver without disgust. That same level of detached concern, void of emotions, then permits a physician to listen empathically without becoming emotionally involved (Fox and Lief 1963). Thus, the standard of care for professional or clinical empathy is neutral empathy that requires turning off one's own humanity to be able to practice detached concern void of emotions.

In returning to the chapter's opening narrative of a Black mother who feared for her life, Dominique, while surviving postpartum hemorrhage, the Black mother was seeking emotional connection and attachment with the postpartum nurse. In maintaining fidelity to professional standards of care, the nurse responded appropriately and accurately. Yet, the nurse acted in a manner that reinforced obstetric racism while maintaining the professional standards of care. According to Davis, intentionally causing pain occurs when health care professionals fail to appropriately manage pain or alleviate or reduce Black suffering. The failures to respond occur within the context of health care professionals holding racialized beliefs about pain immunity and providing care that is void of empathy for Black people's physical suffering. When interpreting the response of postpartums nurses to the Black mother's suffering through and survival beyond postpartum hemorrhage, the postpartum nurse's performance is a manifestation of neutral empathy which is required to reproduce acts of obstetric racism. The postpartum nurse is a symptom of larger systemic and structural problems in medicine and in obstetrics care.

Neutral empathy values and prioritizes intellectual and institutional knowledge over patient experiential, emotional, cultural, and spiritual knowledge, reinforcing both testimonial and hermeneutical injustice (Fricker 2007; Scott 2021; Lyndon et al. 2023). The accurate and precise practice of neutral empathy in the provision of obstetric care also requires shutting off one's own humanity to be able to actively participate in the violation of Black women's humanity and the perpetuation of Black women's suffering. Ideologies of anti-Black racism and misogynoir dating back to antebellum theories and writings from Southern physicians, physician-scientists, and scientists established that Black people were deserving of chattel slavery given their subhuman and non-human characteristics, as discussed in chapter 1. The denial of Black people's innate worth as human beings, or their dignity, is both justified and reinforced by anti-Black racist and anti-Black misogynistic ideologies.

The operationalization of nineteenth-century antebellum ideologies about Black men, women, and children, and twentieth-century definitions of neutral empathy mandates the denial of Black dignity and humanity. Therefore, the system of obstetric care is designed not to facilitate SACKRED, emancipatory, and liberating births. Instead, the institutionalization, professionalization, and financialization of obstetric care are to maintain hierarchies of human value, knowing, and knowledge that favor white femininity and white motherhood, when white women serve as the default woman (Bray and McLemore 2021). And the lack of accountability and justice in addressing obstetric quality and patient safety violations persists given the absence of measurement selection and monitoring strategies that capture empathy, dignity, humanity, and racism, prior to the development and validation of the first and only patient-reported experience measure of obstetric racism©, also known as the PREM-OB Scale® (Scott 2018; Scott 2019a; Scott 2019b; Scott 2021; Scott and Davis 2021; White VanGompel et al. 2022; Lyndon et al. 2023; Scott and Lusero 2023).

In 2020, I designed and led the SACRED Birth During COVID-19 Study to develop and validate the first and only patient- and community-informed instrument to evaluate obstetric quality of care (University of California San Francisco (UCSF) n.d.). At that time, social networks, as one quality domain, was the umbrella term used to include kinship ties. The quality domain of social networks was also tethered to the autonomy domain, as one combined obstetric quality domain, autonomy and social networks. Subsequent rereadings and preliminary data analysis of the 2019 focus group transcripts led to a renaming of the patient-identified quality domains. Based on the expressions, expectations, and experiences of thirty-six Black mothers navigating childbirth within hospitals, Black patient, community, and content experts supported the decision to dissociate social networks from the autonomy domain and renamed that domain Kinship, the seventh and final domain of the SACKRED Birth framework. Focus group data from 2019 provided evidence showing how, when, why, and with whom Black mothers created and leveraged different kinship formations and forces to address the other six quality domains in the framework.

For the first time, the 2020 SACRED Birth During COVID-19 study applied Black women-defined frameworks to the evaluation of obstetric quality and patient safety for, by, and with over 900 Black mothers and birthing people as Black women, queer, and non-binary patient experts, Black women community experts, Black women content experts, and 6 non-Black allied women content experts. The theorized quality care domains that emerged from the 2019 Black feminist hermeneutic phenomenology of pregnancy, labor, birth, and postpartum in the United States as a Black woman included: (1) Safety and accountability; (2) Autonomy & Kinship (3) Communication and information exchange; (4) Racism; (5) Empathy and humanity; and (6) Dignity in Blackness and holistic care (Scott 2018; Scott 2019a; Scott 2019b; UCSF n.d.). The validation science yielded three independent yet related scales as part of a suite of instruments named the patient-reported experience measure of obstetric racism©, also known as The PREM-OB Scale® suite (White VanGompel et al. 2022):

- Humanity has thirty-one items measuring safety, accountability, autonomy, communication, and empathy.
- Kinship: nine items measuring hospital recognition and involvement of social relationships between birthing people and their child or support system.
- Racism: twelve items measuring anti-Black racist & misogynoir in service provision.

We evaluated the association between a non-retained item evaluating empathy (a survey question that was excluded or removed from the final validated survey after evaluating different psychometric properties of the survey items using item response theory and confirmatory factor analysis) and patient-reported experience measures of obstetric racism across all three subtypes, using the three validated measures. The non-retained item that measures empathy, as defined by Black mothers and birthing people and demonstrated by hospital clinicians and staff, reads as follows: The hospital made me feel that because my baby and I survived birth, my experiences in labor, birth, and postpartum did not matter. Black mothers and birthing people who agreed or strongly agreed with the non-retained empathy item were more likely to experience hospital acts of obstetric racism across all three subtypes: > 6x anti-Black racism and misogynoir; ~6x disrupted kinship; and >8x dehumanization. Prior to conducting a literature review for existing measures of empathy and humanity or developing de novo survey items, we supported Black mothers to provide shared meanings and measures of empathy and humanity. Black mothers described empathy and humanity (meaning) as the ability and willingness of hospital clinicians and staff to:

- understand their feelings as Black women, to enter into and become one with the lived experiences of Black women, to "feel with" Black women navigating U.S. society, and especially U.S. hospitals and health systems during any pregnancy-related concern, question, event, condition, or outcome;
- be fully present and truly see, listen, believe, and trust what Black women are saying and feeling (Trust Black Women n.d.) about the joys and sufferings of pregnancy labor, childbirth, postpartum, parenting, lactation, and

infant feeding, bonding, and attachment without judgment or a need to control, but rather with genuine curiosity, concern, and compassion;
- recognize the difference between empathy and sympathy, and that empathy involves expressing care and concern for Black women and a desire for their well-being, without "feeling into" the emotional world of Black women, "feeling sorry for," rather than feeling sorry with (empathy);
- to treat Black women, Black queer and non-binary people, Black bodies, Black births, Black babies, Black lives, and their given and chosen kin of Black women and birthing people with tenderness or tender love that Black communities so often don't experience within hierarchal systems and structures of power and domination;
- practice cultural humility and value, pursue, and prioritize knowledge outside of one's self, discipline, or institution such as patient experiential, emotional, spiritual, and cultural knowledge;
- acknowledge, affirm, and amplify the humanity of Black women, Black men, Black girls, Black boys, and Black gender-expansive adults, children, and youth throughout the perinatal life course by:
  - attempting to understand birthing preparation and planning needs, preferences, priorities, expressions, expectations, and experiences within the context of their whole life, history, experience, and cultural, spiritual, mainstream, and experiential knowledge, including prior experiences and interactions with the health care system and hospital;
  - being curious, without judgment, to discover and understand how the care experience aligned or differed from the care expectation; and
  - acknowledging, affirming, and amplifying the diverse, inclusive, and expansive breadth and depth of identities, lived experiences, types of expertise, knowledge, wisdom, power, expressions, interests, skills, families, partners, communities, and so on within and across the African Diaspora.

Black mothers expressed that empathy shows up in clinical and social interactions, communication, consent, decision-making, and documentation of health care information in patient handoffs, patient sign-outs, and electronic or paper health records (measures) as follows:

- empathy in action from partner/family/support person: partner cried when patient cried;
- empathy in action from hospital clinicians/staff: Midwives and nurses step outside of their professional and into the personal, "feeling with" the patients and community support persons;
- empathy in actions (in general): supportive, very compassionate, like emotionally available and appropriately responsive "mother's or father's care"—parental care that nourishes and nurtures;

- empathy in action: looks like a good, thoughtful, mindful, curious, compassionate, concerned, conscientious listener without judgment, retaliation, or exploitation;
- absence of empathy in action: behaviors interpreted as non-responsive, void of emotion, harshness, hard-heartedness, and hostile, second-guessing patient's request for an epidural or any support or service (denial of the patient's pain and the patient's capacity/autonomy what they need and when they need it); and
- absence of empathy in action: lack of compassion regarding birth expectations and rationale (total disregard, dismissal, and devaluation).

Three dominant themes manifested from the meaning-making of the quality of empathy as measured by the lived experiences of Black mothers in Oakland and Los Angeles and their desire for more authentic, empathetic, and humanistic connections with hospital administrators, clinicians, and staff:

- Demonstration of empathy and humanity (also referred to as humanistic health care) violations, protections, and affirmations;
- Racial, ethnic, or sociocultural concordance between Black mothers and hospital administrators, clinicians, and support staff;
- Parent-child separation at or after childbirth occurring within the hospital, without involvement of family policing systems.

Black mothers described the quality of care in terms of demonstrating the presence or absence of empathy and humanity in the provision of obstetric care. Empathy and humanity in action manifest as genuine and repeated attempts by hospital administrators, clinicians, and staff to understand Black mothers based on their expressions of their expectations and experiences as Black women both in community and hospital settings. Black mothers expected hospital administrators, clinicians, and staff to see, hear, believe, and trust them by "feeling with them" (and not feeling sorry for) the multiplicity of ways that Black women show up in the world, within the context of their whole lives beyond their bodies and births, leveraging their cultural, spiritual, experiential, and mainstream knowledge.

For the purposes of meaning-making and knowledge production from Black mothers' expressions, expectations, and experiences of empathy and humanity during childbirth hospitalization in this chapter, I used both new and existing excerpts from focus group dialogues and individual narratives from previous chapters. This chapter demonstrates the absence of a holistic Black woman-person-focused empathy and humanity framework and praxis in the contemporary professionalization of obstetrics care and in the everyday design, delivery, evaluation, and training of obstetrics care in the U.S.

In response to thirty-six Black mothers in Oakland and Los Angeles who experienced at least one live hospital birth from 2017 to 2019, chapter 7 provides a blueprint for a Black woman-person focused model of obstetrics care for immediate adoption by all U.S. birthing hospitals and OBGYN residency and fellowship training programs. The first step toward curating a culture and practice of empathy and humanity in obstetrics care is for hospitals to recruit, develop, and coach a workforce that loves their job and commits to showing up, being both enthusiastic and fully present to do the job. In being fully present, Black mothers expected hospital clinicians and staff who work in the hospital-based birth industry to be both competent and compassionate, and not only desperate to make ends meet.

According to Imani, during a discussion with me and Simone during the Oakland focus group, "If you're going to be there, love your job and be into your job. Just basically be there. If you're going to have that like in those type of jobs—if you're going to have that kind of job where you're working with people with pain medication, you need to really love your job and really do your job the right way. Not just having a paying job and you take a paycheck." Given the ongoing, ubiquitous, and national epidemic of denying, dismissing, and diminishing Black pain and suffering in the emergency department (Todd et al. 2000; Goyal et al. 2015) and postpartum units after cesarean births (Badreldin et al. 2019), the public and the profession of obstetrics can no longer deny the power of the medical mob mentality to intentionally cause Black pain or to stand by and do nothing to stop Black suffering as the trifecta of violence in the form of obstetric racism (Davis 2018; Davis 2019; Davis 2020), structural racism (Jones 2000; Chambers et al. 2018; Chambers et al. 2020; Chambers et al. 2021; Chambers et al. 2022), and institutionalized racism (Jones 2000), grounded in racialized beliefs about pain immunity in Black bodies, especially Black reproducing bodies.

In integrating and synthesizing data from chapter 2 with data from this chapter, one must begin to wonder about the character of people designing, leading, evaluating, and financing the structures and systems in place that allow for the absence of empathy and humanity toward Black and Brown people to permeate, fester, and grow within most areas of medicine and obstetrics. When an entire hospital system, based on both statistical and clinical significance, responds to evidence of higher patient-reported postpartum pain scores from Black and Hispanic postpartum mothers by administering significantly fewer doses of morphine each day during postpartum hospitalization to Hispanic and Black women (Badreldin et al. 2019), the problem is not due to a few bad actors. When an entire health system responds to Black and Hispanic postpartum women with significantly higher patient-reported pain scores and lower doses of opioid administration by hospital clinicians and staff during hospitalization by distributing significantly lower numbers of opioid prescriptions to Hispanic and Black women upon discharge, in comparison to white postpartum women with lower reported pain scores and higher doses of opioid administration (Badreldin et al. 2019), the entire health system commits culpable negligence.

Based on these data, the health system failed Black and Hispanic women, their newborns, their existing children, and their given and chosen kin. Inaction in the face of need is institutionalized racism (Jones 2000). Thus, I use terms such as state-sanctioned violence or state-sanctioned acts of obstetric racism. At the time of writing this chapter, the profession of obstetrics published an article on the last day of Black Maternal Health Week, April 17, 2024, denouncing the term and denying the existence and evidence of obstetric violence (Chervenak et al. 2024). The silence from the profession of medicine, the specialty of obstetrics and gynecology, and the subspecialty of maternal-fetal medicine since April 17, 2024, remains very loud.

By the time I was writing the final edits to this chapter, three Black women scholars and one allied white woman scholar representing expertise and experience in anthropology, sociology, nursing, public health, history of science, medical humanities, medicine, feminist studies, women, race, and gender studies, published a guest editorial in an academic journal, led by a prolific Black woman nurse scientist as Editor-in-Chief, they offered a necessary, timely, and critical response to Chervenak et al's clinical opinion as "both emotionally charged and damaging to provider–patient relationships" (Davis et al. 2024, 1). I would also add that Chervenak et al's clinical opinion also contributes to the diminishing credibility of the specialty of obstetrics and gynecology as a psychologically safe, scientifically based, culturally relevant and responsive, data-driven, ethically sound, humanistic, and equity aspiring profession, in its current configuration.

Black mothers' expectations for a more empathetic and humane hospital-based workforce place a necessary and urgent demand on the profession of obstetrics and gynecology and hospital leadership in human resources and professional development, including more upstream in nursing and medical education, to prioritize soft skills in the selection process. From the Oakland discussions, Simone offered insight to be mindful in assuming racial or socio-cultural concordance between patients and hospital clinicians automatically transcends into increased empathy and humanity.

> And then I had another overnight nurse. She was Black as well but she didn't even really interact with me. She checked on the baby like twice and that's it. She was like in and out. Some of the nurses be like be ready to go. Like they wouldn't want to have a relationship with you, you know. Yeah, they were just

> ready to just do the job but not being—like why would you get a job like that and not love your job. Not care about your job. Not really just that's—it just sometimes it makes you feel it's all for just a paycheck—the nice paycheck.

Black mothers felt ignored or unworthy when hospital clinicians and staff, particularly nurses, provided standard care void of any enthusiasm, interest, or emotional connection. Not one expectation expressed by a Black mother for curating empathy and humanity in the provision of obstetric care included the possession or pursuit of a degree, title, or technical skill by hospital birth workers. Instead, Black mothers yearned for opportunities, options, choices, and optimal conditions for rapport building, human connection, and humane, non-robotic interactions and communications. With the guidance of quality patient expert Simone, the SACKRED Birth framework offers specific criteria for recruiting or developing a nurse (and physician) workforce that embodies empathy and humanity in their bedside attitude, language, and behavior.

> Well when you love your job you come in with a whole different persona, like you're smiling. You're asking questions, you're very attentive, you are just present. You're there. Anything—you're even looking into a person's eyes like when they going through like you really want to understand. Understand the pain and understand are you in pain. Is there anything—ask other questions afterwards. And you just don't get that. Like okay, bye.

Black mothers' expectation for a re-imagining of the souls of hospital-based perinatal administrators, clinicians, and support staff actualizes diversification (representation), inclusion (participation), belonging (psychological safety and connectedness), and democratization (availability to all people) of the birth workforce in community and hospital settings. Restoration of humanity in the provision of obstetric services to human beings by human-beings holds great potential for vital shifts in the norms and narratives of obstetric and perinatal care. During the Oakland focus group, Ayana and Jada exchanged perspectives and recommendations on what the care provided by these re-imagined souls of the hospital-based perinatal workforce would feel like to Black mothers and birthing people.

> *Ayana:* I think there just needs to be more understanding and not just think of us as like just that we're angry or just overexaggerating like—
>
> *Jada:* Yes.
>
> *Ayana:*—like they need to—
>
> *Jada:* Listen.

Ayana: Yeah, and bond with us how they would want somebody to bond with their daughter or with someone in their family because they just come in and they're like, oh, no, you're fine, oh, this is typical, oh, this is normal, like you don't know that, this is my pregnancy, I'm experiencing this, not you.

The call-and-response rhythm of the above conversation between Ayana and Jada revealed a pattern of focus group interaction and influence that culminated in a conformity of thought. The convergence of thought called for the hospital birth workforce to "feel with" Black women as Black women navigate attacks against their humanity before, during, and after their childbirth hospitalization. Black mothers are "calling in" the hospital perinatal workforce to focus on their experience of care, not just technicalities of providing the care. The practice of neutral empathy, detached concern, and objectivity, including the transition from paper to electronic records, compels nurses and physicians to be driven by checking off boxes and not by curating curiosity and care-based relationships.

In chapter 5, I utilized Chantelle's narrative to both name and explain different intersecting levers weaponized by physicians as mechanisms of subordination to exert reproductive dominance over Black mothers in interactions, consent, and decision-making. In this chapter, I allowed myself to feel with Chantelle as she recognized and interrogated the humanity and vulnerability of physicians whose language and behavior perpetuate and sustain obstetric racism (and obstetric violence), as demonstrated by Chervenak et al.'s public defiance and dismissal of obstetric violence in the *American Journal of Obstetrics & Gynecology*.

> Yeah, I wanted to speak on that too because if technically you're supposed to—or you can be pregnant for 40 weeks, right, or up to 42 weeks. I just feel like this, you get pregnant in a natural—for most people, you get pregnant in a natural way. You carry this baby in a natural way. And your onset—and the onset of your pregnancy is all—it's like—it's something you don't control. So why should you try to control when a baby comes out. Now, for health risks or issues like that, yes, we got to take certain precautionary, but a lot of times a young mom or a foreign mom or somebody that is not from this country, that don't speak the right languages or there's language barriers, there's culture barriers, there's financial barriers, there's all these things in play, you hear this doctor who is a professional who you're entrusting, and so you feel like, oh, well, they're a doctor, they know best, but they're just a person that went to school maybe longer than you or they went to school to study something you didn't study and so they're considered an expert so you trust them, but they are human—they're human so they can make human error and human mistakes and I just feel like there should be—oh, man, it's—me and my women, we'd like to have kids. We like to have kids. I just got a little real passionate about that,

> but I just really feel that you should not try to control something that is natural supposed to happen unless there is something—and what that trust thing is if he says like, oh, you got preeclampsia or you got high blood pressure or you got this or got that, you're like, oh, I do, oh, shoot, and so you just trust the doctor. And the doctor say, oh—the doctor said you got to do this or do this or do that, you go with it. But that's maybe not what you needed to do.

Even in the midst of evaluating the horrors enacted against the Black reproducing and birthing bodies by the hospital administrators, clinicians, and staff, Chantelle recognized the humanity and vulnerability of the perpetrators and sustainers of obstetric racism, "*they're* [doctors] *considered an expert so you trust them, but they are human—they're human so they can make human error and human mistakes.*" The challenge is that Black mothers are asking to be seen and treated as a human being with an innate sense of worth deserving of grace, support, and second chances from a group of individuals conditioned to being mistreated by the system as well. For example, the pipelines to promotions and advancements within bureaucratic institutions like hospitals and academic health centers sometimes require prioritizing likeability and respectability over liberation and disruption. Many times, one must turn off one's humanity and sacrifice emotional connections to achieve certain levels of mainstream (institutional) visibility and power. Thus, systems and structures incentivize neutral empathy and detached concern, even in situations that call for the system to express genuine remorse, regret, or both.

Consider the opening Black birth narrative where Dominique did not experience the usual postpartum bleeding after childbirth. In that situation, the postpartum nurse never explained to Dominique that the absence of blood after any birth is unusual. Nor did the postpartum nurse offer Dominique a plan on what to do if there was a sudden onset of a significant bleed, given the absence of post-birth bleeding for two days. On day two, the patient ambulates and then survives a terrifying ordeal of blood loss so significant, she had to be temporarily placed outside of her room for the removal of blood and clean-up. Never did the postpartum nurse practice vulnerability and honor her own humanity by stating that she had never experienced this specific scenario. By acknowledging her own limitations in professional practice and experience to herself and then to the patient, the postpartum nurse could have leaned into "feeling with" Dominique, not to perpetuate fear, but to acknowledge a shared humanity, shared vulnerability, and shared loss of control.

In line with Dominique, Gabrielle spoke up about ways the specific postpartum nurse and other nurses could improve upon their clinical knowledge, skills, awareness, and experience by making sure nurses learn from Dominique's experience. The interest and commitment to system-level acts of transformation as inspired and developed by, for, and with Black mothers and their children, in the company of their sister Black mothers, permeated each focus group in Oakland and Los Angeles.

> I feel like okay, so you know how she [the postpartum nurse] had said she [the impacted Black mother as the patient] wasn't bleeding and stuff like that. She [the postpartum nurse] said all my years I never seen this or whatever. I feel like anything that they haven't seen they need to jot down and put it in the book. Absolutely anything you haven't seen so there can't be no [more harm]—and start teaching on what happened. Like right now like her [the impacted Black mother] baby's two right now. They should be having stuff going on. Well this happened and we'll be prepared for [the next time] I don't think they jot down what new thing [happens] about anything.

The absence of empathy and humanity in that situation is 100% preventable and requires checks and balances within and across the profession and the health system to mandate life-long learning beyond pathology and pathology-risk-centric patient safety bundles and huddles. Furthermore, the postpartum nurse's detached concern caused her to deny and dismiss Dominique's ongoing fears and confusion, reinforcing a disregard for a Black mother's right to both emotional and physical safety. The imminent threat to Dominique's life may have been resolved, but Dominique still required the postpartum nurse, postpartum charge nurse, house nurse supervisor, attending physician, and the entire health system to acknowledge and affirm her humanity. The incident occurred two years prior to the focus group, and the unresolved emotional harm enacted against the Black mother remained present and palpable.

Although the standard of care was achieved based on the clinical response to the obstetric emergency of a postpartum hemorrhage, the standard of care also resulted in a violation of emotional safety, empathy, and humanity. The postpartum nurses and hospital team failed to express both regret and remorse in response to Dominique's feelings of disappointment and dismissiveness. An expression of regret in this situation focuses on missed opportunities in having the postpartum nurse offer an additional explanation about the unusual absence of postpartum bleeding and an alternative path forward in the event of an emergency such as delayed or secondary postpartum hemorrhage, including a discussion of the incidence, etiologies, and clinical courses. In contrast, an expression of remorse in this situation involves acknowledging the harm done to or experienced by Dominique, independent of intention or outcome. Harm is harm. Neutral empathy and detached concern justify the current patient safety paradigm that prioritizes "being safe," as defined by the system, over "feeling safe," as defined, valued, and shaped by patient and community experiential, spiritual, and cultural knowledge (Lyndon et al. 2023). As described in detail in chapter 1, anti-Black racist and anti-Black misogynistic antebellum ideologies that characterized Black people as subhuman and nonhuman reinforce a standard of obstetric care grounded in neutral empathy and detached concern, especially toward Black humanity and Black people's suffering.

The lack of empathy and humanity as the standard for obstetric care manifests in performing routine, repetitive procedures such as starting an intravenous line (IV) for the administration of fluids and medications during childbirth hospitalization or prolonged observations in hospital settings. As Davis shared in narratives throughout her book *Reproductive Injustice* (Davis 2019), hospital clinicians and staff can engage in acts of obstetric racism during routine IV placement. A few Black mothers in the Oakland focus group recalled their experiences of repeated IV attempts even with the best of the best nurses.

LaToya: I actually had the same—that too. This lady, she comes—actually, I take that back. I did see one Black person in the beginning when you go in and you—it's not the room.

Angie: The triage.

Latoya: The triage. It's not the rooms or whatever. You go in there's a like—she was supposed to put the IV in here but this lady, which was a White lady, came and was like oh, no I'm the—everybody was like oh, she's the best. Which was all the other White lady, well she's the best. Well I'm going to tell you she couldn't even get it in. It took [forever] and she didn't get it in. Somebody else had to come after her and get it in. Like four pokes to get the IV in for all the medication and stuff like that. That actually was really horrible. So, they ended up putting it right here in the corner. But they said they didn't want it there in the corner because it's got the bend. Well that was understood but she poked me so many times I had a bruise for like [weeks].

Dr Scott: Did anyone—and I've heard this several times. Did anyone offer to get another nurse or anesthesiologist to help with an IV. . . .you said the ones kept trying and trying?

LaToya: Try, yeah, I tried [asking for another nurse]. She was like shaking and stick it stick it stick it in. After the second time. . . . After the third time the blood person went and got somebody else the third time.

Dr. Scott: Okay. You do know you could ask for that person to go get a more senior person or an anesthesiologist.

LaToya: She just kept on like oh, you know, if they [don't] go in, I'll have to go get somebody else.

Imani: Yeah, me too. Like she poked me so many times and switched the arms to do it. And she kept—I think she kept going through the vein or something. Like going through the vein instead of actually getting it in there.

A more holistic approach to multiple attempts at IV placement involves the incorporation of empathy and humanity. Instead, Black mothers felt that the repetitive behavior was motivated, not by concern or compassion for the patient, but served to validate the clinician's self-worth and uphold the clinician's domination over the patient. Davis defines this type of repetitive behavior that reinforces power relations, differentials, and dynamics as medical abuse (Davis 2020). Likewise, the routine and repetitive IV placement can also be felt or experienced as intentionally causing pain when medical and nursing professionals fail to appropriately manage pain, due to racialized beliefs about pain immunity and the absence of empathy for Black people's physical suffering, leading to a lack of internal motivation to alleviate or reduce Black suffering.

Imagine incorporating empathy and humanity in the routine practice of IV placement, especially when multiple attempts or "pokes" are required with no offering of different options, including taking a break, finding a different clinician, using the handheld vein finder or ultrasound-guided IV access, or using a different route for medication administration (e.g., by mouth, under the tongue, muscle, or rectum). A dominant overarching theme and phenomenon throughout obstetrics is the denial of the existence and exacerbation of Black women's pain and suffering, independent of pregnancy, medical comorbidity, birth modality, and geography.

> *Dr. Scott:* In this moment, right now, what do you want your hospital to know about your experience with your birth?
>
> *Kenya:* That we are not exaggerating our pain.

For hospitals across the United States that continue to operate freely without any sanctions or delayed reimbursements while simultaneously denying an entire group of people based on race and sex, Black pregnant and postpartum women and gender-expansive individuals, optimal care and treatment for pain speaks volumes to the proliferation of anti-Black racism and misogynoir within all facets of society, especially in U.S. birthing hospitals. For one Black mother in Oakland, her birthing experiences in different settings—home, hospital, and birthing center—gave her many insights into the harms of birthing in hospitals and the joys of birthing in community with midwives. Chanelle's expertise, experiences, and perspectives on Black women's experiences within the larger discourse on birth as a battle, a business, and a movement of magic, restoration, liberation, and power added rich textures and nuanced layers of analyses to the Oakland focus group discussions.

> I just feel like at the birthing center every aspect of giving birth is what the focus is. And the mother is the main focus because she is the one who is going to get this baby here. Yes, we're exterior supports, but actually it's going to come from within. And the birthing center, it was just like a magical experience from beginning to end, and I can't say that at the hospital I felt I was in a magical place. I just felt like I was in a place of business, and they were doing what they do. And I was another number. They let you bond with your baby more so than the hospital [at the birthing center]. My baby never went nowhere. Like they let you bond.

One of the strategies for U.S. birthing hospitals to curate a culture and practice of empathy and humanity is to simultaneously consider institutional and patient—community or population level factors that interact to shape access to and utilization of care. Since 2017, I have included a patient-centered access to care framework, developed and characterized by a group of scholars in the UK (Levesque et al. 2013), in my scholarship. To date, the Levesquian definition of patient-centered access to care as well as the topology allows for a more comprehensive, organized, sophisticated yet simple approach to analyzing population and system level factors that intersect to create a continuum of care access. Levesque and co-authors defined access as a continuum of opportunities, options, and choices to reach and obtain appropriate health care services in situations of perceived need for care, dependent on the following possibilities or optimal conditions: (1) identification of healthcare needs; (2) reaching healthcare resources; (3) obtaining or using health care services; and (4) offerings of services appropriate to the needs for care (Levesque et al. 2013).

The UK-based authors conceptualized access as "resulting from the interface between the characteristics of persons, households, social and physical environments (patient—community factors) and the characteristics of health systems, organizations and providers" (institutional factors) (Levesque et al. 2013, 4). The five dimensions of institutional and structural accessibility include: (1) approachability; (2) acceptability; (3) availability and accommodation; (4) affordability; and (5) appropriateness. The five corresponding patient-community abilities at the population level that interact with the dimensions of institutional accessibility to generate access include: (1) ability to perceive; (2) ability to seek; (3) ability to reach; (4) ability to pay; and (5) ability to engage. When making meaning of a Black mother's expression, expectation and experience in seeking gender affirming care on L&D, one can better appreciate the relationship between empathy, equity, and humanity and the necessity of operationalizing all three concepts in securing high-quality, culturally appropriate, affirming, and safe care (Levesque et al. 2013).

In chapter 5, a Black mother in Los Angeles, Zaria, reflected on her experience of requesting a switch from a male nurse to a female nurse. Around the concept of informed refusal within the communication and information exchange domain, Zaria's narrative demonstrated how hospital clinicians and staff can remain engaged, connected, and attentive to patient needs even within the context of informed refusal of a male nurse when a patient desires gender-affirming care. For the purposes of this chapter, Zaria's narrative provides an opportunity to explore how the capacity for a hospital to provide gender-affirming care impacts patient-centered access to care continuum, leading to care fulfillment and activation and actualization of empathy and humanity. Application of the Levesquian patient-centered access to care framework allows the identification and explanation of system-level factors and corresponding patient level factors that contribute to care fulfillment, delay, or denial (Levesque et al. 2013).

> Originally, it was one nurse, and they switched shifts. And it was a guy. And I was like I don't want a guy in here. So they switched it up with this black nurse, and she was amazing. Like—She checked on me a lot. Even though I told her, no, you can't check me, it's hurting, but she still was like how are you feeling, are you in pain, what do you need, how can I help you. She literally came and sat in the room like basically her whole entire shift. Like, I went to sleep, I woke up, she was there. She was, like, I'm not going anywhere. Like, if you need anything, let me know. And when I was ready to push, the doctor wasn't there, and they had to page the doctor. And she was, like, the doctor is going to be coming in, like, ten minutes, but you can start pushing now. Like, I'm going to help you. Like, she didn't make me wait for the doctor to get there and start pushing.

According to the patient-centered access to care topology, acceptability describes one of five institutional accessibility dimensions involving cultural and social factors that influence the likelihood for patients and community members to accept certain characteristics of the service (e.g., sex, race, age, or social group of health care professionals, the beliefs associated with the medical industrial complex) and the perceptions of appropriateness for persons to seek care (Levesque et al. 2013). The authors described an example in which societal norms or laws disallow casual physical contact between unmarried men and women. Such sociocultural norms would then impair the acceptability of care and the acceptability to seek care among women if health care professionals are mostly men. Thus, gender discordance between health care professionals and patients creates structural inequities in service design, causing certain health services to be inaccessible and underutilized (or not utilized at all) due to a lack of acceptability to patients and community members (Whitehead 1992). Likewise, the ability to seek health care is greatly informed by multiple interrelated factors: concepts of personal autonomy (free will), agency (power to make decisions), self-efficacy (belief in self to achieve a goal), capacity to choose to seek care, and knowledge about health care options and individual rights (Levesque et al. 2013).

The UK authors offered another example that focuses on sex discrimination against women regarding the initiation of care or abuse and neglect, obstructing structurally minoritized and marginalized individuals and communities from seeking care. Health equity in access means providing patients and communities with opportunities, options, and resources to achieve the highest level of health for all, based on individual and community-level needs, independent of their social, economic, demographic, or geographic circumstances. In 2014, Dr. Camara Phyllis Jones defined health equity as the assurance of optimal conditions for all people, a perpetual process whereby systems and structures are required to value everyone equally, rectify historic inequities, and distribute resources according to need. Applying health equity, empathy, and humanity to patient and community abilities to seek health care recognizes that different groups hold different norms and narratives of appropriateness and quality (Jones 2014).

Zaria reflected on the hospital's empathic and humanistic response to her request for a gender-affirming birth attendant at the birthing hospital, which provided 24/7 access to both OBGYN physicians and nurse midwives on the L&D unit, "And also, I asked them was there a man doctor that was on shift and they told me yes, and I explained to them like I don't want a man looking in my vagina. And they were so like—they took it not offensively. Like I said, they found the nearest midwife and she delivered my baby perfectly fine." When contextualizing institutional acceptability and patient-community ability to seek health care within concepts of health equity, empathy, and humanity, the hospital clinicians and staff in Los Angeles and Oakland abandoned detached concern and neutral empathy. Instead, the hospital charge nurses and nursing staff at two different hospitals in different geographic locations in Northern and Southern California, respectively, chose to "feel with" Black mothers, normalizing and validating their expectations and needs, and then creating optimal conditions for them to experience the birth they desired and dreamed of, respectively, and not a coerced and forced birth with a male nurse or male OBGYN attending physician based on the initial service design on L&D.

Accordingly, racial, ethnic, or cultural concordance between Black mothers and hospital clinicians offers the possibility of advancing empathy, humanity, and equity while simultaneously preventing or mitigating hospital acts of obstetric racism. Black mothers preferred to be cared for by hospital clinicians, nurses, and support staff who shared the same or similar racial, ethnic, socioeconomic, residential, and/or demographic background. Racial, ethnic, or cultural concordance can serve as a facilitator of optimal birth preparation and experience. Brianna's narrative remains one of the more powerful manifestations of the SACKRED birth framework and model of care for childbirth hospitalization, across all seven patient-identified quality care domains.

In chapter 2, the reader learned of Brianna's 100 percent all Black women star-studded hospital team of clinicians and support that cared for her in a way that she experienced safety and accountability as feeling love and loved. In this chapter, Brianna's narrative begins on her birthday, one week before her estimated due date. As a result of noticing a change in the usual pattern of her baby's movements, she took an unexpected trip to L&D triage for decreased fetal movement, which then turned into a hospitalization to induce labor.

> On my birthday. I wasn't due for another week but it was just like everybody's like maybe she's just chilling because it's your birthday. I was like, no, I'm going to the hospital. And it was the first time I ever had to go for any reason. But it was like something's not right. So, they hooked her up to do monitoring and she woke up and started moving. But then she started having delayed (overlapping). So, basically it just means that her heart rate is slowly going down and slowly coming back up. Not like the quick one that they expect. So, they were like okay, with the combination of those issues like you need to stay. But I did stay overnight. I didn't just do the two-hour thing. And they said if it happens again while you're in here you should probably stay. But my triage nurses and my doctor, they were all Black women. So, I felt really comfortable. They took their time and explained all of the steps. And then they even took the time throughout the night to explain all my options for induction. Because they knew that if I stayed, I was going to be induced. They explained—I wanted to have a natural birth. I didn't want any meds, or anything. And so, I just explained that to them. But I had a whole night to kind of explain that to them. And they took their time to explain to me all my options about how to do that. Not to start with Pitocin but to do the—I did everything. It was three days (overlapping). I went to Hospital #2. And during my—I was there for three days laboring. And all of my—every shift was full of Black women.

A celebration of the heterogeneity of Black women's humanity and lived experiences recognizes and affirms that each Black mother is different, with different care needs, priorities, preferences, and aspirations. At the same time, many Black mothers desire concordance, trusting that a shared history or experience facilitates the activation of empathy and humanity, resulting in improved quality and equity in obstetrics care. The focus group dialogue between me and Yolanda, a Black mother in the Oakland focus group, showed how racial and gender concordance between her and her obstetrician improved the level of hospital attention and responsiveness to her care needs. In the presence of her Black woman obstetrician, the hospital nurses performed well, at the level of the Black mothers' expectation. In contrast, the hospital nurses responded in a delayed manner in the absence of the Black woman obstetrician. One could argue that the hospital nurses provided better quality of care based on the hierarchy of power between the nurses and the obstetrician. At the same time, one must consider why a Black woman OBGYN physician gave her personal mobile number to her pregnant Black patient. Moreover, Yolanda kept the mobile number of her Black woman OBGYN and was astute enough to recognize the perfect moment in the postpartum period to activate the power to restore dignity to her hospital care experience.

> *Yolanda:* Mine actually I gave birth at [Hospital No Name]. I started in the Hospital 2 here and then moved to Richmond area. And then she was—friend knew her personally so she was kind of like, you know, normally there. But when she was there, the nurses—everybody was on their toes. But when she left it was a different story.
>
> *Dr. Scott:* Wow.
>
> *Yolanda:* So, I had a different experience when she was there. So, I kept on calling her because I had her personal number. So, I had to text her a couple of times so I can get the help that I need. So, I felt alone because like—and the next day they were so different when she showed up in the morning. Everybody was like oh, what are we doing. Let's take care of her.

The actions of both the Black woman OBGYN and Yolanda align with what Davis names racial reconnaissance, the Herculean effort made by Black women to avoid or mitigate racist encounters, including being hypervigilant about procedures and finding providers (Davis 2020; Davis, Varner, and Dill 2021; Davis 2022a; Davis 2022b). Interestingly, Yolanda's actions in response to feeling ignored and neglected were not to seek a hospital nurse supervisor or to exit her room to identify a second nurse on the floor in the hallway. Instead, she notified a trusted advocate located outside the hospital to restore dignity, hold the hospital team accountable, and activate the six quality domains described by the AHRQ and the National Academy of Medicine, formerly known as the Institute of Medicine (IOM): safe, effective, patient-centered, effective, efficient, and equitable care (IOM 2001; AHRQ 2022).

In chapter 1 and earlier in this chapter, I briefly described the components of the PREM-OB Scale® and provided a general overview of the process of psychometric validation (Scott 2018; Scott 2019a; Scott 2019b; Scott 2021; Scott and Davis 2021; White VanGompel et al. 2022; Lyndon et al. 2023; Scott and Lusero 2023). More details are available in chapter 8. For this chapter, I focused on a particular analysis conducted by me and my research team from the 2020 SACRED Birth Study (UCSF n.d.). We examined the association between three subtypes of obstetric racism (humanity, kinship, and medical-kinship) and Black mothers who reported they would seek out a Black physician, midwife, doula, lactation educator, or nurse to be part of their hospital birth team if they could re-do their 2020 hospital birth (White VanGompel et al. 2022). The study sample included 806 Black mothers and birthing people who experienced labor, birth, and immediate postpartum from January 1, 2020, to December 31, 2020, across 348 hospitals within thirty-four states and Washington, DC. Black mothers and birthing people who agreed or strongly agreed with "wanting racial or cultural concordance in the re-do of their 2020 hospital birth" were more likely to experience hospital acts of obstetric racism, across all three subtypes:

- six times more likely to experience anti-Black racism and misogynoir
- approximately six times more likely to experience disrupted kinship (biological or social) between the Black mother and their baby, partner, family, or any other community support person(s)
- more than eight times more likely to experience dehumanization, including violations of safety and accountability, autonomy, communication and information exchange, and empathy and humanity

Quality and patient safety experts must reconcile the challenge that positive outcomes can exist within the context of harmful experiences. When the spectrum of safety frameworks defines safety only as the absence of a physical injury, and when safety meanings, measures, and monitoring strategies prioritize pathology-centered individual "bodily" performance outcomes, then positive outcomes coexist with harmful experiences (Lyndon et al. 2023). Restoring empathy and humanity in the provision and performance of health and human services in obstetric care offers a possibility for improving quality, reducing costs, and addressing anti-Black racism and misogynoir.

In Chapter 2, Gabrielle, a Black mother in Oakland, recalled her harmful experience with an older white nurse who lacked empathy in the provision of obstetric care and repeatedly asserted her domination and control over Gabrielle. In response, Gabrielle shared her demands for the powers that define, value, shape, and finance the hospital birth workforce.

> I just want—More color. Well, I feel like if you see someone more [people] of color and women. If you're familiar with someone that's like, you know, your color or something. You know, I'm not being a racist, but just open up to them

> more. I look like you. I think it's much better in my opinion. It was I could only relate to one lady that was Vietnam, because I'm from [inaudible] because she kind of helped me later. She became like a mom. So, I was always happy when she starts her P.M. shift. I'm like yes, God, she's here, because I can relate to her. It [seeing myself in staff] makes me feel like I'm safe. And it's safety.

Gabrielle offered a clear and concise strategy for diversifying and democratizing the hospital birth workforce by simultaneously increasing representation, participation, and leadership among people of color and women.

Restoration of empathy and humanity in obstetric care by diversifying and democratizing the workforce facilitates the curation of a culture and practice of emotional safety. The presence and proliferation of emotional safety also create the possibility for trust and transparency between Black mothers and individual hospital clinicians and support, and Black mothers and U.S. birthing hospitals. Transformative healing for all within and across U.S. birthing hospital systems can occur over time, starting first with individuals, families, and communities experiencing the most harm and loss of human lives. Another Black mother in the Oakland focus group, Rhonda, explained the importance of racial, social, and cultural concordance in curating a more empathetic and humanistic care experience.

> I think for me it was same color. Same color, same persona, same background. Just somebody on my level per se. My doctor, she is a woman of color and she's from Oakland. And she was really good. She's a doctor at Hospital 1. So, she really—she's one of those doctors that personalized every one of her patients. Like she knows me—like we've become closer. And so, you know, we exchange about our different children—where they go to school. And she just makes you feel like you're not at the doctor's office, you know. So, I think she was cool.

Shared racial, ethnic, and sociocultural perspectives, traditions, and experiences offer one strategy to activate psychological safety and connectedness in U.S. birthing hospitals. Racial, ethnic, and sociocultural concordance holds endless possibilities for benefiting Black patients, communities, clinicians, and staff by addressing structural inequities and injustices disproportionately impacting Black communities that the hospital workplace rarely, if ever, addresses publicly (e.g., anti-Black racism, misogynoir, mass incarceration, police brutality, redlining, and involvement of family policing systems). Hospital executives and administrators may not comprehend the kinship bonds that can form between patients and nursing staff that bring pleasure to both individuals. Narratives can bridge the gap between misunderstanding driven by unbelief and understanding driven by empathy or shared humanity.

In chapter 3, Ayana's interactions and rapport with a Black woman nurse curated feelings of love and being loved. Racial and gender concordance between Ayana and her hospital nurse combined with an empathetic and humanistic bedside manner reassured Ayana that she and her family were valued, wanted, and cared for in that hospital room.

> I had a Black woman. She was with me the time that I checked in and then her shift was over at like 5:30. And she was so sad because right when her shift ended like everything started happening. I was starting to push—everything. So, she clocked out, she came back to my room and she stayed for two hours off the clock. And then she was off the next day and she came up here to visit me on her off day just to meet this baby girl and, you know, just to say hi to my family. Because she was like really involved in my family all day. So, she was so nice.

While writing this book in 2024, the entire country continued to bear witness to U.S. birthing hospitals serving as modern-day arenas of unmitigated torture and terror enacted against Black reproducing bodies, based on system-wide inaction to stop Black pain and suffering, as documented in existing qualitative data presented in this research (collected in 2019) and quantitative studies described in chapter 2 and above (Todd et al. 2000; Goyal et al. 2015; Badreldin et al. 2019). Capacity building is needed to disrupt inaction in the hospital birth workplace and to spark a more empathetic, humane, equitable, just, and accountable response to preventing or mitigating workplace violence, in any form, against Black mothers and birthing people, Black babies, and their given and chosen kin. The hospital birth workplace and birth workforce need leadership, investments, operations, and infrastructure to support sustainability and scalability to diversify and democratize the workplace and workforce. Likewise, disruptions and innovations are needed to further develop workforce "soft skills" in providing empathy-focused, humanistic care. These transformations are crucial to addressing the manufactured maternal health crisis for all, starting with existing and future Black mothers and gender-expansive parents.

In the Oakland focus group discussion, Maya shared the privilege and power of being cared for by two Black women travel nurses from Atlanta. The quality of care provided by these two Black nurses activated and actualized safety and accountability, patient autonomy, communication and information exchange, Black woman-person focused, empathetic, and humanistic care.

> and I'll say with Hospital 3, they were good. I had traveling nurses, two Black sisters from Atlanta. I loved them, Nurse 1 and Nurse 2. I called them Nurse1

Nurse 2 from Atlanta. And I just remember them. It was like they was like my big sisters or something. You know, it's like they had been knowing me. But just that they were my color—you know, they were—they knew what—they knew what I come from because they came from similar so we could just relate. You know, if I was saying something—I feel like that was very important because these are moments that only happen when they happen and you can't rewrite the moment. And so, to have people of your culture or your—or you share some similar background, it just make you feel safe, comfortable, received, accepted, no judgment. Yeah, and it was just a lot of laughter in the Hospital 3 birth.

Another example of a Black woman-person focused model of services that prioritizes anti-Black racism and activating belonging for Black mothers navigating harmful systems and structures is the California Black Infant Health Program (BIH), offered through the California Department of Public Health (CDPH) (BIH n.d.; CDPH n.d.). BIH aims to elevate the health of Black mothers and babies by activating the power of pregnant and parenting Black women to make healthy decisions for a better and brighter future. BIH achieves its goals through the implementation of evidence-informed interventions using group socialization combined with client-centered planning, goal setting, and service referrals for BIH participants and their families. Measures of BIH success include life skills enhancement, stress reduction, and improved social support among Black mothers, according to the BIH website (BIH n.d.).

Felicia: I would say just thank God for BIH.

Dr.Scott: BIH?

Felicia: Melanin Moms. My—I call them my maternity sisters. I love them so much. There are a couple of them that are here today.

Toni: We love you, too.

Felicia: Jasmine: my sister downstairs. Without that group—there's things that we encountered during our pregnancies that we couldn't or didn't feel comfortable telling other people. You know, so they were all—even—all of us have had our babies now, the six of us, you know, and we are still tight. We meet up with our babies and everything. And—some key words that I think of (inaudible) loving, understanding, just available. You know, each of us have gone through something where we've been there for each other, like, I'm going to come get you or come over, or it's just supported or key words like that, so.

Bearing witness to the transformative healing impact of California BIH during a focus group session with no past or present connection stirred up emotions in me then in 2019 and now five years later. Bringing forth the powerful truths of Black mothers in Los Angeles and Oakland from a focus group transcription to text in a book manuscript is an act of testimonial justice and hermeneutical justice (Fricker 2007; Scott 2021; Lyndon et al. 2023). More importantly, translating the stories of poor quality and unsafe obstetric care into strategies to prevent and mitigate the harms of birthing while Black in hospital spaces embodies all three responses to obstetric racism: racial reconnaissance, refusal, and resistance (Davis 2020; Davis, Varner, and Dill 2021; Davis 2022a; Davis 2022b).

> *Dr. Scott:* What things made it easier or harder for your birth preferences to be heard or recognized?
>
> *Toni:* I think Black Infant Health helped with feeding and birthing plan. Now, whether or not that birthing plan was followed, just the initial, you know, preparation of having that and then, being educated on certain things that I think made it a little bit easier in retrospect. Because it's, you know, kind of telling you something that you probably wouldn't otherwise think about. Like, not wanting Pitocin. You know what I mean? Or like, you know, just different like, what medications or what don't you want or what do you want? And I tried to make sure that my husband was aware of this, that and, you know, my mom also. To this day I kind of hate that I kind of don't remember if they followed the birthing plan exactly. I know I gave birth on my back. So, I'm like, well that didn't happen. But I think that that really helped in regard to going in. Like knowing this is what I absolutely do not want. But something else is okay.
>
> *Dr. Scott:* And what did Black Infant Health mean to you again, in relationship to your birth?
>
> *Jasmine:* A lot. Now, that helped me think about me. Like she spoke of the affirmations—like things like that. That was like one of the best things that happened to my pregnancy. Being able to talk to other women who were pregnant. Listen to other people's not necessarily personal stories. But just, you know, helpful things. You never know. Somebody else's story could be therapy to you. It could be like the most minimal thing, but it's therapy to you because somebody else is sharing it with you. The videos. The videos, even though they weren't like other Black women—I think they were still very helpful. Especially in the regard where you have to like talk about your takeaway. Like what you get from it.
>
> *Felicia:* I would just like to say, it is very, very nice to be amongst a lot of beautiful Black strong women.

Investments in implementing, spreading, and scale of California BIH within and across U.S. states beyond the west coast would serve as political and structural prevention and mitigation strategies against anti-Black racism and misogynoir in U.S. maternal, perinatal, child, and infant health. California BIH implementation embodies all three responses to obstetric racism. At the individual, interpersonal, and community levels, California BIH not only improves outcomes but also improves the lived experiences of Black mothers and their children by activating and actualizing safety and accountability, kinship, and empathy and the humanity of Black mothers, Black babies, Black families, and Black communities. California BIH represents state and federally funded political and structural interventions for addressing the primary causes and drivers of the manufactured Black maternal health crisis.

As recommended by another Black mother in Los Angeles, Aaliyah, interventions like BIH need to be made accessible to as many Black pregnant and postpartum women and people who desire to participate.

> So, our community is misinformed and mislead. Because as a Black woman, you're strong, you got this, you got other kids. And it's like, if you say you need help. You need help. Yeah, you need help. And they're like, they're just dismissing it. So, they're not rallying against you. Because your mom who's in your house is great. But I feel that we've gotten away from that community. So, I said, where do we go? Most people don't know about the Black Infant Health. There should be somewhere we go. Like, it should be a localized, a centralized where we come together. Because there's so many of us going through this. No matter your age. But we're all African American women. And there's no centralized place to go.

Even successful state programs like California BIH could benefit from improving accessibility to and utilization by additional eligible Black women by addressing structural and institutional dimensions of accessibility: approachability, acceptability, availability and accommodation, affordability, and appropriateness (Levesque et al. 2013). For previous and existing California BIH participants, psychological safety and connectedness flourish despite the harmful conditions of birthing while Black in U.S. hospitals.

Given the impact of California BIH, widespread implementation in 2024 may not appeal to certain states with recent legislation to terminate programs and services like BIH. Many states have decided to turn back time and govern their states using antiquated and oppressive policies that could restore antebellum and Jim Crow ideologies and conditions. At the time of writing this chapter in my birth city and state of Nashville, Tennessee, at least ten states had introduced, passed, and implemented legislation that mandates restricting diversity, equity, and inclusion (DEI) initiatives: Alabama, Florida, Idaho, Indiana, North Carolina, North Dakota, Tennessee, Texas, Utah, and Wyoming. Some of the anti-DEI policies prohibit the use of state funds in supporting diversity-based programs, activities, and offices on the campuses of colleges and universities, as well as diversity-based training or development programs in private workplaces (Alfonseca 2024).

For experts in DEI-related industries, organizations, and associations who purport to be driven by data and evidence, then anti-DEI policies and strategies are grounded in false science and reinforce anti-Black racist and anti-Black misogynistic antebellum ideologies and practices. Passing anti-DEI legislation contradicts the will of the people who would most likely benefit from investments and infrastructures in implementing and scaling DEI data-driven initiatives. For example, in the psychometric validation of the PREM-OB Scale®, we also examined the association between subtypes of obstetric racism (humanity, kinship, and racism) and Black mothers and birthing people reporting they want more Black mother-parent focused information and support about lactation, breastfeeding, or chestfeeding literature. Black mothers and birthing people who agreed or strongly agreed with the statement were more likely to experience hospital acts of obstetric racism, across all three subtypes of obstetric racism analyzed in the PREM-OB Scale® suite:

- two times more likely to experience anti-Black racism and misogynoir (racism subtype)
- more than 2.5 times more likely to experience disrupted kinship (biological or social) between the Black mother and their baby, partner, family, or any other community support person(s) (kinship subtype)
- more than two times more likely to experience dehumanization, including violations of safety and accountability, autonomy, communication and information exchange, and empathy and humanity (humanity subtype)

The third dominant theme within the empathy and humanity quality domain is parent-child separation at or after childbirth initiated by a hospital clinician, without reliance on or involvement of traditional family policing systems. Black mothers expressed concern and experienced harm when hospital clinicians and staff made unilateral decisions to separate babies from Black mothers or Black fathers for prolonged periods of time, with no regard for the impact on the parent, child, or parent-child bonding and attachment. Even when maintaining fidelity to the standardization of care in hospitals for pregnant persons and newborns, hospital clinician and staff decision-making can create a disproportionate, predictable, and preventable amount of unnecessary anxiety and fear within parents and families. For Black parents and families with a shared history of chattel slavery combined with disproportionate rates of mass incarceration, the impact of missing Black children, utilization of CPS, and destruction and destabilization of Black human connections, families, and communities feels like a state-sanctioned genocide. The trifecta of violence enacted against Black reproducing bodies,

Black births, and Black lives in the form of obstetric racism (Davis 2018; Davis 2019; Davis 2020), structural racism (Jones 2000; Chambers et al. 2018; Chamber et al. 2020; Chambers et al. 2021; Chambers et al. 2022), and institutionalized racism (Jones 2000) continues without local, state, regional, or national mandates, accountability, or oversight around recognition, reflection, reporting, responding, resource allocation, and reconciliation. Decisions by hospital systems, administrators, clinicians, and support staff that usually uphold harmful language and behavior as "hospital policies and rules" need to be rigorously interrogated and interpreted within the context of the criminalization, subjugation, stigmatization, and punishment of the reproducing Black body, Black pregnancy, and Black motherhood.

Dominique: I felt like, you know, they had student—probably like eight people in the room. And they asked my husband to wait out[side]. I'm like I need to have him [here with me] And they were all like—first, you know before they laid me down, I'm like I need to have him in the room right now. Because it's all like white and I don't see anything that I'm familiar with and she [the student] was in there at that time. So, I was like have him in here. They were like oh, you have to wait a little. I had to scream and start crying like I need to have my husband right here like right now. So, he came in a little earlier. And then after the baby was born, actually, they had to take her away because they had me on a diet for so long that she didn't have any sugar. So, she was shaking when she came out. So, I was mad about that so I started crying. Because I asked him, I want [him] to follow her. I don't want them to mix up my baby or anything. Just go, as soon as she came out. So, I started crying because I was . . .why was I on a diet this whole time. So, the first night I didn't sleep with her. I gave birth at 10:30 and I didn't see my baby until like 6 p.m.

Dr. Scott: Like eight something hours after?

Dominque: Yes, 6 p.m. And I started crying because I had to breast feed her.

Dr. Scott: Right.

Dominique: And then there was no bond, or anything. So, I was like I'm going to get up and walk to her room. And they came and they drive me there and everything. The whole time I was crying. Because she was all hooked up and everything and she had to spend the night there. And the first thing that they tried to give her was formula. . ..oh, she needs this sugar right now. And then I said why did you guys have me on a diet for so long if she needed that sugar.

Dr. Scott: Did you get a response to the questions?

Dominique: No, they were responding that well this is what she needs. And I was like I don't even want that formula.

Neutral empathy and detached concern seem appropriate and "professional," only in the context of turning off one's emotions and humanity to inflict a particular type of violence that leaves no physical scars. When the pursuit and performance of safety centers on leaving no scars behind, then predators and perpetrators of violence must design and utilize psychological forms of torture to harm their prey. Reflecting on the impact of clinician and staff interactions and communications felt by Dominique, as described in her narrative, the magnitude of neutral empathy and detached concern warrants a type of investigation as an intervention to address manifestations of obstetric racism and violations of obstetric quality when defined for, by, and with Black mothers and birthing people, and their given and chosen kin. A proposed intervention would include assessing the clinical burden of obstetric racism throughout the health system and the gap in addressing multi-level manifestations of obstetric racism in clinical practice (e.g., interactions and communications), consent and decision-making, delivery of care (e.g., phone, video, home visit, facility visit, 1:1 care, or group care), and documentation and dissemination of health care information in patient handoffs, patient sign-outs, and paper or electronic health records. In this situation, and perhaps, like many similar or worse cases around the U.S., the denial of neutral empathy and detached concern as types of inaction in the face of need is, therefore, the evidence of institutionalized racism intersecting with manifestations of obstetric racism. Mobilizing administrative leaders, board members, philanthropists, insurance companies, purchasers of insurance, policymakers, clinicians, and support staff, in partnership with patients, caregivers, and community leaders, to conduct a system-wide diagnostic of the symptoms and signs of obstetric racism is a bold action forward in the face of need, and represents the antithesis and antidote to institutionalized racism.

Prior to the development and validation of the PREM-OB Scale® suite (White VanGompel et al. 2022), no existing performance indicator of safety included disruptions in kinship relations and attachments as evidence of violations in obstetric quality and safety. Dominique's story reads like a Hollywood movie chronicling the kidnapping and trafficking of Black babies under the guise of a birthing hospital. What may seem ridiculous to hospital executives, boards of directors, administrators, lawyers, clinicians, social workers, and support staff is an authentic and valid fear for Black mothers and Black families in the world today. "Obstetric racism," as defined by Dána-Ain Davis, Ph.D., is both an event and framework that explains how U.S. maternal health systems devalue, dehumanize, control, and abuse Black women and their babies in ways that track along histories of anti-Black racism and eugenics. "The current quality and patient safety paradigm lacks the historical contextualization and contemporary implications of obstetric racism as a well-defined, measurable, predictable, preventable never event," Karen A.

Scott, MD, MPH, FACOG, during a November 2023 workshop convened by AcademyHealth and supported by The Commonwealth Fund to examine the impact of *Dobbs* on health and equity (Cassil, Decosta, and Simpson 2024, 21). We must interrogate and reconcile "being safe" as defined by systems and "feeling safe" as defined by patient experiences and community wisdom. We delay or deny accepting the reality that for patients, caregivers, and families the patient experience is the same as patient safety (Cassil, Decosta, and Simpson 2024). Then we create and perpetuate epistemic and testimonial injustice (Fricker 2007; Scott 2021; Lyndon et al. 2023), and thereby cover up the realities of harm and hurt happening daily throughout obstetric units across U.S. hospitals.

Coerced or forced parent-child separation, independent of the intent or involvement of family policing systems in hospital settings, conjures up cellular and ancestral memories and responses from generations of enslaved Black mothers being torn apart from their Black babies at birth, on the auction block, and in the fields. The Black mother's cries for safety, security, and protection guaranteed by having her husband in the operating room at her side "*Because it's all like white*," and not the student, would activate an emotional response in any emotionally available and intelligent human who has also known the benefits of psychological safety and connectedness. The ongoing terror described by Dominique and other Black mothers in the Oakland and Los Angeles in prior chapters, and the lack of motivation by hospital clinicians and staff to ameliorate a Black mother's suffering, can easily be mapped onto Davis' dimensions of obstetric racism: neglect, dismissiveness, disrespect, intentionally causing pain, medical abuse, and coercion (Davis 2018; Davis 2019; Davis 2020; Davis, Varner, and Dill 2021). Excluding patient-reported experiences of harm as defined by obstetric racism from standardized safety meanings, measures, and monitoring strategies is immoral, unethical, unjust, inhumane, void of empathy, and racist. As stated by Dr. Camara Jones in 2000, "Inaction in the face of need is institutionalized racism." (Jones 2000).

Contextualizing and integrating mixed data from Black mothers' stories and the PREM-OB Scale® suite (White VanGompel et al. 2022; Lett et al. 2023) is a structural solution to achieve a higher level of data transparency, accuracy, and precision in the evaluation of obstetric care design and provision to Black mothers and birthing people. Study findings from this Black feminist hermeneutic phenomenology methodology demonstrate the value of interpreting mixed data within quality frameworks of health equity, obstetric racism, empathy, and humanity as defined by, for, and with Black women patient, community, and content experts. The powerful consequence of the chosen methodology is the ability to more clearly see that the design and provision of obstetric care void of diversity, inclusion, psychological safety, empathy, humanity, and emotional connections creates and proliferates harm in the form of callous and inhumane care and care experiences for pregnant and postpartum Black mothers. The study design, results, and implications for the use of the PREM-OB Scale® suite are discussed in chapter 8.

At the time of co-designing and co-facilitating the 2019 focus groups with Black women-owned and/or led community organizations in Oakland and Los Angeles, a paucity of information existed on conceptual frameworks and measurements of patient dignity in obstetrics or childbirth from U.S.-based researchers and institutions. Most of the existing literature dating back to 1966 on patient dignity or dignity in healthcare existed outside of the U.S. and focused on terminally or critically ill patients or older patients navigating cancer, chronic disease, palliative care, and psychiatric care. The most recent peer-reviewed literature on patient dignity published in the era of post-2020 COVID-19 explored the association between patient dignity and patient satisfaction and equity and dignity. Two scholars (Schiller 2016; Lowe 2014) published articles exploring dignity in childbirth in the United States. In writing this chapter, I found a study published in the UK (Ekpenyong et al. 2021) that more closely aligned with the research questions, aims, and methodology of my Black feminist hermeneutic phenomenology of pregnancy, labor, birth, and postpartum while Black and woman. The UK scholars in nursing applied an integrative review methodological approach to systematically identify relevant articles between 2008 to 2019 that examined the association between quality of care and patient and nurse perceptions of dignity, outside of the end-of-life paradigm, in community and hospital settings in European countries. Based on the inclusion criteria, fourteen relevant articles were included in the review. Study findings identified four broader themes and ten subthemes that impact patient dignity. The four broader themes included: autonomy, healthcare delivery factors, organizational factors, and the meaning of dignity. The ten subthemes included dependence/independence, choice, staff attitudes, communication, privacy, structure of services, staff shortages, physical environment, respect, and person-centered care (Ekpenyong et al. 2021).

Study findings from our temporal-spatial analysis of the lived experiences of Black mothers in Oakland and Los Angeles navigating community and hospital settings from the onset of labor to hospital discharge revealed patient-defined meanings and measures for Dignity in Blackness and Holistic care. Thus, we prioritized and relied upon the experiential, emotional, spiritual, and cultural knowledge and ways of knowing held and utilized by Black mothers to develop our conceptual framework for recognizing, measuring, and monitoring the association between the quality of obstetric care and the dignity of Black mothers in U.S. community and hospital settings.

Black mothers described dignity (meaning) as a state or quality of existence as a human being worthy of honor and respect. Black mothers also described a type of dignity manufactured by society and forced onto all Black people, whereby society assigns a social value or worth based on a hierarchy of qualities determined by racism, sexism, gender oppression, gender phobia, xenophobia, and class exploitation (e.g., social worth). Black mothers define dignity in Blackness as possessing innate value for and to self and love of self, combined with the following intrinsic qualities and abilities:

- innate power, strength, and inner will
- self-pride, self-respect, and self-confidence
- integrity—having an internal sense of right and wrong, having morals, values, boundaries, and standards

Black mothers assert that they have a right to access and utilize holistic care in the form of a SACKRED birth, as part of the hospital's obligation to recognize and protect their dignity in Blackness (meaning) (Scott 2018; Scott 2019a; Scott 2019b):

- SACKRED birth is a radical attitude and vision toward human births, specifically Blackness, Black bodies, and Black births, that regards all birth activities as fundamentally normal, healthy, spiritual, magical, transformative, erotic, communal, emancipatory, and power-activating.
- SACKRED birth encourages diverse and inclusive birth pleasures, practices, care, spaces, options, partners, communities, and experiences.
- The SACKRED birth movement advocates for safer, respectful, dignified, high-quality "participatory" birth care, conditions, experiences, and outcomes and improved workforce diversification, development, sustainability, and restoration of Black Midwifery and Black Doula as part of its campaign.

Black mothers believe that dignity shows up in clinical and social interactions, communications, consent, decision-making, and documentation and dissemination of health care information in patient handoffs, sign-outs, and electronic and paper health records (measures) as follows:

- oral or written acknowledgment, affirmation, and/or incorporation of their faith, religion, spirituality, rituals, and traditions into their birth plan and experience, as well as provision of hospital perinatal care, supports, and services;
- self-praise or self-recognition of personal achievement—"I did that";
- resilience and resistance—self and family advocacy, innate power and will: "I had to get strength to build my dignity" in preparation for hospital births;

- authenticity and transparency—hospital culture of practice supports open communication and information exchange between hospital clinicians and staff, and permits Black women to be "real woman," to be human with their perfect imperfections;
- protection and preservation of human dignity—Black mothers and birthing communities are "afforded every option," receive "thorough explanations," have access to "a midwife or birth attendant of their choosing," obtain information, education, and sufficient time to make decisions, and have access to and utilization of preferred support person(s) during the entire hospitalization to serve as advocates, regardless of socioeconomic status and relational or political capital;
- increased availability, patience, support, respect, listening (to learn and not to respond), and transparency;
- sense of loss and discomfort (denial of dignity)—general "lacking," "c-section takes your womanhood," "none-existent" (dignity is non-existent and completely absence in hospital birth experiences), lack of time, patients, care and respect, absence of morality, ethics, and boundaries; and
- loss of autonomy (denial of dignity)—"felt cheated by emergency," felt "exploited," had "no choice, no options," "no choices/lack of choices on birthing positions."

Two dominant themes manifested from the meaning-making and knowledge production from the lived experiences of thirty-six Black mothers in Oakland and Los Angeles and their desire for hospital administrators, clinicians, and staff to acknowledge, affirm, and protect their innate worth, or dignity, as Black mothers and birthing people, their Black babies, and their given and chosen kin.

- affirmations and activations of human worth in the quality of care
- denials and violations of human worth manifesting as gaps in Black women-focused birth resources about birth options and resources/strategies to access birth options

After reading and feeling with Black mothers as they endure dignity affirmations and violations during pregnancy, childbirth hospitalization, and postpartum, I began to critically reflect on the book's totality, and this chapter's role in offering a blueprint for a holistic model of childbirth hospitalization. In a matter of hours, I would be moved to tears by the enormity of harm manifested as gaps in services and resources that denied or violated the dignity of Black mothers. At the same time, a rush of emotions followed by tears would overcome me as I read the outpouring of tender loving care extended to Black mothers and their given and chosen kin. In wanting to highlight exemplars of honoring the human worth of the Black reproducing body, I decided to identify the common themes revealed within hospital affirmations and activations of dignity in Blackness, as reported by Black mothers in Oakland and Los Angeles. Four themes emerged as manifestations of dignity activations or affirmations across hospital spaces, phases, places, and individual clinicians of care:

- Facility design space
- Postpartum phase
- Operating room culture
- Hospital clinician actions and behavior

Black mothers described manifestations of dignity based on the quality of clinical attention, recognition, and responsiveness. Clinical manifestations of dignity during social and clinical interactions, communications, consent, decision-making, and documentation and dissemination of health care information in patient handoffs, patient sign-outs, and paper and electronic health records included asking culturally appropriate, relevant, and clarifying questions, making eye contact, and listening to Black women and birthing people during the labor and birth process. To enhance community meanings and measures of dignity in Blackness, the definition is expanded to define dignity as a fundamental and universal right and value of a member of the human race, our "human dignity." In comparison, "social dignity" is seen as the product of the interaction between individuals and society, with its culture and tradition (Jacobson 2009). According to the Italian version of the Patient Dignity Inventory (PDI), dignity can be measured by examining patients' perception of and attitude about three factors: (1) loss of self-identity and social role; (2) anxiety and uncertainty about the future; and (3) loss of personal autonomy at the intersection of health service provision and violation of human rights (Di Lorenzo et al. 2017). Similar to existing literature on patient dignity frameworks, meanings, and measures, the focus is on evaluating and restoring patient dignity in end-of-life and palliative care.

At the time of study design, implementation, data analysis, data interpretation and triangulation, and chapter writing from 2018 to 2024, no quality instrument existed for the purposes of measuring or monitoring patient dignity in Blackness and holistic care during the provision of hospital-based obstetric services. In developing an obstetric quality measurement of patient dignity, survey items must evaluate patient experiences of distress, demoralization, anxiety, depression, hopelessness, and loss of functional aspects of life. Integrating dignity meanings and measures from Black mothers and existing literature adds more specificity by including hospital language and behavior that acknowledges, affirms, amplifies, and prioritizes historical context, identity formation, and heterogeneous expressions of Blackness, Black womanhood/personhood, Black femininity, Black birth, Black motherhood/parenthood, and Black lactation. When re-examining the literature, individual excerpts, focus group dialogue, and the content in the previous chapters, I decided to focus on sharing text that can guide hospital executives, physicians, nurses, researchers, evaluators, funders, insurance companies, quality and safety professionals, and improvement and implementation scientists and practitioners to re-imagine and then design a new hospital-based model of obstetric care. The remainder of the chapter will provide recommendations for curating a culture, practice, and space of holistic and humanistic care in childbirth hospitalization that acknowledges, affirms, activates, and amplifies dignity in Blackness. Each recommendation was generated by thirty-six Black mothers in Oakland and Los Angeles during the 2019 focus group sessions, and organized into four themes: facility design space of care, postpartum phase of care, operating room place of care culture, and individual clinician actions and behaviors.

First, hospital policies and space design can contribute to a culture and practice of holistic and humanistic hospital-based care by affirming and activating dignity in Blackness and Black kinship. Considering the timing of the focus group activities in 2019, hospitals had yet to weaponize visitation policies to further isolate and subjugate pregnant and postpartum mothers and individuals. For Michelle, a Black mother in Los Angeles, birthing with the freedom to surround herself with as many of her loved ones affirmed her dignity in Blackness and actualized her desire for a holistic, family-focused birth.

> Yeah, I was lucky, too. Because Hospital 1 rooms are pretty big. And I guess they had changed their policy maybe a year or whatever before I came. So they were, like, you can have as many people as you want in there. I'm, like, cool. So my mom was there and my sister and my aunt. But I also had my little brother and my nephew who were probably about 12—11, 12 at the time. Yeah, they had to leave when I started pushing. The adults could stay. They made the kids step out when I started pushing. But, yeah, we were just one big happy family chilling.

Another example of human and community-centered design is the incorporation of images and messages along with practical skills-building sessions to facilitate the mechanics and benefits of human milk feeding to babies. Hospitals do have the capacity to promote breast/chest/body feeding using patient and community-friendly and focused strategies. During one of the focus group sessions in Los Angeles, I asked Zaria for permission to ask a follow-up question for her to identify and describe the hospital feature or characteristic that caused her to know, feel, believe, and/or trust that the hospital was pro-breastfeeding. In asking Zaria a clarifying question, with her consent, I facilitated her participation and partnership in the development of a Black mother-focused and driven meaning of a breast-chest-body-friendly feeding facility. Zaria immediately responded with a list of actionable, measurable, and modifiable items for any hospital to adopt, test, and scale if acceptable, appropriate, feasible, and sustainable.

> They had little stickers. Yeah, and there's like posters that tell you, like, the stages of milk and how much. And they actually came in and literally took my boob and showed me how to put it in his mouth and how to get him to properly latch. There were, like, little—like little informational thingies that they have posted. And they didn't—they told me—there's a sign that they don't give the babies pacifiers in the beginning. Yeah. So it's—I forgot what it said, but he literally didn't [use a pacifier]—he still doesn't use them right now. Yeah, I had an appointment to see the lactation nurse before I even left the hospital.

Second, evaluation of the postpartum phase of care in hospital settings is crucial to addressing the manufactured U.S. maternal health crisis that disproportionately impacts Black mothers and gender-expansive parents. Over half of all pregnancy-related deaths in the United States occur 7 days up to one year postpartum, with 25 percent of lives lost happening on the day of childbirth or within postpartum day 7 (Trost et al. 2022). Despite evidence showing Black women as the largest demographic abandoning hospital births for community and home births (Hoyert 2023), 98 percent of all U.S. births still occur in hospital settings (NASEM 2020), and 88 percent of all U.S. births in 2021 were attended by physicians (U.S. Government Accountability Office 2023). The mounting evidence continues to demonstrate persistent failures in achieving and sustaining high quality and safe(r) pregnancy, childbirth, and postpartum care outcomes and experiences for all mothers and birthing people, particularly Black mothers and birthing people. Black mothers spoke at length about the interactions, meaningful support, and sharing of information, options, and resources during the postpartum period that affirmed, activated, and actualized dignity in Blackness and holistic care. In the Los Angeles focus group, Toni remarked about the additional attention her postpartum nurse gave regarding post-birth vulvo-vaginal care, healing, and any signs or symptoms of pain, infection, or bleeding,

> You know what I'm saying. Beyond physical but mentally. Sometimes, you know, the guys, they don't pay attention to that part of us after we have the children or whatnot. So the nurse was very adamant about, you know, what signs to look for, you know, with me, and I appreciate that part. That after-care part. It—it was—it was—I didn't expect it to be that thorough.

Most postpartum models of care prioritize disease surveillance, management, and mitigation during birth and beyond, reinforcing the medicalization, professionalization, pathologization, and commodification of the Black reproducing body and Black birth. Consequently, my co-author and I developed a 12-Step Black Woman-Person First Approach to postpartum care, titled "Building and Bridging Black Futures Beyond Birth Model," a more humane and holistic model of culturally affirming and clinically responsive care (Scott and Davis 2022). Inspired by the lived experiences of Black mothers navigating oppressive postpartum health systems and structures, our hope was to provide guidance for bridging the gap between systemic and structural intent and patient and community impact in postpartum care optimization, particularly for Black women, girls, gender-expansive individuals, and their communities who experienced childbirth in hospital settings (Scott and Davis 2022). During her L&D triage visit, Kiara experienced neutral empathy and detached concern about her painful, regular contractions, leading to violations of all six quality domains defined by AHRQ and NAM (IOM 2001; AHRQ 2022), reproduction of diagnostic lapse and neglect, dismissiveness, and disrespect from Davis' obstetric racism (Davis 2018; Davis 2019), and reproduction of anti-Black racism and misogynoir combined with violations of bodily and decisional autonomy, communication and information exchange, empathy and humanity, and dignity in Blackness and holistic care based on the SACKRED Birth framework. When reflecting on her immediate postoperative and postpartum care experience, Kiara spoke highly of her nurse based on improved higher quality care provided to her and her baby, compared to the care provided to her, her baby, and her mother in L&D triage and the operating room.

> I feel like after birth they definitely—they did a great job as far as like caring for me and my baby, giving me the rest I need. They did come in there a little too much for me, but I wasn't complaining because they was coming like to help with her. And after having a C-section, I was just like in a lot of pain. The nurse made sure that she came in and made me start walking. Like she made me stand up at 5:00 in the morning and I had her at 9:00 the night before. So, at 5:00, she was like I need you to stand. I started walking with the catheter in. So, I was in no pain when I got home. So, they definitely helped with that. Yeah, for the most part, I think they were pretty great as far as their care after birth and just making sure that she was fine. She latched great so I didn't need help with that. They checked all of that. I had a Black lactation consultant come in and she was just like you don't need no—she was like—because I think the—well, actually no, she was a midwife and they were saying they were going to send a lactation consultant to come in. And she was like oh, no, you don't need that, here, let me show you. She was really helpful. She just really—she helped out a lot.

Kiara's reported experiences of dignity-affirming postoperative and postpartum care highlighted common features of nursing care. A Black woman-person focused dignity-affirming nurse demonstrates an appropriate level of readiness and responsiveness that meets or exceeds patient expectations. The impact of Black woman-person focused dignity-affirming nursing care is experienced by the Black mother as helpful, resourceful, and reassuring. Dignity-centered nursing and physician care, even during the postpartum phase of hospitalization, must always offer information such as indications, risks, benefits, and alternatives, assess for comprehension, and facilitate voluntariness. Postpartum care always requires continuous consent, including checking and recording the patient's vitals.

In Ebony's narrative below, a Black mother from the Los Angeles focus group, she simply desired peace and rest for herself and her baby. She accepted and activated her own human right to informed consent or informed refusal, and therefore she affirmed her own human worth.

> Can I say, like, I do feel like there was a time when I was given—right after I gave birth to my baby in the hospital, there was just too much going on. I wanted them to leave me alone for a little bit and it was the very first time I was staying in the hospital that I actually spoke up about that. And I denied some services. She [hospital postpartum nurse] was all so, you're saying you're going to deny me to check your vitals right now. I said yeah, I just fell asleep, I just put my baby to sleep, and I just need rest right now. I'm not going to be rude, but—it was the first time I spoke up about that and I denied them giving him a bath. I told them I'll give him a bath at home, he didn't [have] one. And I just felt good about that because it's the first time I felt comfortable enough to speak up to say I don't need that.

Third, Black mothers tapped into prior experiences in the operating room (OR) where the culture, practices, and people accepted and affirmed their human worth during a cesarean or abdominal birth. These data may represent the first insights into the quality of care in the OR on L&D in U.S. hospitals, based on the lived experiences of Black mothers. Although prior evidence has established a relationship between patient safety culture and patient outcomes, evaluating safety culture in the OR receives little to no interest or investment and usually deploys surveys and questionnaires as part of data collections. (Pimentel 2021; Hansen et al. 2012; Najjar et al. 2015; Nwosu et al. 2022).

The epitome of a Black woman-person-focused, dignity-affirming model of OR etiquette manifested in the intimate details of Simone's cesarean birth, which was discussed in previous chapters as manifestations of the SACKRED Birth framework for the safety and accentuality domain in chapter 3 and the kinship domain in chapter 6. In this chapter, Simone's narrative highlights the exemplary behavior of a Black male anesthesiologist in affirming and actualizing dignity in Blackness and holistic care in the L&D OR.

> ...but where I felt like I was heard was during the OR. They definitely made me feel safe. I was nervous being my first time having a baby, but they definitely—they all made me feel at home and safe. They checked in with me. So, my—is it an anesthesiologist? He was a Black male. He definitely—he assured me everything was going to be fine. He would touch me, say can you feel here, can you feel there, can you breathe, and I'm like I can breathe. He asked me—you know, they were like do you need blankets, are you cold, feel warm. When they did the spinal, they held me because my mom couldn't be in there with me and her father wasn't there, so I was already really scared.

The immobility of the Black reproducing body due to epidural analgesia, in combination with one or two restraints placed on the lower extremities, tethering the Black mother to the OR table, conjures up images of the slaughtering of animals and shackling of enslaved Africans. Though fully conscious, and hopefully with full consent, Black mothers are at the mercy of the entire room of physicians, nurses, support staff, including medical students, and anyone else who comes into the OR. Therefore, humanizing the OR for all, particularly for Black mothers, gender-expansive individuals, and their given and chosen kin, is critical to curating an OR culture and practice of obstetric quality and patient safety rooted in dignity and holistic care. Reassurance with frequent check-ins brought comfort and peace to Simone. A gentle touch after consent further affirms her dignity. Offering blankets and being fully present and attentive to Simone's emotional, cultural, and physical needs and safety matter most.

What may be routine and normal for a few may, in fact, be new and extraordinary for most. The continuation of Simone's narrative highlights the power of authenticity and vulnerability with accountability. Each intentional interaction and gesture performed by the OR nurse conveyed to Simone that the OR team, as representatives of the larger health system, recognized and valued her humanity and the sanctity of that moment. In her most vulnerable position, Simone felt "love, loved, cared for and safe." Before she brought forth life into the world, she encountered love.

> *Simone:* When they did the spinal, they held me because my mom couldn't be in there with me and her father wasn't there, so I was already really scared—being that my mom couldn't be in the room with me. So, the nurses hugged me as they did the spinal. So, I just—in that way I guess I felt cared for, loved, and safe in that way. They surrounded me with love and care. And they asked me if

I wanted to—because now Hospital 1 offers an option to where the drape can drop clear—so you can see your baby get pulled out. So, they offered that to me, if I wanted to see her getting pulled out and—sorry if I get a little emotional too. But yeah, and—yeah, they like offered that to me, so—it like—it definitely made my experience a little better.

Dr. Scott: You can cry. It's your birth story.

Simone: I know, but it just gets—it's like always emotional. But yeah, like them being able to just give me that option because I already was just sad that—I would say naturally, but I was sad that I couldn't have her vaginally.

Fourth, Black mothers also offered a blueprint for the specific types of actions and behaviors that serve as affirmations and activations of Black women's human worth, or dignity. When reimagining the role of a holistic and humanistic obstetric physician or nurse that activates dignity in Blackness and holistic care, Black mothers expect bold patient advocacy from their obstetric physician or advanced practice nurse. The expectations of Black mothers from Oakland and Los Angeles displace the onus of speaking up from the patient and family members to the obstetric physician, nurse, or other health professional. Currently, many national campaigns, popularized by credible and prolific organizations in the obstetric quality and patient safety space, demand that patients, family members, and community advocates speak up. According to the thirty-six Black mothers whose voices are amplified in this book, health providers, particularly OBGYN physicians, hold the power to speak up the most and the loudest against harms. Black mothers demand that obstetric providers leverage their power to speak up and protect the autonomy, humanity, and interests of pregnant and postpartum Black mothers and people.

Angie (Oakland): I also feel like your care provider definitely should advocate. I feel like advocating for yourself is very important and educating yourself, but I feel like if you're going to that care provider, you're with, what, your doctor for nine, ten months, that that's a relationship you built over time, your care provider should also be advocating for you. So, when you can't speak for yourself and you're in pain, your doctor should be saying, no, listen this is the plan, this is what's going on, this is what—this is what she told me she wants, so this is what we're going to do.

Mariah (Los Angeles): My specialist—if I had not been high risk and been anemic and needed the specialist to follow me, then he would not have had a voice in me trying for the vaginal birth. Which means that I could have been another dead African-American from bleeding to death. And that is just really concerning. And traumatizing. And it's just—wow. Unbelievable. Unbelievable.

By naming and activating OBGYN physicians to intervene on their behalf, Black mothers demonstrated a keen awareness and commitment to disrupting power inequities by leveraging the top of hierarchy of human value, knowledge, and decision-making in maternal child health service provision and obstetric quality and patient safety. Black mothers operationalized one of the four tenets of Black feminist praxis, Black women confront and dismantle the "overarching" and "interlocking" systems and structures of domination in terms of racism, class exploitation, and gender oppression (Collins 1990). Black mothers also expressed that they desire and deserve an obstetrician who is available, attentive, responsive, and resourceful. Black mothers' vision for a Black woman-person focused, dignity-affirming obstetrician also included a demand for obstetricians to provide information coupled with explanations. Additional preferred qualities for dignity-affirming obstetricians included being aware of current events affecting different Black communities, having the ability to engage in interesting conversations beyond medicine, and remembering details about patients' families.

Michelle (Los Angeles): So, being it's my first child by myself, I'm boohooing in Hospital 13 by myself. And I'm calling my mom, screaming. He said there's something wrong the baby. Da, da, da. But Doctor 6 was like, see, no. This is why you need to check your bed manner. Don't worry about it. There's another test that we can do to make sure that there's nothing else. Yeah. You know, we can fix this. Or it can, you know, fix on its own and da, da, da. So, after that, I never went to that [other] doctor again by myself. Even though I had to go monthly. But every time I would get something from this doctor, I would say okay, can you send that to Doctor 6. And then, I'd be like, Doctor 6, so, what do you think about these results? You know, what is our next step? Is there stuff that I need to be worried about? He said, I should be worried about this. What do you think? And he's like, no. It's okay. You'll be fine. I guess his bedside manner is really good. he's really hip. And he's not like some doctors. So, some doctors are just like want to give you like information and that's it. He like breaks it down and—oh yeah, home girl, so did you hear about the Lakers? Are you going to name your baby Michael if it's a boy? Like he's really Very personable. And he explains things. And some doctors, you know—You're just a patient to them. So, they don't remember from day to day to day, like. But I felt even if I was just a patient to him that he knew exactly who I was. Like whether it was over the phone. Or email. Or when I came in. He was like, yeah, I was waiting on you. But, you know, stuff like—so, he was very personable. I mean, he remembered like the family history. Like oh, didn't I—wasn't you here with your sister? Like—oh and how old is this baby now. Like, he was

> very personable. And I feel like he understood me. Because he was my color. So, he understood where[as] this specialist was not of my color. But Doctor 6 was more like educating [me] at the same time. But [also] culturally aware.

When setting the expectations for hospital obstetric team norms, holistic and humanistic care for Black mothers begins with shifting the hierarchy of presence and power that favors OBGYN physicians to establishing a midwifery first model of care. Black mothers expressed a desire for a change in care so that the first attendant to evaluate pregnant and postpartum patients on L&D would be a nurse midwife with collaborative support from an obstetrician, with exceptions for patients whose concerns, conditions, or complications require higher level, complex, and resource-intensive services. At the time of shift changes, Black mothers envisioned patient handoffs and patient sign-outs would facilitate, with intentionality and authenticity, the honoring of the human worth of the Black mother, her whole life, her whole body, her birth dreams, her pregnancy, her baby, her placenta, and her given and chosen kinship.

> *Brianna (Oakland):* How I felt I was heard? Like a couple things. For one, at Hospital 2 there's a whole staff of midwives that actually run the labor and delivery. Which is amazing because the nurses aren't overworked. The nurses just can come in and check and kind of assist. But the midwives, they have a lot more time I feel like. So, when the shifts would change like I felt like a celebrity. Like the whole staff—the new staff would come in, introduce themselves, get back on the same page about what I want, what we're doing, what the last people did. The prior shift would introduce the new shift. And it was crazy like. Like it was just like I couldn't believe it. I was like is this real like. And they all looked like me too. So, it was like I'm home. They could have been horrible but like I can't complain because everyone is so amazing. Like I was crying like the whole time just happy like—I felt safe because everybody would explain everything. Nobody—I never felt like anyone was being rushed like they needed to go and see someone else or talk to someone else. Everyone was talking to me. Like they were present and in the moment.

Transforming the culture and practice of patient handoffs, patient sign-outs, and patient safety huddles to prioritize human worth, or dignity in Blackness, mandates the demarginalization of the social worth of Blackness in relation to the medicalization, professionalization, pathologization, and commodification of birth. Requiring hospital clinicians and staff to interact, communicate with, and care for Black mothers in a humanistic and holistic manner begins by teaching hospital teams to believe in, accept, and affirm the human worth of Black people.

Brianna (Oakland): 'I think the most important part of my experience was that every medical professional took their time to explain every step, every procedure that was happening, every medication that was administered, all of my options and I never felt rushed. Those things were like the key. Those were the things that made me feel safe. There was no talking amongst themselves and me not being having been included.'

The existing model of obstetric care that exists in most hospitals reinforces antebellum ideologies rooted in anti-Black racism and misogynoir. Diversification (representation) in the workplace by merely promoting and advancing the only Black physician, nurse, or administrator, or the small number of Black health care professionals with social and political capital as alumni or legacy hires, will not dismantle oppressive institutional ideologies and practices. An insider Black community rule and mantra is, "All skin folk ain't kin folk," a quote by Zora Neale Hurston. Diversification without interrogation, deconstruction, and disruption simply reproduces anti-Black racism and misogynoir in different, more insidious yet impactful ways. Curating a humanistic and holistic culture and practice of obstetric care requires infrastructure and investments to hold all accountable for securing and proliferating spaces of inclusion and belonging, or authentic and equitable participation in leadership with the assurances of psychological safety and connectedness. Consequences for facilitating exploitation, extraction, erasure, or exclusion of individuals with the least power in influencing hospital policies and procedures, such as patients, family members of patients, community advocates and leaders, and support staff (e.g., registrars, clerks, environmental services, chaplains, technicians, culinary services), must be put into place.

Toni (Los Angeles): Because a lot of—once again, my family is out of state. I did a lot—I did too much by myself. And so, the information that I did receive, I received from the nurses. So, I will say a very big thank you to the nurses because they helped—gave me a lot—all the information that I would not have known. They are excellent. Above and beyond. I mean from the delivery to recovery. Like I said, I had my baby and I said I'm not leaving because I didn't feel well. They said, okay. Let us know—when you're ready. I didn't feel rushed, I didn't feel kicked out. So, I thoroughly enjoyed my experience there.

The minimum change to prevent and mitigate ongoing harms committed against the humanity of Black mothers, their babies, their partners, including their given and chosen kin is to mandate professional language and behavior during the provision of obstetric care that affirms and activates the human worth, not social worth, of all Black people. Initially, I planned to use the word *accept* or *believe* in the human worth of Black lives and Black people until I remembered that all licensed health care professionals pass a series of written and/or oral examinations, certifications, and re-certifications and complete multiple licensure and credentialing applications based on professional facts and norms that may not be accepted or believed by every licensed professional. Compliance with professional norms in health and human services does not guarantee belief in professional norms. Compliance means conformity to standards of practices, protocols, or procedures as determined by a set of actions or behaviors (repeated behaviors) used to evaluate performance. Therefore, Black mothers desire, deserve, and demand the elevation of the standards of professional conduct for any licensed or certified professional that serves or supports pregnant and postpartum people in hospital settings, including but not limited to physicians, nurses, social workers, mental health specialists, dieticians, phlebotomists, chaplains, and more.

Shanice (Los Angeles): So, I would like to say thank you to [inaudible] during my hospital tour, everything, all the birthing options, how to use each, the ball, the peanut, you could squat like this. Let us know, like everything. Everything that they said I was going to get, I got. And even like I delivered two days before Thanksgiving. They were like, you ready to go home? I'm like, no. Okay, well, we'll keep you here though—if you let us know, but, you know, they'll give you this extra day but—we're going to need this room. Okay. You know. And then, they even let like set up the room. For some reason, my child's father wanted to have her in the middle of us. And then, he slept on the couch. Like we rearranged the room. And the nurse is like, okay, well you comfortable? All right. Good for you. So, I was like, yes. Thank you. But everything good. And they even, I would say—called afterwards and I think I told—they set up my baby's first appointment for the next Monday afterwards.

Mariah (Los Angeles): Very quickly—the last nurse on my team that actually delivered the twins, I call her my personal cheerleader. I pushed both of the babies out within a ten-minute time frame, and she's like this is unheard of.

Dr. Scott: That's why I kept asking eight-pound twins. You was like boom boom. That's amazing.

Mariah: She just—I'll never forget—she locked eyes with me, and she was like you can do this. And she was just like this is just one moment in time. You have the rest of your lives about these babies. Give it all you got. Push. And I was like okay. And I pushed. So she was amazing. Yeah.

Dr. Scott: Beautiful. Anyone else?

Simone (Los Angeles): I have chills.

The Black birth narratives of Shanice and Mariah demonstrated the impact of hospital language and behavior on care experiences of Black mothers. Feeling seen, heard, valued, and safe emanated from both encounters. The hospital team offered many birth options that activated patient choice and autonomy and followed up with services and supports that were available and aligned with hospital offerings. Such alignment between hospital offerings and patient experiences facilitates congruency between intention and impact. The hospital offerings ("the menu") planted a seedling of hope. The alignment ("the experience") nourished and nurtured a beautiful bouquet of safety, trust, belonging, and joy. When I asked Black mothers in Los Angeles to name the changes they desired to see implemented throughout U.S. birthing hospitals, the recommendations included succinct and simple solutions.

> *Shanice:* Be available. Especially for first-time moms.
>
> Ebony: I don't want to have to repeat my no. The first no is a no. Yeah, listen to me.
>
> *Tiara:* Please get walking monitors so that I can walk instead of having to sit in this bed. And anesthesiologist, listen to me when I say I'm in pain. And you qualify it as just—oh, you're just having pressure.
>
> *Kenya:* Be gentle. Sensitivity training is very necessary.

In the psychometric validation of the PREM-OB Scale®, the co-authors and I examined the association between patient-reported experiences of obstetric racism and patient-reported experiences of hospital staff availability and attentiveness when Black mothers and birthing people perceived a need for help. Black mothers and birthing people who agreed or strongly agreed with the statement were less likely to experience hospital acts of obstetric racism, based on the three valid scales and subtypes of obstetric racism analyzed in the PREM-OB Scale® (White VanGompel et al. 2022):

- 87% fewer acts of anti-Black racism/misogynoir.
- 90% fewer acts of disrupted kinship.
- 97% fewer acts of dehumanization.

By focusing on specific hospital actions and behaviors during the provision of care and the corresponding impact on how Black mothers feel and think about themselves as human beings, I hope the reader obtains guidance on simple changes to affirm the dignity of the Black reproducing body. The vitriol against Black women is so pervasive that systems and structures normalize violence of any type against Black women.

Imagine a Black mother feeling loved because a hospital L&D nurse chose to be fully present, attentive, responsive, and supportive. Having a nurse act as a nurturer and caregiver, like a vision of a Black mother, if she needs assistance in taking a shower or changing her bottoms, feels like love.

> *Rhonda (Oakland):* And they all told me like, you know, if you want to get the epidural, you know, it's good and—it wasn't more—like they—to me my nurses showed me a lot of love compared to what I thought it was going to be, so I'm excited about that.
>
> *Dr. Scott:* So that's what I was going to ask you, like what—as I hear you talk about all the support, and stuff, what did that mean to you and from what you're saying, is it love?
>
> *Rhonda:* Yeah.
>
> *Dr. Scott:* If you could speak a little bit more to like what all that attention and support from different folks and having a nurse who was a childhood friend, like how did that make you feel?
>
> *Rhonda:* It made me—it made me not feel worried anymore versus like I said I didn't know who was going to be in the room and I didn't want like his family and my family like all fighting to be in there because like this was his first girl on their side and it was the first girl on our side in 17 years. So, like everybody wanted to be there and I just—one of the nurses that I had, she was a travel nurse, but she became so loving to me. Like I loved her to death.
>
> *Dr. Scott:* What was loving? Like tell me what she did?
>
> *Rhonda:* I can't even remember the lady name, but she was an older lady. She was more so like a mom to me. She came in every time I called, every time like my stuff was beeping or I—just anything like and it was more—what made me even more loving about her is because like she wasn't even my nurse on some of the days, and she would come in and ask me do I need this, do I—you know, do I want to take a shower, do I need shower stuff. So that made me feel good because I wasn't prepared to have her. And just knowing that they actually cared that much to, you know, ask me every day do I want to take a shower, to ask me every day do I need help like changing my bottoms because I was having an illness crisis as well as having my daughter. All that love made me feel really good to know that I had them as a backbone if anything to go wrong.

Not one Black mother commented on the hospital ranking, parking, location, room decor, colors, lighting, food, bed, furniture, sheets, or gown. In some instances, Black mothers expressed not liking certain hospitals to the extent of expressing no desire to give birth at certain hospitals, for unknown reasons. One such example is a Black mother who cried for hours in protest against giving birth at Hospital 2 in Oakland until she experienced the care.

> *Tiffany (Oakland):* Can I chime in on that real quick? So, like I said I gave birth at Hospital 2 and I was totally against Hospital 2. Like I cried for like three hours because I didn't want to give birth at Hospital 2, but like I said from the time I got there, they was like so supportive for me. I felt like they was more so my family than my actual family. Like I said, when my 37 weeks hit that day and they started my induction, they gave me so many different options. They told me I could walk around. They told me I could go where I wanted to go in the hospital, I just needed to be back at the checking times. They also told me that if I felt like I had a boo-boo and I'm like down the hall, to don't like try to walk back, like stop the nearest nurse or whatever and just get a wheelchair so that they could wheel me back. They also told me like—because a lot of people be like you can't eat, you can't eat. She was like no, eat what you want to eat, don't listen to everyone.

Once again, Black mothers described feeling supportive and cared for by hospital nurses in a manner reminiscent of familial connections. Tiffany felt special based on the quality of the interactions and exchange of information with hospital nurses. Hospital offerings included different options for laboring, such as walking around the hospital, including guidance on when to return for regular check-ins. Hospital nurses also considered the possibility of human defecation, which also feels similarly to the pressure of a crowning baby's head. More reassuring to the patient was the hospital culture and practice of supporting eating throughout labor. Affirming the human worth, or dignity, of a Black mother did not require any technical skill. Affirming a Black mother's dignity manifested as offering comprehensive, relevant, and responsive information and guidance on birthing options, facilitating mobility, and encouraging nourishment during labor.

> *Tiffany (Oakland):* She told me like—I was like I just really need to take a shower. So, she, you know, hooked me up to the shower. When I got out of the shower, I was in so much pain to where like I was just like on all fours on the bed or whatever. And she brought in the ball, and I was kind of like bouncing on the ball for a second but then it was like hurting too much. So, she was like just stay on all fours, like if you're okay, if the baby is about to come, you're fine, don't get nervous, people have their baby on all fours all the time. There was a—one—there was another nurse, a travel nurse, too, she was my age too, and me and her had became cool because she was my night nurse for the

> last couple days. And she wasn't even like on my side, but she came over to help me and I felt really loved for that too. And she just kept saying, you'll be okay, like you'll be okay. And like just that there and like her dad was on the way coming, but just that, having that moment the day of my induction it felt really, really well and really good for me because like my family wasn't there. My mom had came because she took off work, but the baby didn't come. And I didn't want my mom to take off the second day and then she didn't come again. So, my mom was on the phone the whole time while I was giving birth, but just having that—having her there and like those two nurses for the—for the most part was like everything. And they told me like, you know, whatever way she come is the way she come, because I was begging like just please give me a C-section, like I don't want to do this no more. And she was just like, no, you're going to be fine, just keep breathing, things going to work out, you know. And she just kept saying keep praying, God got you, and all of that and all of that. I was playing my gospel music, and every time they came in, it was just, you know, wonderful. And Nurse 3 came in and was dancing and stuff like trying to make me laugh and just trying to take all my stress away. So, like all of that made me feel really, really good, especially because I didn't have my family there. So, it was more so—and I was totally against Hospital 2, but I support Hospital 2.

Initially, Tiffany expressed a strong dislike for Hospital 2. However, her patient-reported experiences of her hospital birth revealed a model holistic hospital birth, full of empathy, humanity, and dignity. The nurse recognized and responded to Tiffany's pain with compassion, grace, patience, and tenderness. A second nurse shared racial and cultural concordance with the patient, facilitating the activation of another familial or chosen kinship bond. The hospital nurses encouraged Tiffany, allaying her fears and anxiety with constant reassurance. The visitations by the nurses from different sides of the hospital manifested as genuine concern and love to Tiffany. The hospital nurses carefully and tenderly curated a cocoon of love, safety, protection, laughter, and praise including the incorporation of faith through music and prayer. Incorporating play, laughter, and dancing served as stress prevention and mitigation. Although obstetric care in the U.S. was never designed to facilitate the emancipation and liberation of Black births through Black reproducing bodies, the narratives of Black mothers prove the existence of a remnant of hospital systems, teams, and individual clinicians and support staff dedicated to serving Black communities with empathy, humanity, and dignity.

Chapter 8

Emancipating Black Reproducing Bodies and Black Births

Based on the lived experiences of thirty-six Black mothers in Oakland and Los Angeles, I developed a new theoretical framework for emancipating and liberating the full power, potential, and promise of Black reproducing bodies and Black births in hospital settings. The SACKRED Birth framework offers guiding principles that shape attitudes, values, intentions, skills, conditions, practices, and behaviors in relation to Black Mothers and Black births, birth care, birth spaces, birth work, and birth partners. SACKRED Birth also celebrates sexuality, sexual pleasure, and birth as affirming aspects of human life and development. As a radical attitude toward human births, specifically Blackness, Black bodies, and Black births, SACKRED Birth regards all birth activities as fundamentally normal, healthy, spiritual, familial, magical, transformative, erotic, communal, emancipatory, and power activating. When considering the role of equity and justice, SACKRED Birth encourages diverse and inclusive birth pleasure, practices, care, spaces, options, partners, communities, and experiences and flourishes in the absence of structural barriers and burdens such as shame, stigma, and stigmatization. The SACKRED Birth framework mobilizes a movement for community advocates and hospital champions to support and promote safer, respectful, dignified, high(er) quality "participatory" birth care, conditions, experiences, and outcomes, as well as improved workforce diversification, development, sustainability, and restoration of Black Midwifery care and Black Doula support models as part of its campaign (Scott 2018; Scott 2019a; Scott 2019b).

In 2020, I recruited and mobilized a new team of patient, community, and content experts as the Principal Investigator, and designed and led the SACRED Birth in the time of COVID-19 study to acknowledge, affirm, activate, and amplify the voices, lived experiences, wisdom, and humanity of Black mothers and birthing people, Black women-led community-based organizations (BWCBOs), and Black women scholars (Scott 2019a; Scott 2019b; Davis and Scott 2020; UCSF n.d.). The goal of the SACRED Birth study was to test a new survey tool designed in 2019 and owned by me, the Patient Reported Experience Measure of obstetric racism©, also known as the PREM-OB Scale® suite. My team of Black women patient, community, and content experts included and compensated over 900 Black women across different disciplines, generations, and states, including Black women artists, activists, and advocates from fifteen community organizations and six non-Black women scholars. We completed six fundamental steps in making a novel measure and applied a Black feminist praxis across each step: (1) Determine the theoretical framework that was developed or adapted by a Black woman patient, community, or content expert; (2) Develop a preliminary conceptual model; (3) Review existing measures to start developing an item bank; (4) Design new items if needed; (5) Review the item bank with patient, community, and content experts; and (6) Pilot test and perform psychometric analysis. The specific details outlining the conceptual model, methods, results, and discussion were published in *Birth* journal in March 2022, and made available to the public via open access (White VanGompel et al. 2022).

My research team and I remain forever grateful to the 806 Black mothers and birthing people, across 348 birthing hospitals in the United States and 34 states including Washington DC, who completed the initial survey (White VanGompel et al. 2022; UCSF n.d.). Characteristics of the SACRED Birth study participants were similar to the U.S. Black population, with increased representation from individuals with a higher level of education. Despite Black women being one of the most formally educated demographics in the United States, our study findings demonstrated that one in three households had a total income of $25,000 or less (before taxes), despite higher levels of education. The PREM-OB Scale® suite offers three independent valid measures, Humanity, Kinship, and Racism, that characterize the impact of the quality of hospital-based services on patient experiences through the perspectives of Black mothers and birthing people. Each score varied significantly by socioeconomic factors previously shown to be associated with experiences of racism, including income and education levels. One key finding is that each score did not vary by reported clinical characteristics (including maternal body mass index, gestational age, and mode of delivery), demonstrating that the PREM-OB Scale® suite measures obstetric racism independent of clinical risk. Therefore, the prioritization of clinical outcomes as quality and safety indicators to evaluate hospital performance is not an evidence-based measure of hospital performance in preventing and mitigating racism, specifically obstetric racism (White VanGompel et al. 2022).

Study findings of 806 Black mothers and birthing people who experienced labor, birth, and immediate postpartum across 348 hospitals within thirty-four states, including Washington, DC, from January 1, 2020, to December 31, 2020, revealed deeper insights into the association between childbirth hospitalization in the United States and obstetric racism. We asked a series of questions that were not retained in the validated instrument to help us better under the lived experience of birthing as a Black mother or gender-expansive parent throughout the U.S. Black mothers and birthing people who agreed or strongly agreed with the statement were more likely to experience hospital acts of obstetric racism, based on the three subtypes of obstetric racism analyzed in Racism, Kinship, and Humanity. Black mothers and birthing people who agreed or strongly agreed with the following statement were more likely to experience hospital acts of obstetric racism: *I wish I had more information and support about lactation, breastfeeding, or chest feeding that was specific to Black mothers and birthing people.* Based on the three subtypes of obstetric racism, Black mothers and birthing people were:

- Two times more likely to experience hospital acts of racism (anti-Black racism and misogynoir).
- More than 2.5 times more likely to experience hospital acts of disrupted kinship.
- More than two times more likely to experience hospital acts of dehumanization.

Black mothers and birthing people who agreed or strongly agreed with the following statement were more likely to experience hospital acts of obstetric racism: *I would seek out a Black physician, midwife, doula, lactation educator, or nurse to be part of my hospital birth team, if I could re-do my 2020 hospital birth.* Based on the three subtypes of obstetric racism, Black mothers and birthing people were:

- Nearly three times more likely to experience acts of racism (anti-Black racism and misogynoir).
- Three times more likely to experience hospital acts of disrupted kinship.
- Nearly three times more likely to experience hospital acts of dehumanization.

Black mothers and birthing people who agreed or strongly agreed with the following statement were more likely to experience hospital acts of obstetric racism: *The hospital made me feel that because my baby and I survived birth, my experiences in labor, birth, and postpartum did not matter.* Based on the three subtypes of obstetric racism, Black mothers and birthing people were:

- More than six times more likely to experience hospital acts of racism (anti-Black racism and misogynoir).
- Nearly six times more likely to experience hospital acts of disrupted kinship.
- More than eight times more likely to experience hospital acts of dehumanization.

Black mothers and birthing people who agreed or strongly agreed with the following statement were more likely to experience hospital acts of obstetric racism: *I felt the hospital staff were available and paid attention to me when I needed help.* Based on the three subtypes of obstetric racism, Black mothers and birthing people were less likely to experience hospital acts of obstetric racism:

- 87 percent fewer hospital acts of racism (anti-Black racism and misogynoir).
- 90 percent fewer hospital acts of disrupted kinship.
- 97 percent fewer hospital acts of dehumanization.

In our 2023 open access publication, we evaluated the association between experiences of obstetric racism and the presence of a community support person during labor, birth, and immediate postpartum (Lett et al. 2023). A community support person was defined as any person without hospital affiliation or alignment who accompanied a Black mother or birthing person during hospitalization for labor, birth, or postpartum. Birthing with a community support person significantly decreased hospital acts of obstetric racism based on three independent scores or subtypes of obstetric racism as measured by the PREM-OB Scale® suite: humanity, kinship, and racism. The reduction in hospital acts of obstetric racism remained significant even after controlling for the effect of the relationship status of the Black mother or birthing person. Marriage or partnership among Black mothers and birthing people did not sufficiently mitigate obstetric racism. Thus, the physical presence of a community support person is far more impactful than marriage or partnership as a prevention or mitigation strategy against hospital acts of obstetric racism (Lett et al. 2023). In building interpersonal or community levels of resistance, based on our study, we recommend Black mothers and gender-expansive parents, and their given and chosen kin to build an in-person and/or virtual birth safety team of community support persons who are not affiliated or aligned with the hospital. We also recommend assigning each community support person on your birth safety team one of the following roles: emotional support, active bystander, notetaker, meal/snack prep, playlist of music and movies/TV shows, aromatherapy and essential oils specialist, and oral or written communicator of words of affirmation, and whatever else Black mothers and gender-expansive parents desire and deserve (Lett et al. 2023; McCain 2019, 7).

To date, the PREM-OB Scale® suite remains the first and only patient and community-driven quality improvement (QI) measure that monitors and evaluates the presence, permeation, and magnitude of obstetric racism for use in hospital perinatal improvement and implementation initiatives (Scott 2019a; Scott 2019b; Davis and Scott 2020; NASEM 2020; Scott and Davis

2021; White VanGompel et al. 2022; Lett et al. 2023; Scott and Lusero 2023; Cassil, DeCosta, and Simpson 2024; Davis et al. 2024). The primary aim of the PREM-OB Scale® suite is to transform obstetric quality and patient safety culture in hospital settings by providing equitable, dignified, and humane care to Black mothers, birthing people, and their families through evidence-based awareness, action, and accountability. The hospital policies and practices that govern the quality of care provided during labor, birth, and immediate postpartum care can now be evaluated by Black mothers and birthing people through the application of the PREM-OB Scale® suite. With these data, state perinatal quality collaboratives, health plans, public health departments, hospitals, scientists, funders, community organizations, and the public can now quantitatively measure, monitor, and modify harmful language and behavior enacted against Black mothers and birthing people by hospital systems, teams, and individual clinicians and staff members during childbirth hospitalization. These scores of humanity, kinship, and racism can also be applied to other data analytics to better characterize and address the dual burden of obstetric racism and any other quantifiable phenomena such as labor induction rates within a hospital, eviction rates within a city, rates of police-related shootings in a county, or the rate of maternity unit closures within a state.

The PREM-OB Scale® suite explicitly uncovers obstetric racism during service provision in hospital settings during labor, birth, and postpartum care (White VanGompel et al. 2022; Lett et al. 2023; Scott and Lusero 2023). These data provide a roadmap to diagnose obstetric racism in service provision and to dismantle, design, and transform interactions, communications, counseling, decision-making, and documentation and dissemination of information during patient handoffs, patient sign-outs, electronic health records, peer reviews, maternal morbidity and mortality reviews, fetal infant mortality reviews, patient complaints or grievances, employee performance improvement plans, or depositions.

Below I offer a list of multi-level strategies at the structural, institutional, and disciplinary level to facilitate application of obstetric racism, the SACKRED Birth framework, and the PREM-OB Scale® suite in mainstream knowledge. Because Black mothers and gender-expansive parents, their babies, or their given or chosen kin did not create nor magnify the problem, I purposefully did not include individual patient-level actions.

On April 12, 2023, I shared the following structural level recommendations for advancing accountability and transformation in research and data sovereignty during an online series of popcorn presentations for Black Maternal Health Week, hosted by Black Mamas Matter Alliance. I felt compelled to share it again in the body of the last chapter of my book as a seven-point plan to fight back against the manufactured epidemic of obstetric racism in U.S. hospitals and health systems, and to emancipate and liberate Black reproducing bodies and Black births in U.S. hospitals (Scott 2023).

At the structural level, I recommend:

- Endorsement of obstetric racism as an adverse event by dominant quality, safety, accreditation, and insurance companies.
- Development, testing, and evaluation of a patient and community obstetric safety hotline, which can serve as a prototype system for collecting narrative and structured data (mixed data) about the quality and safety of childbirth hospitalization using the narratives mapped onto the dimensions of obstetric care and the domains of the SACKRED Birth framework and the PREM-OB Scale® and quality scores generated from implementation of the funded and publicly accessible PREM-OB Scale®, using the Health Care Safety Hotline of the AHRQ as a model (Schneider et al 2016).
- Development of a civil and criminal liability regime to address obstetric racism, taking into account the U.S. legal system.
    - Expanding the definition of gender-based violence as defined by the Violence Against Women Act (VAWA) to include obstetric racism, following Venezuela (Borges 2017).
- Implementation and utilization of the PREM-OB Scale® suite as a validated systems-level measure to connect provider reimbursement to the value of care during hospital births and use payment to drive systems change, meaning providers get paid based on their patient's birth experience AND outcome.
- *Ethics:* Funding, supporting, and amplifying Black women and Black people-led community initiatives that unapologetically and radically activate the power, potential, passion, and promise, not pathology, of Black lives and livelihoods, to better align ethics with equity and justice-grounded actions.
- *Knowledge:* Operationalization of Black women's and people's theories in naming, defining, and examining the challenges and solutions. Demand historical contextualization and contemporary implications of different types and levels of oppressions, such as medical misogynoir and obstetric racism, and different types and levels of individual and community resilience AND resistance to flatten the hierarchy of knowing and knowledge.
- *Leadership:* Examination of leadership's proximity to the outcomes of interest and to the communities most impacted, and how proximity, positionality, and power impact the 4Ts: Truth, Trust, Transparency, & Transformation to flatten the hierarchy of leadership or disrupt and reorganize leadership.
- *Science:* Prioritization of methods of data collection, analysis, and interpretation of BOTH narratives and numbers that illuminate the nuances, diversity, beauty, complexity, and power of Black women's and Black people's humanity, ingenuity, and innovation to innovate and transform science.
- *Measurement selection and monitoring strategies:* Implementation of measurement, monitoring, and mitigation strategies that best uncover the problems and create solutions as defined for, by, and with Black patients,

community, and content experts to innovate and transform measurement selection and monitoring strategies:

  - Outcome-only measures evaluate the physical performance of the Black birthing body in response to the quality of care as well as generations and centuries of violence, control, injustice, and dominance.
  - Thus, the over-reliance and misuse of clinical outcome-only measures as performance indicators create a false narrative of quality and safety AND fail to capture hospital performance based on how well or how poorly hospitals see, hear, believe, support, want, and celebrate Black people.
- *Data quality and accessibility:* Interrogation of data sources and types, and how data is collected, stored, analyzed, interpreted, utilized, triangulated, and shared. Examination of how structural data infrastructures and practices reinforce power inequities and oppression as part of addressing data quality and accessibility.
- *Community participation and partnership:* Acknowledgment, affirmation, activation, and amplification of community participation and partnership with equitable compensation and resources without structural and institutional barriers, such as "work first—pay later or never" reimbursement practices.

At the institutional level, I recommend:

- Design and implementation of a comparative effectiveness research study to test the clinical effectiveness and efficacy of a clinical intervention (e.g., incorporation of the birth plan in the electronic health record, incorporation of the birth plan in the implementation of patient huddles, or both) in reducing hospital acts of obstetric racism using the PREM-OB Scale® suite as a primary patient-focused outcome and to provide comparative information to the healthcare providers, patients, payers, and policymakers.
- Implementation of the PREM-OB Scale® suite to supplement existing data collection and analysis of outcome, process, and structural measures during improvement or implementation initiatives impacting Black mothers and gender-expansive parents.
- Implementation of the PREM-OB Scale® suite to publicly demonstrate institutional commitment to advancing Black-centered racial justice & perinatal equity in hospital-based birth services, support, and care through actions, accountability, and oversight.
- Implementation of the PREM-OB Scale® suite to improve communication and capacity building in understanding, describing, measuring, and modifying how hospital systems, teams, and individual clinicians and support staff contribute to quality and safety violations as defined by the analytic frameworks and phenomena of obstetric racism and SACKRED Birth.

- Exploration and participation in a civil and criminal liability movement to address obstetric racism, taking into account the U.S. legal system.
  - Endorsing the expansion of the definition of gender-based violence as defined by the Violence Against Women Act (VAWA) to include obstetric racism (Borges 2017).
  - Supporting your clients or larger communities navigating obstetric racism and other forms of mistreatment and discrimination to file a discrimination with the Office of Civil Rights (Office of Civil Rights 2020).
  - Referring your clients or larger communities to Elephant Circle navigating obstetric racism, obstetric violence, and other forms of mistreatment and discrimination to file a discrimination with the Office of Civil Rights (Elephant Circle n.d.).
  - Application of the SACKRED Birth Framework, obstetric racism, and AHRQ's quality domain during a narrative analysis of a Black patient experience as a method for evaluating the quality of hospital-based obstetric care across three different obstetric quality and patient safety frameworks.

At the disciplinary level, I recommend:

- Inclusion of *SACKRED Birth: Mobilizing a New Quality Paradigm in Obstetric Care* on the reading list for undergraduate, graduate, postgraduate, and continuing education courses in social sciences, medical humanities, feminist studies, Black feminist studies, misogynoir, anti-racism, nursing, medicine, public health, social epidemiology, social work, comparative women's and gender studies, legal studies, civil rights, improvement and implementation science, measurement science, research justice methodology, participatory action research methodology, and hermeneutic phenomenology.
- Mandating every graduating medical student or resident physician who matched into a residency training or fellowship program, respectively, in the field of obstetrics to read *SACKRED Birth.*
- Integration of obstetric racism, the SACKRED Birth framework and the PREM-OB Scale® suite as a core competency evaluation tool as approved and authorized by the Council on Resident Education in Obstetrics and Gynecology (CREOG) (ACOG n.d.)
  - Specifically, in Unit 1 General Considerations, Section III Patient Care, Item E, educate and train OBGYN residents to provide direct care and/or referral for patients who are victim to the following situations including a seventh phenomenon, obstetric racism, and refer patients or family survivors of obstetric racism to community partner organizations such as Birthing Cultural Rigor to access the PREM-OB Scale® suite.

- Specifically, in Unit 2 Obstetrics, Section II Antepartum Care, Item D, educate and train OBGYN residents to counsel the pregnant patient on the warning signs of the following events, including hospital acts of obstetric racism and violations of the SACKRED Birth framework as an adverse pregnancy events.
- Specifically, in Unit 2 Obstetrics, Section II Antepartum Care, Item E, educate and train OBGYN residents to recognize and support diverse socioeconomic, family, and environmental factors affecting access to care and pregnancy outcomes, including exposure to hospital acts of obstetric racism and violations of obstetric quality and patient safety using the SACKRED Birth framework or the PREM-OB Scale® suite.
- Specifically, in Unit 2 Obstetrics, Section IV Postpartum Care, and create a new item C, educate and train OBGYN residents to recognize obstetric racism and counsel the pregnant patient on the warning signs of the following events, including hospital acts of obstetric racism and violations of the SACKRED Birth framework as an adverse pregnancy events.

A second product of the 2020 SACRED Birth Study was the development of the first Virtual Quality Improvement Prioritization by Affected Communities (VQPAC) (Scott et al. 2021) is an adaptation of the Research Prioritization by Affected Communities (RPAC) protocol (Franck et al. 2018). The aim of VQPAC was to facilitate community participation in prioritizing perinatal improvement (QI) recommendations across the original six theorized patient-identified domains of the SACRED Birth, where Kinship was tethered to Autonomy, and previously referred to as social networks (Scott 2018; Scott 2019a; Scott 2019b). The six foundational domains serve as the foundation for the validated Patient Reported Experience Measure of Obstetric Racism© (PREM-OB Scale® suite). The VQPAC applied a Black feminist ethnographic methodology to describe different forms of resistance and resilience that twenty-four Black women leaders from fifteen Black women community-led organizations leaders across northern and southern California adopt to recognize and respond to the dimensions of obstetric racism and power inequities that emerge from supporting Black mothers and birthing people during hospital births. Implementation of the VQPAC protocol utilized a web-based video conferencing tool and presentation software for interactive real-time input. The components of the VQPAC included: (1) preparation; (2) facilitated group work to generate a list of potential techniques and topics (Session 1); (3) interim analysis by the same two Black women researchers; (4) facilitated group work to prioritize topics (Session 2); and 5) summary analysis using reflexive thematic analysis. We used both inductive coding and theoretical coding in this analytic approach (Scott et al. 2021).

The VQPAC participants supported Black women and people experiencing pregnancy, birth, and lactation, ranging in age from twenty-eight to seventy-two years, with experience supporting a Black mother during a hospital birth in California (n = 15), previous hospital births in California (n = 13), no prior QI experience (n = 10), prior perinatal QI experience (n = 7), and other QI experience (n = 3). Twenty of the twenty-four participants completed the demographic survey. VQPAC implementation occurred over 6 x 2-hour virtual sessions and supported twenty-four community leaders to identify seventy-four and prioritized forty-four potential perinatal QI topics across the PREM-OB Scale® suite domains. Then they further prioritized QI topics down to the top two mitigations for each domain in the SACRED Birth framework (see table 8.1) (Scott et al. 2021).

As stated in prior chapters, what may seem ridiculous and/or routine to hospital executives, boards of directors, administrators, lawyers, clinicians, social workers, and support staff may, in fact, be new and extraordinary or an authentic and valid fear for Black mothers and Black families in the world

Table 8.1 Top Twp Perinatal Quality Improvement Priority Areas by SACKRED Birth Domains

SACKRED Birth Quality Domain	*Perinatal Quality Priorities and Mitigations against Obstetric Racism*
Safety & Accountability	Shame, Stigma, Love, Grace, and Dignity: Birthing While Black
	Patient/Community Feedback in EHR Language and Patient Handoff
Autonomy & Social Capital/Kinship	Black Birthing Rights in Hospital Settings
	Black Women's/People's Autonomy: Asset vs Threat
Communication & Information Exchange	Pre-Escalation Steps Prior to Calling Hospital Security
	Use of Mediation with a Professional and Community Representative External to Hospital
Racism	Redesign and expansion of care team
	Anti-Racism Community Advisory & Accountability Board/Taskforce
Empathy & Humanity	Human Resources Accountability Metric: What is your Why? and Empathy-specific Competency Based Screening/Interviews
	SACRED Birth Assessment/Checklist for Black People Focused Care
Dignity in Blackness & Holistic Care	Explicit Informed Consent/Refusal for Every Cervical Exam
	Racial Equity Caucus for the Restoration of Dignity in Blackness for patients, community, clinicians, staff, and physicians with hospital

today. Based on meaning-making and knowledge production from thirty-six Black mothers' expressions, expectations, and experiences of navigating hospitals and health systems throughout the greater Oakland and Los Angeles communities, the opportunities for a Black woman-person focused holistic healing, truth, reconciliation, repair, and recovery can be found within and among Black patient, community, and content experts, and not only within existing patient safety bundles. The VQPAC protocol offers hospitals a novel method for generating rapid, in-depth knowledge of socio-cultural QI priorities from Black women community leaders who support Black mothers and birthing people during hospital births. Within this Black feminist hermeneutic phenomenology of California Black mothers' expressions, expectations, and experiences of childbirth hospitalization and the VQPAC recommendations from California Black women birth workers, advocates, mothers, leaders, and activists, obstetric quality and patient safety systems, structures, teams, and individuals possess clear resources, recommendations, and references to better name, recognize, measure, monitor, prevent, and mitigate obstetric racism beyond pathology centered—risk reduction strategies described in existing QI safety bundles.

Current quality measures lack accuracy, precision, relevance, and rigor to optimally examine the quality, value, and safety of birthing while Black. We must continuously re-examine the seven pain points previously named and described in the list of structural level recommendations as performance indicators for the implementation, spread, and scale of Black women and people-first AND focused community-led accountability and transformation in obstetric quality and patient safety: ethics, knowledge, leadership, science, measurement selection and monitoring strategies, data quality and accessibility, and community participation and partnership (Scott 2023). Through the intellectual thoughts and political activism of Black women and people as patient, community, and content experts, we call upon you to inquire, invest, implement, impact, and innovate with us to end obstetric racism.

The alternative is inaction. And, well, you already know what Dr. Jones said back in 2000: "Indeed, institutionalized racism is often evident as inaction in the face of need" (Jones 2000, 1).

References

Abdullah, Afi Samelia. 1998. "Mammy-ism: A Diagnosis of Psychological Misorientation for Women of African Descent." *Journal of Black Psychology* 24(2): 196–210.

Accapadi, Mamta Motwani. 2007. "When White Women Cry: How White Women's Tears Oppress Women of Color." *College Student Affairs Journal* 26(2): 208–215.

Agency for Healthcare Research and Quality (AHRQ) Patient Safety Network (PSNet). 2019. "Adverse Events, Near Misses, and Errors." September 7, 2019. Accessed September 25, 2022. https://psnet.ahrq.gov/primer/adverse-events-near-misses-and-errors.

Agency for Healthcare Research and Quality (AHRQ) Patient Safety Network (PSNet). n.d.(a). "Glossary." Accessed September 25, 2022. https://psnet.ahrq.gov/glossary-0.

Agency for Healthcare Research and Quality (AHRQ) Patient Safety Network (PSNet). n.d.(b). "Patient Safety 101: The Fundamentals 101, What is Patient Safety?" Last updated August 1, 2024. Accessed September 25, 2022. https://psnet.ahrq.gov/patient-safety-101.

Agency for Healthcare Research and Quality (AHRQ). 2022. "Six Domains of Healthcare Quality." Last updated December 2022. Agency for Healthcare Research and Quality, Rockville, MD. Accessed April 2, 2024. https://www.ahrq.gov/talkingquality/measures/six-domains.html.

Agrò, F. E., F. Salvinelli, M. Casale, and S. Antonelli. 2003. "Temporomandibular Joint Assessment in Anaesthetic Practice." *British Journal of Anaesthesia* 90(5): 707–708.

Alfonseca, Kiara. 2024. "Map: The Impact of Anti-DEI Legislation." ABC News. April 5, 2024. Accessed May 7, 2024. https://abcnews.go.com/US/map-impact-anti-dei-legislation/story?id=108795967.

Alliance for Innovation in Maternal Health (AIM). n.d. "Patient Safety Bundles." Accessed July 21, 2024. https://saferbirth.org/patient-safety-bundles/.

Altman, Molly R., Talita Oseguera, Monica R. McLemore, Ira Kantrowitz-Gordon, Linda S. Franck, and Audrey Lyndon. 2019. "Information and Power: Women of Color's Experiences Interacting with Health Care Providers in Pregnancy and Birth." *Social Science & Medicine* 238: 112491–112491.

Alves, Isabella. 2018. "Women's Empowerment Helped Pave Way for Modern Childbirth." Associated Press. Accessed August 4, 2024. https://apnews.com/general-news-d052aa450fb145a9be3bc04e90f0151f.

The American College of Obstetricians and Gynecologists (ACOG) Committee on Patient Safety and Quality Improvement. 2003. "Patient Safety in Obstetrics and Gynecology." ACOG Number 447 (Replaces No. 286, October 2003). Reaffirmed 2019. Accessed August 22, 2024. https://www.acog.org/clinical/clinical-guidance/committee-opinion/articles/2009/12/patient-safety-in-obstetrics-and-gynecology.

The American College of Obstetricians and Gynecologists (ACOG). n.d. "Council on Resident Education in Obstetrics and Gynecology (CREOG) Educational Objectives 13th Edition." ACOG. Accessed July 28, 2024. https://www.acog.org/education-and-events/creog/curriculum-resources/creog-educational-objectives.

American College of Obstetricians and Gynecologists (ACOG). n.d. "Labor Induction." Last updated June 2022. Accessed August 18, 2024. https://www.acog.org/womens-health/faqs/labor-induction.

American Medical Association (AMA). 1847. "Chapter 2 Consent, Communication & Decision Making: Informed Consent." *Code of Medical Ethics,* edited by AMA Council on Ethical and Judicial Affairs (CEJA). Accessed May 4, 2024. https://code-medical-ethics.ama-assn.org/chapters/consent-communication-decision-making.

American Midwifery Certification Board (AMCB). 2021. 2021 Demographic Report. Accessed May 2, 2024. https://www.amcbmidwife.org/docs/default-source/reports/demographic-report-2021.pdf?sfvrsn=cac0b1e8_2.

Ancient Song Doula Services. n.d. "About Ancient Song." Accessed August 11, 2024. https://www.ancientsongdoulaservices.com/about.

Angood, P., E. Colchamiro, A. Lyzenga, and M. Marinelarena. 2009. National Quality Forum (NQF) Patient Safety Terms and Definitions. National Quality Forum. Accessed May 2, 2024. https://www.qualityforum.org/topics/safety_definitions.aspx.

Apfelbaum, Jeffrey L., Carin A. Hagberg, Richard T. Connis, Basem B. Abdelmalak, Madhulika Agarkar, Richard P. Dutton, John E. Fiadjoe, Robert Greif, P. Allan Klock, David Mercier, et al. 2022. "American Society of Anesthesiologists Practice Guidelines for Management of the Difficult Airway." *Anesthesiology* 136: 31–81. https://doi.org/10.1097/ALN.0000000000004002.

Aring, Charles D. 1958. "Sympathy and Empathy." *Journal of the American Medical Association* 167(4): 448–452.

Associated Press. 2017. "Opioid Epidemic Shares Chilling Similarities with Past Drug Crises." Stat News. October 29, 2017. Accessed August 8, 2024. https://www.statnews.com/2017/10/29/opioid-epidemic-shares-chilling-similarities-with-past-drug-crises/.

Attanasio, Laura B., and Rachel R. Hardeman. 2019. "Declined Care and Discrimination During the Childbirth Hospitalization." *Social Science & Medicine* 232: 270–277.

Badreldin, Nevert, William A. Grobman, and Lynn M. Yee. 2019. "Racial Disparities in Postpartum Pain Management." *Obstetrics & Gynecology* 134(6): 1147–1153.

Bailey, Moya. 2016. "Misogynoir in Medical Media: On Caster Semenya and R. Kelly." *Catalyst: Feminism, Theory, Technoscience* 2(2): 1–31.

Bailey, Moya. 2021. *Misogynoir Transformed: Black Women's Digital Resistance*. New York, NY: New York University Press.

Bailey, Moya, and Trudy. 2018. "On Misogynoir: Citation, Erasure, and Plagiarism." *Feminist Media Studies* 18(4): 762–768.

Beach, Mary Catherine, Somnath Saha, Jenny Park, Janiece Taylor, Paul Drew, Eve Plank, Lisa A. Cooper, and Brant Chee. 2021. "Testimonial Injustice: Linguistic Bias in the Medical Records of Black Patients and Women." *Journal of General Internal Medicine: JGIM* 36(6): 1708–1714.

Beauchamp, Tom L. 2007. "History and Theory in 'Applied Ethics'." *Kennedy Institute of Ethics Journal* 17(1): 55–64.

Bernhardt, Boris C., and Tania Singer. 2012. "The Neural Basis of Empathy." *Annual Review of Neuroscience* 35(1): 1–23.

Berry, D. R. 2017. *Their Price for Their Pound of Flesh: The Value of the Enslaved from Womb to Grave in the Building of a Nation*. Boston, MA: Beacon Press.

Betancourt, Joseph R., and Angela W. Maina. 2004. "The Institute of Medicine Report 'Unequal Treatment': Implications for Academic Health Centers." *The Mount Sinai Journal of Medicine* 71(5): 314–321.

Biblegateway. n.d. "Bible Book List: 1 John Chapter 14, Verse 8." Accessed August 14, 2024. https://www.biblegateway.com/passage/?search=1%20John%204%3A18&version=KJV.

Birthing Cultural Rigor. n.d. "Our Services: Our 4T Model of Inquiry, Improvement, Implementation, and Impact." Accessed May 7, 2024. https://www.birthingculturalrigor.org/services.

Black Infant Health (BIH). n.d. "About Us." Accessed August 20, 2024. https://blackinfanthealth.org/about-us/.

Black Women Birthing Justice (BWBJ). n.d. "Black Women Birthing Justice: Who We Are." Accessed August 16, 2024. https://www.blackwomenbirthingjustice.com/who-we-are.

Black Women Scholars and Research Working Group for the Black Mamas Matter Alliance. 2020. "Black Maternal Health Research Re-Envisioned: Best Practices for the Conduct of Research with, for, and by Black Mamas." *Harvard Law & Policy Review* 14: 393–415.

Blumgart, Herrman L. 1964. "Caring for the Patient." *New England Journal of Medicine* 270(9): 449–456.

Bonaparte, Alicia D. 2014. "Physicians' Discourse for Establishing Authoritative Knowledge in Birthing Work and Reducing the Presence of the Granny Midwife." *Journal of Historical Sociology* 28(2): 168–194. https://doi.org/10.1111/johs.12045.

Borges, Maria TR. 2017. "A Violent Birth: Reframing Coerced Procedures during Childbirth as Obstetric Violence." *Duke Luke Journal* 67: 827.

The Boring Bug. 2017. "What is the Difference Between Option and Choice?" November 15, 2017. Accessed May 7, 2024. https://boringbug.com/2017/11/15/the-difference-between-options-and-choices/#:~:text=Choices%20are%20the%20decisions%20we,which%20something%20is%20chosen%20from.

Bostick, Nathan A., Robert Sade, John W. McMahon, and Regina Benjamin. 2006. "Report of the American Medical Association Council on Ethical and Judicial Affairs: Withholding Information from Patients: Rethinking the Propriety of 'Therapeutic Privilege'." *The Journal of Clinical Ethics* 17(4): 302–306.

Bowie, Courney. 2011. "The Most Dangerous Place for Black Children..." American Civil Liberties Union (ACLU) News & Commentary. February 25, 2011. Accessed August 15, 2024. https://www.aclu.org/news/smart-justice/most-dangerous-place-black-children.

Boyle, Peter. 2023. "What's Your Specialty? New Data Show the Choices of America's Doctors by Gender, Race, and Age?" Association of American Medical Colleges (AAMC). January 12, 2023. Accessed May 2, 2024. https://www.aamc.org/news/what-s-your-specialty-new-data-show-choices-america-s-doctors-gender-race-and-age-.

Braun, Kathrin, Svea Luise Herrmann, Sabine Könninger, and Alfred Moore. 2010. "Ethical Reflection Must Always Be Measured." *Science, Technology, & Human Values* 35(6): 839–864.

Bray, Stephanie R., and Monica R. McLemore. 2021. "Demolishing the Myth of the Default Human That is Killing Black Mothers." *Frontiers in Public Health* 9: 675788.

Bridges, Kiara M. 2020. "Racial Disparities in Maternal Mortality." *New York University Law Review* 95: 1229–1318.

Bueter, Anke. 2022. "Bias as an Epistemic Notion." *Studies in History and Philosophy of Science* 91: 307–315.

Byrd, W. Michael, and Linda A. Clayton. 2001. "Race, Medicine, and Health Care in the United States: A Historical Survey." *Journal of the National Medical Association* 93(3): 11S–34S.

California Department of Public Health (CDPH). n.d. "Black Infant Health: About Us." Last updated April 23, 2024. Accessed May 8, 2024. https://www.cdph.ca.gov/Programs/CFH/DMCAH/BIH/Pages/default.aspx.

Cameron, Susan, and Imani Turtle-Song. 2002. "Learning to Write Case Notes Using the SOAP Format." *Journal of Counseling & Development* 80(3): 286–292.

Cassil, Alwyn, Danielle DeCosta, and Lisa Simpson. 2024. "A New Paradigm for Equitable Measurement: Using Racism – Not Race – As A Risk Factor." In *Documenting the Ripple Effects of Dobbs on Health, Equity, and Health Services Research*. AcademyHealtth.

CDC. 2017. "Severe Maternal Morbidity." Last modified May 15, 2024. Accessed August 3, 2024. https://www.cdc.gov/maternal-infant-health/php/severe-maternal-morbidity/index.html.

CDC. 2021. "About Maternal Mortality Review Committee." Last modified May 15, 2024. Accessed August 4, 2024. https://www.cdc.gov/maternal-mortality

/php/mmrc/index.html#:~:text=What%20to%20know,recommendations%20for%20preventing%20future%20deaths.

CDC. 2022. "Four in 5 Pregnancy-Related Deaths in the U.S. are Preventable." Last reviewed September 19, 2022. Accessed September 25, 2022. https://www.cdc.gov/media/releases/2022/p0919-pregnancy-related-deaths.html.

CDC National Center for Health Statistics (NCHS). 2022. Home Births in the U.S. Increase to Highest Level in 30 Years. Last updated November 17, 2022. Accessed May 3, 2024. https://www.cdc.gov/nchs/pressroom/nchs_press_releases/2022/20221117.htm.

CDC. n.d. "Frequently Asked Questions About Vitamin K Deficiency Bleeding." Last updated May 15, 2024. Accessed May 2, 2024. https://www.cdc.gov/vitamin-k-deficiency/faq/index.html.

Center for Medicare & Medicaid Services (CMS). n.d. "Quality Measurement and Quality Improvement." Accessed August 5, 2024. https://www.cms.gov/Medicare/Quality-Initiatives-Patient-Assessment-Instruments/MMS/Quality-Measure-and-Quality-Improvement-.

Chambers, Brittany D., Brianne Taylor, Tamara Nelson, Jessica Harrison, Arielle Bell, Allison O'Leary, Helen A. Arega, Sepehr Hashemi, Safyer McKenzie-Sampson, Karen A. Scott, et al. 2022. "Clinicians' Perspectives on Racism and Black Women's Maternal Health." *Women's Health Reports* 3(1): 476–482.

Chambers, Brittany D., Helen A. Arega, Silvia E. Arabia, Brianne Taylor, Robyn G. Barron, Brandi Gates, Loretta Scruggs-Leach, Karen A. Scott, and Monica R. McLemore. 2021. "Black Women's Perspectives on Structural Racism Across the Reproductive Lifespan: A Conceptual Framework for Measurement Development." *Maternal and Child Health Journal* 25: 402–413.

Chambers, Brittany D., Helen Arega, Solaire Spellen, Silvia E. Arabia, Darcy Stanley, Anu Manchikanti Gomez, Linda Franck, Rachel Berkowitz, Sky Feuer, Laura Jelliffe-Pawlowski, et al. 2018. "Pregnant Black Women's Experiences of Racial Discrimination." *American Journal of Obstetrics & Gynecology* 218(1): S569.

Chambers, Brittany D., Silvia E. Arabia, Helen A. Arega, Molly R. Altman, Rachel Berkowitz, Sky K. Feuer, Linda S. Franck, Anu M. Gomez, Kord Kober, Tania Pacheco-Werner, et al. 2020. "Exposures to Structural Racism and Racial Discrimination Among Pregnant and Early Post-partum Black Women Living in Oakland, California." *Stress and Health* 36(2): 213–219.

Charmaz, Kathy. 2016. *Constructing Grounded Theory: A Practical Guide Through Qualitative Analysis*. Los Angeles, CA: Sage.

Cheah, Irene Guat Sim. 2019. "Economic Assessment of Neonatal Intensive Care." *Translational Pediatrics* 8(3): 246–256.

Chervenak, Frank A., Renee McLeod-Sordjan, Susan L. Pollet, Monique De Four Jones, Mollie R. Gordon, Adriann Combs, Eran Bornstein, Dawnette Lewis, Adi Katz, Ashley Warman, et al. 2024. "Obstetric Violence is a Misnomer." *American Journal of Obstetrics and Gynecology* 230(3): S1138–S1145.

Childs, Erica Chito. 2005. "Looking Behind the Stereotypes of the 'Angry Black Woman' an Exploration of Black Women's Responses to Interracial Relationships." *Gender & Society* 19(4): 544–561.

Cimino, James J., Ziran Li, and Chunhua Weng. 2018. "An Exploration of the Terminology of Clinical Cognition and Reasoning." *AMIA Annu Symp Proc* 2018: 321–329.

Civil Rights Congress. 1951. *We Charge Genocide: The Crime of the Government Against the Negro People.* William L. Patterson (ed.). New York, NY: International Publishers.

Collins, Patricia Hill. 1990. "Black Feminist Thought in the Matrix of Domination." *Black Feminist Thought: Knowledge, Consciousness, and the Politics of Empowerment* 138(1990): 221–238.

Collins, Patricia Hill. 1996. "What's in a Name? Womanism, Black Feminism, and Beyond." *The Black Scholar* 26(1): 9–17. https://doi.rg/10.1080/00064246.1996.11430765.

Collins, Patricia Hill. 2004. *Black Sexual Politics: African Americans, Gender, and the New Racism.* New York, NY: Routledge.

Collins, Patricia Hill, and Sirma Bilge. 2000. *Intersectionality.* Hoboken, NJ: John Wiley & Son.

Committee on Quality of Health Care in America, Institute of Medicine. 2001. *Crossing the Quality Chasm: A New Health System for the 21st Century.* Washington, DC: National Academies Press.

Cooper, Iman. 2015. "Commodification of the Black Body, Sexual Objectification and Social Hierarchies During Slavery." *Earlham Historical Journal* 7(2): 21–41.

Cooper, Jeffrey B., David M. Gaba, Bryan Liang, David Woods, and Laura N. Blum. 2024. "The National Patient Safety Foundation Agenda for Research and Development in Patient Safety." Medscape. August 12, 2024. Accessed May 2, 2024. https://www.medscape.com/viewarticle/408064_3?form=fpf.

Cooper, Lisa A., Debra L. Roter, Rachel L. Johnson, Daniel E. Ford, Donald M. Steinwachs, and Neil R. Powe. 2003. "Patient-Centered Communication, Ratings of Care, and Concordance of Patient and Physician Race." *Annals of Internal Medicine* 139(11): 907–915.

Cooper Owens, Deirdre. 2017. *Medical Bondage: Race, Gender, and the Origins of American Gynecology.* Athens, GA: University of Georgia Press.

Crenshaw, Kimberle. 1991. "Race, Gender, and Sexual Harassment." *Southern California Law Review* 65: 1467.

Crowther, Susan, and Gill Thomson. 2023. "Introduction: Situating Hermeneutic Phenomenology as Research Method in Health, Social Care, and Education." In *Hermeneutic Phenomenology in Health and Social Care Research,* Susan Crowther and Gill Thompson (eds.), pp. 1–20. New York, NY: Routledge Taylor & Francis Group.

Dalton, E. D., Ivanka Pjesivac, Scott Eldredge, and Laura Miller. 2020. "From Vulnerability to Disclosure: A Normative Approach to Understanding Trust in Obstetric and Intrapartum Nurse-Patient Communication." *Health Communication* 36(5): 616–629. https://doi.org/10.1080/10410236.2020.1733225.

Dankwa, Serena O. 2023. "Desiring Queer Motherhood and Mothering Ourselves." *Journal of African Cultural Studies* 35(2): 165–175. https://doi.org/10.1080/13696815.2023.2186380.

Da Silva, Denise Ferreira. 2007. *Toward a Global Idea of Race.* Minneapolis, MN: University of Minnesota Press.

David, Richard J., and James W. Collins, Jr. 1997. "Differing Birth Weight Among Infants of U.S.-Born Blacks, African-Born Blacks, and U.S.-Born Whites." *New England Journal of Medicine* 337(17): 1209e14. https://doi.org/10.1056/NEJM199710233371706.

Davis, Dána-Ain. 2018. "Obstetric Racism: The Racial Politics of Pregnancy, Labor, and Birthing". Medical Anthropology. Published online December 8, 2018. Accessed May 5, 2024. https://doi.org/10.1080/01459740.2018.1549389.

Davis, Dàna-Ain. 2019. *Reproductive Injustice: Racism, Pregnancy, and Premature Birth.* New York, NY: NYU Press.

Davis, Dána-Ain. 2020. "Reproducing while Black: The Crisis of Black Maternal Health, Obstetric Racism and Assisted Reproductive Technology." *Reproductive Biomedicine & Society Online* 11: 56–64.

Davis, Dána-Ain. 2022a, May 13. A Grammar of Obstetric Racism. Paper presented at the Sarah Parker Redmond Center for the Study of Race and Racialisation, University College of London (Live).

Davis, Dána-Ain. 2022b, October 26. Traumatic Repercussions: Black Birthing People and Obstetric Racism. Paper presented at the AFIN International Virtual Conference on Female Reproductive Health. Women Between Invisible Disease and Impossible Well-Being, Universitat Autònoma de Barcelona (Virtual).

Davis, Dána-Ain, Cheyenne Varner, and LeConté J. Dill. 2021. "A Birth Story." Anthropology News website. August 27, 2021. Accessed August 11, 2024. https://www.anthropology-news.org/articles/a-birth-story/.

Davis, Dána-Ain, and Karen A. Scott. 2020. "Translating Obstetric Racism into a Patient-Reported Experience Measure." Social Sciences Grand Rounds Humanities and Social Sciences Department University of California San Francisco (UCSF). July 24, 2020. Accessed August 22, 2024. https://humsci.ucsf.edu/social-science-grand-rounds.

Davis, Dána-Ain, Monica J. Casper, Evelynn Hammonds, and Wendy Post. 2024. "The Continued Significance of Obstetric Violence: A Response to Chervenak, McLeod-Sordjan, Pollet et al." *Health Equity* 8(1): 513–518.

Declercq, Eugene, and Laurie Zephyrin. 2021. "Severe Maternal Morbidity in the United States: A Primer." Commonwealth Fund. Accessed August 3, 2024. https://doi.org/10.26099/r43h-vh76.

Dekker, Rebecca. 2013. "American Obstetrics in the 1950's." Evidence Based Birth Evidence That Empowers. Accessed August 4, 2024. https://evidencebasedbirth.com/american-obstetrics-in-the-1950s/.

Dekker, Sidney. 2017. *Just Culture: Restoring Trust and Accountability in Your Organization.* Third Edition. Boca Raton, FL: CRC Press.

Di Lorenzo, Rosaria, Giulio Cabri, Eleonora Carretti, Giacomo Galli, Nina Giambalvo, Giulia Rioli, Serena Saraceni, Giulia Spiga, Cinzia Del Giovane, and Paola Ferri. 2017. "A Preliminary Study of Patient Dignity Inventory Validation Among Patients Hospitalized in an Acute Psychiatric Ward." *Neuropsychiatric Disease and Treatment* 13(2017): 177–190.

Dictionary. n.d. "Chattel Slavery." Accessed May 7, 2024. https://www.dictionary.com/browse/chattel-slavery.

Dominquez, Tyan Parker. 2011. "Adverse Birth Outcomes in African-American Women: The Social Context of Persistent Reproductive Advantage." *Social Work in Public Health* 26(1): 3–16. https://doi.org/10.1080/10911350902986880.

Dominquez, Tyan Parker, Emily Ficklin Strong, Nancy Krieger, Matthew W. Gillman, and Janet W. Rich-Edwards. 2009. "Differences in the Self-Reported Racism Experiences of US-Born and Foreign-Born Black Pregnant Women." *Social Science and Medicine* 69(2): 258–265. https://doi.org/10.1016/j.socscimed.2009.03.022.

Donaldson, Molla S., Janet M. Corrigan, and Linda T. Kohn, eds. 2000. *To Err is Human: Building a Safer Health System*. Vol. 6. Washington, DC: National Academies Press.

Doyle, Kathleen. 2023. "The Queen Mary Psalter." In *The Book by Design: The Remarkable Story of the World's Greatest Invention*, P. J. M. Marks and Stephen Parkin (eds.), p. 64. Chicago, IL: University of Chicago Press.

DuBois, W. E. Burghardt, ed. 1906. The Health and Physique of the Negro American. Report of a Social Study Made Under the Direction of Atlanta University; Together with the Proceedings of the Eleventh Conference for the Study of the Negro Problems, Held at Atlanta University, on May 29th, 1906. Atlanta, GA: Atlanta University Press, 1906. https://ajph.aphapublications.org/doi/pdf/10.2105/AJPH.93.2.272.

DuBois, W. E. Burghardt. 2003. "The Health and Physique of the Negro American." *American Journal of Public Health* 93(2): 272–276. https://doi.org/10.2105/ajph.93.2.272.

Duke Health. n.d. "Duke Heath Stands Against Racism, Bias, and Hate." Accessed August 5, 2024. https://www.dukehealth.org/diversity-equity-and-inclusion/Duke-health-stands-against-racism.

Edmonds, Brownsyne Tucker, Sacha Sharp, and Valencia P. Walker. 2023. "Mitigating Misogynoir: Inclusive Professionalism as a Health Equity Strategy." *Clinical Obstetrics and Gynecology* 66(1): 14–21.

Eichelberger, Kacey Y., Kemi Doll, Geraldine E. Ekpo, and Matthew L. Zerden. 2016. "Black Lives Matter: Claiming a Space for Evidence-Based Outrage in Obstetrics and Gynecology." *American Journal of Public Health* 106(10): 1771–1772.

Ekeke, Paris, Dara D. Mendez, Toby D. Yanowiitz, and Janet M. Catov. 2020. "Racial Differences in the Biochemical Effects of Stress in Pregnancy." *International Journal of Environmental Research and Public Health* 17(19): 6941.

Elephant Circle. n.d. "Filing Discrimination Complaints." Accessed August, 22, 2024. https://www.elephantcircle.net/ocr.

Emanuel, Linda, Don Berwick, James Conway, John Combes, Martin Hatlie, Lucian Leape, James Reason, Paul Schyve, Charles Vincent, and Merrilyn Walton. 2008. "What Exactly Is Patient Safety?" In A*dvances in Patient Safety: New Directions and Alternative Approaches (Vol. 1: Assessment)*, Kerm Henriksen, James B. Battles, Margaret A. Keyes, and Mary L. Grady (eds.). Rockville, MD: Agency for Healthcare Research and Quality. Accessed May 2, 2024. https://www.ncbi.nlm.nih.gov/books/NBK43629/.

Firoz, Tabassum, Doris Chou, Peter von Dadelszen, Priya Agrawal, Rachel Vanderkruik, Ozge Tunçalp, Laura A. Magee, Nynke van Den Broek, Lale Say, and Maternal Morbidity Working Group. 2013. "Measuring Maternal Health: Focus on Maternal Morbidity." *Bulletin of the World Health Organization* 91(10): 794–796. https://doi.org/10.2471/BLT.13.117564.

Ford, Chandra L., and Collins O. Airhihenbuwa. 2010. "The Public Health Critical Race Methodology: Praxis for Antiracism Research." *Social Science & Medicine* 71(8): 1390–1398. https://doi.org/10.1016/j.socscimed.2010.07.030. Epub 2010 Aug 11.

Forgiarini, Matteo, Marcello Gallucci, and Angelo Maravita. 2011. "Racism and the Empathy for Pain on Our Skin." *Frontiers in Psychology* 2: 108.

Forna, Amiatta. 2002. "Racism as Distraction: Aminatta Forna Writes About Toni Morrison." Georgetown University Medical Humanities Media and Scholarship. Accessed April 5, 2024. https://medicalhumanities.georgetown.edu/media-and-scholarship/media/racism-as-distraction/.

Fox, Renee, and Harold Lief. 1963. "Training for "Detached Concern." In *The Psychological Basis of Medical Practice,* H. Lief (ed.), pp. 12–35. New York, NY: Harper & Row.

Franck, Linda S., Monica R. McLemore, Norlissa Cooper, Baylee De Castro, Anastasia Y. Gordon, Schyneida Williams, Shanell Williams, and Larry Rand. 2018. "A Novel Method for Involving Women of Color at High Risk for Preterm Birth in Research Priority Setting." *JoVE (Journal of Visualized Experiments)* 131(2018): e56220.

Fricker Miranda. 2007. *Epistemic Injustice: Power and the Ethics of Knowing.* Oxford: Oxford University Press.

Gathercole, Rebecca. "The Sheppard-Towner Act." Discovering The 1920s, February 21, 2024. Accessed May 08, 2025. https://dh-wordpress.ramapo.edu/discovering1920s/blog/2024/02/21/sheppard-towner-act/.

Goode, Keisha, and Barbara Katz Rothman. 2017. "African-American Midwifery, a History and a Lament." *American Journal of Economics and Sociology* 76(1): 65–94.

Goode, Keisha La'Nesha. 2014. "Birthing, Blackness, and the Body: Black Midwives and Experiential Continuities of Institutional Racism." CUNY Academic Works. https://academicworks.cuny.edu/gc_etds/42.

Goodwin, Michele. 2014. "Fetal Protection Laws: Moral Panic and the New Constitutional Battlefront." *California Law Review* 102: 781–876.

Goodwin, Michele. 2017. "How the Criminalization of Pregnancy Robs Women of Reproductive Autonomy." *Hastings Center Report* 47: S19–S27. https://doi.org/10.1002/hast.791.

Goodwin, Michele. 2020. *Policing the Womb: Invisible Women and the Criminalization of Motherhood.* United Kingdom; New York, USA: Cambridge University Press.

Goyal, Monika K., Kuppermann, Natthanial, Cleary, Sean D., Teach, Stephen J., and James M. Chamberlain. 2015. "Racial Disparities in Pain Management of Children with Appendicitis in Emergency Departments." *JAMA Pediatrics* 169(11): 996-1002.

Greene, Beverly. 1994. "African-American Women: Derivatives of Racism and Sexism in Psychotherapy." In *Challenging Racism and Sexism: Alternatives to*

Genetic Explanations, E. Tobach and B. Rosoff (eds.), pp. 122–139. New York, NY: Feminist Press.

Greene, Beverly. 1995. "Addressing racism, Sexism, and Heterosexism in Psychoanalytic Psychotherapy." In *Lesbians and Psychoanalysis: Revolutions in Theory and Practice*, Judith M. Glassgold and Suzanne Lasenza (eds.), pp. 145–159. New York, NY: Simon and Schuster.

Griffin, F. A., and R. K. Resar. 2009. *IHI Global Trigger Tool for Measuring Adverse Events*. 2nd Edition. IHI Innovation Series white paper. Cambridge, MA: Institute for Healthcare Improvement.

Grober, Ethan D., and John M. A. Bohnen. 2005. "Defining Medical Error." *Canadian Journal of Surgery* 48(1): 39.

Grobman, William A. 2012. "Obstetric Patient Safety: An Overview." *American Journal of Perinatology* 29(1): 3–6. https://doi.org/10.1055/s-0031-1285828.

Grove, Robert D., and Alica M. Hetzel. 1968. "Vital Statistics Rates in the United States 1940–1960." National Center for Health Statistics Division of Vital Statistics. Public Health Service Publication no. 1677. Accessed August 4, 2024. https://www.cdc.gov/nchs/data/vsus/vsrates1940_60.pdf.

Hagen, Christy. 2023. "Infant Mortality Rate Sees First Rise in 20 Years." Blog for the National Center for Health Statistics (NCHS). Last updated October 31, 2023. Accessed May 3, 2024. https://blogs.cdc.gov/nchs/2023/11/01/7479/.

Hall, Essie M., and Karen McCurtis Witherspoon. 2015. "How Adopting Stereotypical Roles May Impact Sexual Risk Behavior Among African American College Women." *Journal of Black Sexuality and Relationships* 1(4): 1–22.

Halpern, Jodi. 2003. "What is Clinical Empathy?" *Journal of General Internal Medicine* 18(8): 670–674.

Hamilton, Brady E., Joyce A. Martin, and Michelle J. K. Osterman. 2022. "Births: Provisional Data for 2021." *Vital Statistics Rapid Release*; no. 20, Hyattsville, MD: National Center for Health Statistics. May 2022. Accessed April 8, 2024. https://dx.doi.org/10.15620/cdc:116027.

Hamilton, Jameaka Latrice, Diane Shumbusho, Devin Cooper, Tara Fletcher, James Aden, Larissa Weir, and Erin Keyser. 2021. "Race Matters: Maternal Morbidity in the Military Health System." *American Journal of Obstetrics and Gynecology* 224(5): 512e1–512e6.

Hansen, Terry Leonid, Kyle Goerl, Reginald Fears, Tim Nguyen, Traci Hart, and Paul Uhlig. 2012. "Observations of Pre-operative Teamwork and Communication during the Implementation of a City-Wide Surgical Safety Checklist." *Kansas Journal of Medicine* 5(4): 117-133.

Hardeman, Rachel R., Eduardo M. Medina, and Katy B. Kozhimannil. 2016. "Structural Racism and Supporting Black Lives—the Role of Health Professionals." *New England Journal of Medicine* 375(22): 21132115.

Hardeman, Rachel R., and J'Mag Karbeah. 2020. "Examining Racism in Health Services Research: A Disciplinary Self-Critique." *Health Services Research* 55(5): 777–780. https://doi.org/10.1111/1475-6773.13558.

Hardeman, Rachel R., J'Mag Karbeah, and Katy B. Kozhimannil. 2020. "Applying a Critical Race Lens to Relationship-Centered Care in Pregnancy and Childbirth:

An Antidote to Structural Racism." *Birth* 47(1): 3–7. https://doi.org/10.1111/birt.12462.

Hardeman, Rachel R., Katy A. Murphy, J'Mag Karbeah, and Katy Backes Kozhimannil. 2018. "Naming Institutionalized Racism in the Public Health Literature: A Systematic Literature Review." *Public Health Reports* 133(3): 240–249. https://doi.org/10.1177/0033354918760574.

Harrison, Eona, Faith Mitchell, Leandra Lacy, Kimá Joy Taylor, and Lauren Fung. 2023. "Understanding Training and Workforce Pathways to Develop and Retain Black Maternal Health Clinicians in California." Urban Institute, May 2023. Accessed May 2, 2024. https://www.urban.org/sites/default/files/2023-05/Understanding%20Training%20and%20Workforce%20Pathways%20to%20Develop%20and%20Retain%20Black%20Maternal%20Health%20Clinicians%20in%20California.pdf.

Heidegger, Martin. 2010. *Being and Time*. Translated by Joan Stambaugh. Albany, NY: SUNY Press.

Hill, Shirley A. 2016. *Inequality and African-American Health: How Racial Disparities Create Sickness*. Chicago, IL: University of Chicago Press.

Hoberman, J. 2012. *Black and Blue: The Origins and Consequences of Medical Racism* (First Edition). Berkeley, CA: University of California Press.

Hooker, Angelo B., Anouk Etman, Matthijs Westra, and Wouter J. Van der Kam. 2019. "Aggregate Analysis of Sentinel Events as a Strategic Tool in Safety Management Can Contribute to the Improvement of Healthcare Safety." *International Journal of Quality in Health Care* 31(2): 110–116.

Howland, Renata E., Angley, Meghan, Won, Sang Hee, et al. 2019. "Determinants of Severe Maternal Morbidity and Its Racial/Ethnic Disparities in New York City, 2008–2012." *Maternal and Child Health Journal* 23: 346–355.

Hoyert, Donna L. 2023. "Maternal Mortality Rates in the United States, 2021." National Center for Health Statistics (NCHS) Health E-Stats. Last updated March 16, 2023. https://dx.doi.org/10.15620/cdc:124678.

Illich, Ivan. 1974. "Medical Nemesis." *Lancet* 7(7863): 918–921.

Illich, Ivan. 2003. "Medical Nemesis." *Journal of Epidemiology & Community Health* 57(12): 919–922. https://www.ncbi.nlm.nih.gov/pmc/articles/PMC1732343/pdf/v057p00919.pdf.

IMDb. n.d. "The Business of Being Born." Accessed May 2, 2024. https://www.imdb.com/title/tt0995061/.

Institute of Medicine (IOM). 2001. *Crossing the Quality Chasm: A New Health System for the 21st Century*. Washington, DC: National Academy Press.

Institute of Medicine (US) Committee on Data Standards for Patient Safety. 2004. *Patient Safety: Achieving a New Standard For Care*. Shari M. Erickson, Julie Wolcott, Janet M. Corrigan, and Philip Aspden, eds. Washington, DC: National Academies Press (US).

Institute of Medicine (US) Committee on Quality of Health Care in America. 2000. *To Err is Human: Building a Safer Health System*. Linda T. Kohn, Janet M. Corrigan, and Molla S. Donaldson, eds. Washington, DC: National Academies Press (US).

Institute of Medicine (US) Committee on Understanding and Eliminating Racial and Ethnic Disparities in Health Care. 2003. *Unequal Treatment: Confronting Racial and Ethnic Disparities in Health Care*, Brian D. Smedley, Adrienne Y. Stith, and R. Alan eds. Washington, DC: National Academies Press (US). Accessed May 2, 2024. https://www.ncbi.nlm.nih.gov/books/NBK220358/.

Jacobson, Nora. 2009. "A Taxonomy of Dignity: A Grounded Theory Study." *BMC International Health and Human Rights* 9(2009): 1–9.

Johnson, Akilah. 2022. "America Has a Maternal Mortality Crisis. Biden Push Aims to Change That." *Washington Post.* August 9. 2022. Accessed May 7, 2024. https://www.washingtonpost.com/health/2022/08/08/maternal-mortality-biden/.

Johnson, Rachel L., Debra Roter, Neil R. Powe, and Lisa A. Cooper. 2004. "Patient Race/Ethnicity and Quality of Patient-Physician Communication During Medical Visits." *American Journal of Public Health* 94(12): 2084–2090.

Jolivétte, Andrew, ed. 2015. *Research Justice: Methodologies for Social Change.* Bristol: Policy Press.

Jones, Camara Phyllis. 2000. "Levels of Racism: A Theoretic Framework and A Gardener's Tale." *American Journal of Public Health* 90(8): 1212–1215.

Jones, Camara Phyllis. 2014. "Systems of Power, Axes of Inequity: Parallels, Intersections, Braiding the Strands." *Medical Care* 52(10) (suppl 3): S71–S75. https://doi.org/10.1097/MLR.0000000000000216.

Jones, Jo, and William D. Mosher. 2013. "Fathers' Involvement with Their Children: United States, 2006–2010." *National Health Statistics Reports* (71): 1–21.

Kapaki, Vasiliki, and Kyriakos Souliotis. 2018. "Defining Adverse Events and Determinants of Medical Errors in Healthcare." In *Vignettes in Patient Safety-Volume 3,* Stanislaw P. Stawicki and Michael S. Firstenberg (eds.). London: IntechOpen.

Kerppola, Jenni, Nina Halme, Marja-Leena Perälä, and Anna Maija-Pietilä. 2019. "Parental Empowerment—Lesbian, Gay, Bisexual, Trans or Queer Parents' Perceptions of Maternity and Child Healthcare." *International Journal of Nursing Practice* 25(5): e12755.

Khabele, Dineo, Kevin Holcomb, Ngina K. Connors, and Linda Bradley 2021. "A Perspective on James Marion Sims, MD, and Anti-Black Racism in Obstetrics and Gynecology." *Journal of Minimally Invasive Gynecology* 28(2): 153–155.

Kidd, Ian James, José Medina, and Gaile Pohlhaus. 2017. "Introduction to the Routledge Handbook of Epistemic Injustice." In *The Routledge Handbook of Epistemic Injustice*, Ian James Kidd, José Medina, and Gaile Pohlhaus (eds.), pp. 1–9. Abingdon, NY: Routledge, 2017.

Koerber, Anne, Sangeeta Gajendra, Reginald L. Fulford, Ellen BeGole, and Carla A. Evans. 2004. "An Exploratory Study of Orthodontic Resident Communication by Patient Race and Ethnicity." *Journal of Dental Education* 68(5): 553–562.

Koonin, Lisa M., Atrash Hani K., Rochat Roger W., and Jack C. Smith. 1988. "Maternal Mortality Surveillance, United States, 1980–1985." *MMWR CDC Surveillance Summary* 37(5): 19–29.

Krishnan, N. R., and A. S. Kasthuri. 2005. "Iatrogenic Disorders." *Medical Journal, Armed Forces India (MJAFI)* 61: 2–6.

Larimore, Walter L., and Elizabeth V. Jordan. 1995. "SOAP to SNOCAMP: Improving the Medical Record Format." *Journal of Family Practice* 41(4): 393–398. Gale Academic OneFile. Accessed August 17, 2024. https://link.gale.com/apps/doc/A17527982/AONE?u=tel_oweb&sid=googleScholar&xid=d3bf28c3.

Lauer, Mike. 2016. "Scientific Rigor in NIH Grant Applications." National Institutes of Health. January 28, 2016. Accessed May 8, 2024. https://nexus.od.nih.gov/all/2016/01/28/scientific-rigor-in-nih-grant-applications/.

Lazarou, Jason, Bruce H. Pomeranz, and Paul N. Corey. 1998. "Incidence of Adverse Drug Reactions in Hospitalized Patients: A Meta-analysis of Prospective Studies." *JAMA: The Journal of the American Medical Association* 279(15): 1200–1205. https://doi.org/10.1001/jama.279.15.1200.

Lett, Elle, Marie-Fatima Hyacinthe, Dána-Ain Davis, and Karen A. Scott. 2023. "Community Support Persons and Mitigating Obstetric Racism During Childbirth." *The Annals of Family Medicine* 21(3): 227–233.

Levesque, Jean-Frederic, Mark F. Harris, and Grant Russell. 2013. "Patient-Centred Access to Health Care: Conceptualising Access at the Interface of Health Systems and Populations." *International Journal for Equity in Health* 12(18): 1–9.

Lin, Sunny C., Gmerice Hammond, Michael Esposito, Cassandra Majewski, Randi E. Foraker, and Karen E. Joynt Maddox. 2023. "Segregated Patterns of Hospital Care Delivery and Health Outcomes." *JAMA Health Forum, American Medical Association* 4(11): e234172–e234172.

Loudon, I. 2008. "General Practitioners and Obstetrics: A Brief History." *Journal of the Royal Society of Medicine* 101(11): 531–535. https://doi.org/10.1258/jrsm.2008.080264.

The Lowcountry Digital History Initiative (LDHI). n.d. "Hidden Voices: Enslaved Women in the Lowcountry and U.S. South." Exploitation Through Reproductive Labor. Accessed August 17, 2024. https://ldhi.library.cofc.edu/exhibits/show/hidden-voices/enslaved-women-and-slaveholder/reproductive-exploitation.

Lowe, Nancy K. 2014. "Dignity in Childbirth." *Journal of Obstetric, Gynecologic, and Neonatal Nursing* 43(2): 137–138.

Lyndon, Audrey, Dána-Ain Davis, Anjana E. Sharma, and Karen A. Scott. 2023. "Emotional Safety Is Patient Safety." *BMJ Quality & Safety* 32: 369–372. https://doi.org/10.1136/bmjqs-2022-015573.

MacDorman, Marian F., and Eugene Declercq. 2019. "Trends and State Variations in Out-of-Hospital Births in the United States, 2004–2017." *Birth* 46(2): 279–288.

MacDorman, Marian F., Fay Menacker, and Eugene Declercq. 2010. "Trends and Characteristics of Home and Other Out-of-Hospital Births in the United States, 1990–2006." *National Vital Statistics Reports: from the Centers for Disease Control and Prevention, National Center for Health Statistics, National Vital Statistics System* 58(11): 1–14.

MacLachlan, Alice. 2022. "Tone Policing and the Assertion of Authority." Blog of the APA. May 20, 2022. Accessed April 8, 2024. https://blog.apaonline.org/2022/05/10/tone-policing-and-the-assertion-of-authority/.

Madgett, Katherine. 2017. "Sheppard-Towner Maternity and Infancy Protection Act (1921)." *Embryo Project Encyclopedia.* Arizona State University. May 08, 2017. Accessed May 08, 2024. https://embryo.asu.edu/pages/sheppard-towner-maternity-and-infancy-protection-act-1921.

Manfredini, Daniele, M. B. Bucci, F. Montagna, and L. Guarda-Nardini. 2011. "Temporomandibular Disorders Assessment: Medicolegal Considerations in the Evidence-Based Era." *Journal of Oral Rehabilitation* 38(2): 101–119.

March of Dimes. 2023. "2023 March of Dimes Report Card Shows Modest Improvement in U.S. Preterm Birth Rate, Which Remains at Decade-Long High, Earning Nation D+ Grade." November 16, 2023. Accessed May 3, 2024. https://www.marchofdimes.org/about/news/2023-march-dimes-report-card-shows-modest-improvement-us-preterm-birth-rate.

March of Dimes Peristats. n.d. "2023 March of Dimes Report Card for United States." Accessed May 8, 2024. https://www.marchofdimes.org/peristats/reports/united-states/report-card.

Markakis, K., R. Frankel, H. Beckman, and A. Suchman. 1999. "Teaching Empathy: It Can Be Done." Working Paper Presented at the Annual Meeting of the Society of General Internal Medicine, San Francisco, CA, April 29–May 1, 1999.

Martin, Michael D., Kory J. Wilson, Brian K. Ross, and Karen Souter. 2007. "Intubation Risk Factors for Temporomandibular Joint/Facial Pain." *Anesthesia Progress* 54(3): 109–114.

May, Vivian M. 2014. "'Speaking into the Void'? Intersectionality Critiques and Epistemic Backlash." *Hypatia* 29(1): 94–112.

Mbembe, Achille. 2006. "On the Postcolony: A Brief Response to Critics." *African identities* 4(2): 143–178.

McClain, Dani. 2019. "You're Black and Pregnant. What Should Your Birth Plan Actually Look Like?" Self. November 22, 2019. Accessed May 8, 2024. https://www.self.com/story/black-pregnant-birth-plan.

McClurg, Asha Belle, Kavita Shah, Schiff Arora, Lauren D. Schiff, Erin T. Carey, and Genevieve Scott Neal-Perry. 2022. "Dismantling Structural Barriers: Resident Clinics Refocused on Equity." *Obstetrics & Gynecology* 140(5): 739–742. https://doi.org/10.1097/AOG.0000000000004920

McFarling, Usha Lee. 2022. "'So Much More to Do': A Hospital System's Campaign to Confront Racism – and Resistance to Change – Makes Early Strides." Stata News. August 25, 2022. https://www.statnews.com/2022/08/25/mass-general-brigham-campaign-confront-racism-early-progress/.

McLemore, Monica R. 2018. "What Blame the Mother Stories Get Wrong About Birth Outcomes Among Black Moms." Center for Health Journalism Website. March 14, 2018. Accessed November 4, 2018. https://centerforhealthjournalism.org/our-work/insights/what-blame-mother-stories-get-wrong-about-birth-outcomes-among-black-moms.

Metzl, Jonathan M., and Dorothy E. Roberts. 2014. "Structural Competency Meets Structural Racism: Race, Politics, and the Structure of Medical Knowledge." *The Virtual Mentor* 16(9): 674–690. https://doi.org/10.1001/virtualmentor.2014.16.09.spec1-1409.

Mitchell, Angela, and Kennise Herring. 1998. *What the Blues Is All About: Black Women Overcoming Stress and Depression.* New York: Perigree Book.

Mount Sinani. n.d. "Road Map for Action to Address Racism." Accessed August 5, 2024. https://www.mountsinai.org/about/addressing-racism.

Mullings, Leith. 2005. "Resistance and Resilience: The Sojourner Syndrome and the Social Context of Reproduction in Central Harlem." *Transforming Anthropology* 13(2): 79–91.

Mullings, Leith, Alaka Wali, Diane McLean, Janet Mittchell, Sabiyah Prince, Deborah Thomas, and Patricia Tovar. 2001. "Qualitative Methodologies and Community Participation in Examining Reproductive Experiences: The Harlem Birth Right Project." *Maternal Child Health Journal* 5: 85–93. https://doi.org/10.1023/A:1011397031640.

Murray-García, Jann, and Melanie Tervalon. 2014. "The Concept of Cultural Humility." *Health Affairs* 33(7): 1303–1303. https://doi.org/10.1377/hlthaff.2014.0564. PMID: 25006160.

Najjar, Peter, Allen Kachalia, Tori Sutherland, Jennifer Beloff, Jo Ann David-Kasdan, David W. Bates, and Richard D. Urman. 2015. "A Multidisciplinary Three-Phase Approach to Improve the Clinical Utility of Patient Safety Indicators." *Quality Management in Healthcare* 24(2): 62–68.

National Academies of Sciences, Engineering, and Medicine (NASEM); Health and Medicine Division; Division of Behavioral and Social Sciences and Education; Board on Children, Youth, and Families; Committee on Assessing Health Outcomes by Birth Settings. 2020a. *Birth Settings in America: Outcomes, Quality, Access, and Choice,* Backes EP and Scrimshaw SC (eds.). Washington, DC: National Academies Press (US). Accessed May 3, 2024. https://www.ncbi.nlm.nih.gov/books/NBK555484/.

National Academies of Sciences, Engineering, and Medicine (NASEM); Health and Medicine Division; Board on Health Care Services; Board on Health Sciences Policy; Committee on Temporomandibular Disorders (TMDs): From Research Discoveries to Clinical Treatment. Yost O, Liverman CT, English R, et al., editors. 2020b. *Temporomandibular Disorders: Priorities for Research and Care.* Washington (DC): National Academies Press (US). Accessed May 3, 2024. https://www.ncbi.nlm.nih.gov/books/NBK558001/.

National Center for Chronic Disease Prevention and Health Promotion (U.S.), Division of Reproductive Health. 2023. "Pregnancy Mortality Surveillance System." March 23, 2023. Accessed May 08, 2024. https://stacks.cdc.gov/view/cdc/128166.

National Institute of Health. n.d. "Enhancing Reproducibility through Rigor and Transparency." Updated September 9, 2024. Accessed October 15, 2024. https://grants.nih.gov/policy-and-compliance/policy-topics/reproducibility.

National Partnership for Women and Families. n.d. "More People Giving Birth at Home and In Birth Centers." Press Release. Accessed May 3, 2024. https://nationalpartnership.org/news_post/more-people-giving-birth-at-home-html/#:~:text=Press%20Release,Black%2C%20Indigenous%20and%20Hispanic%20communities.

National Quality Forum. 2006. "Standardizing a Patient Safety Taxonomy." Washington, DC. Accessed September 23, 2022. https://psnet.ahrq.gov/issue/standardizing-patient-safety-taxonomy.

Nwosu, Arinze D. G., Edmund Ossai, Francis Ahaotu, Okechukwu Onwuasoigwe, Adaobi Amucheazi, and Irene Akhideno. 2022. "Patient Safety Culture in the Operating Room: A Cross-Sectional Study Using the Hospital Survey on Patient Safety Culture (HSOPSC) Instrument." *BMC Health Services Research* 22(1): 1445.

Office of Civil Rights. 2020. "Filing a Civil Rights Complaint." Accessed August 22, 2024. https://www.hhs.gov/civil-rights/filing-a-complaint/index.html.

Office of Policy Planning and Research, United States, Department of Labor. 1965. "The Negro Family: The Case for National Action." Stanford University. Accessed August 19, 2024. https://web.stanford.edu/~mrosenfe/Moynihan's%20The%20Negro%20Family.pdf.

Offices of U.S. Congressman Gregory F. Murphy, MD. 2024. "Murphy Introduces Bill to Ban DEI in Medicine." March 19, 2024. Accessed March 19, 2024. https://murphy.house.gov/media/press-releases/murphy-introduces-bill-ban-dei-medicine.

Okwandu, Ijeoma C., Meredith Anderson, Debbie Postlethwaite, Aida Shirazi, and Sandra Torrente. 2022. "Racial and Ethnic Disparities in Cesarean Delivery and Indications Among Nulliparous, Term, Singleton, Vertex Women." *Journal of Racial and Ethnic Health Disparities* 9(4): 1161–1171. Epub July 12, 2021. https://doi.org10.1007/s40615-021-01057-w.

Oluo, Ijeoma. 2019. *So You Want to Talk About Race*. London: Hachette UK.

O'Mahony, Seamus. 2016. "Medical Nemesis 40 Years on: The Enduring Legacy of Ivan Illich." *Journal of the Royal College of Physicians of Edinburgh* 46(2): 134–139.

Oparah, Julia Chinyere, and Alicia D. Bonaparte. 2015. *Birthing Justice: Black Women, Pregnancy, and Childbirth.* New York, NY: Routledge Taylor & Francis Group.

Oparah, Julia Chinyere, Helen Arega, Dantia Hudson, Linda Jones, and Talita Oseguera. 2017. "Of Black Women Birthing Justice." In *Battling Over Birth: Black Women and the Maternal Health Care Crisis*. Amarillo, TX: Praeclarus Press.

Opara, Ijeoma, Jasmine A. Abrams, Kristina Cross, and Ndidiamaka Amutah-Onukagha. 2021. "Reframing Sexual Health for Black Girls and Women in HIV/STI Prevention Work: Highlighting the Role of Identity and Interpersonal Relationships." *International Journal of Environmental Research and Public Health* 18(22): 12088.

Oregon Health & Science University. n.d. "A Brief History of Midwifery in America." Accessed August 4, 2024.

Osler, William. 1910. *Aequanimitas: With Other Addresses to Medical Students, Nurses and Practitioners of Medicine*. Philadelphia, PA: P. Blakiston's Son & Company.

Oyebode, F. 2013. "Clinical Errors and Medical Negligence." *Medical Principles and Practice* 22(4): 323–333.

Park, Shelley M. 2019. "Queering and Querying Motherhood." In *The Routledge Companion to Motherhood*, Lynn O'Brien Hallstein, Andrea O'Reilly, and Melinda Giles (eds.), pp. 63–76. London: Routledge.

Peer, Rafia Farooq, and Nadeem Shabir. 2018. "Iatrogenesis: A Review on Nature, Extent, and Distribution of Healthcare Hazards." *Journal of Family Medicine and Primary Care* 7(2): 309–314.

Penner, Louis A., John F. Dovidio, Tessa V. West, Samuel L. Gaertner, Terrance L. Albrecht, Rhonda K. Dailey, and Tsveti Markova. 2010. "Aversive Racism and Medical Interactions with Black Patients: A Field Study." *Journal of Experimental Social Psychology* 46(2): 436–440.

Pennycoke, Makeda. n.d. "The Power of Sisterhood." Maked Pennycoke. Accessed May 3, 2024. https://makedapennycooke.com/the-power-of-sisterhood/.

Pimentel, Marc Philip T., Stephanie Choi, Karen Fiumara, Allen Kachalia, and Richard D. Urman. 2021. "Safety Culture in the Operating Room: Variability Among Perioperative Healthcare Workers." *Journal of Patient Safety* 17(6): 412–416.

Poehlmann, John R., Gabrielle Avery, Kathleen M. Antony, Aimee Teo Broman, Amy Godecker, and Tiffany L. Green. 2022. "Racial Disparities in Post-Operative Pain Experience and Treatment Following Cesarean Birth." *The Journal of Maternal-Fetal & Neonatal Medicine* 35(26): 10305–10313. https://www.ohsu.edu/womens-health/brief-history-midwifery-america.

Pronovost, Peter J., Christine G. Holzmueller, Christopher S. Ennen, and Harold E. Fox. 2011. "Overview of Progress in Patient Safety." *American Journal of Obstetrics and Gynecology* 204(1): 5–10.

Putnam, Robert D. 1995. "Bowling Alone: America's Declining Social Capital." *Journal of Democracy* 6: 65–78.

Richard, Claude, Yvette Lajeunesse, and Marie-Thérèse Lussier. 2010. "Therapeutic Privilege: Between the Ethics of Lying and the Practice of Truth." *Journal of Medical Ethics* 36(6): 353–357.

Rich-Edwards, Janet, Nancy Krieger, Joseph Majzoub, Sally Zierler, Ellice Lieberman, and Matthew Gillman. 2001. "Maternal Experiences of Racism and Violence as Predictors of Preterm Birth: Rationale and Study Design." *Paediatric & Perinatal Epidemiology* 15(supp 2): 124–135. https://doi.org/10.1046/j.1365-3016.2001.00013.x.

Robbins, Liz. 2011. "Billboard Opposing Abortion Stirs Debate." New York Times City Room. February 23, 2011. Accessed August 15, 2024. https://archive.nytimes.com/cityroom.blogs.nytimes.com/2011/02/23/billboard-opposing-abortion-stirs-debate/.

Roberts, Dorothy. 1997. *Killing the Black Body: Race, Reproduction, and the Meaning of Liberty*. New York, NY: Random House/Pantheon, Vintage 20th Anniversary Edition, 2017.

Roberts, Dorothy. 2011. *Fatal Invention: How Science, Politics, and Big Business Re-create Race in the Twenty-First Century*. New York, NY: New Press/ORIM.

Roberts, Dorothy. 2012. "Prison, Foster Care, and the Systemic Punishment of Black Mothers." *UCLA Law Review* 59: 1474–1500.

Roberts, Dorothy. 2022. *Torn Apart: How the Child Welfare System Destroys Black Families--and How Abolition Can Build a Safer World.* New York, NY: Basic Books.

Rodziewicz, T. L., Benjamin Houseman, Sarosh Vaqar, and John E. Hipskind. 2024. "Medical Error Reduction and Prevention." [Updated 2024 Feb 12]. In StatPearls [Internet]. Treasure Island (FL): StatPearls Publishing; 2024 Jan-. Available from: https://www.ncbi.nlm.nih.gov/books/NBK499956/.

Rönnerhag, Maria. 2020. "Safe Maternity Care: The Perspectives of Childbearing Women and Healthcare Professionals." PhD diss, University of South-Eastern Norway. Accessed August 17, 2024. https://openarchive.usn.no/usn-xmlui/bitstream/handle/11250/2638979/PhD%20Thesis%20R%c3%b6nnerhag.pdf?sequence=8&isAllowed=y.

Ross, Loretta, Erika Derkas, Whitney Peoples, Lynn Roberts, and Pamela Bridgewater, eds. 2017. *Radical Reproductive Justice: Foundation, Theory, Practice, Critique.* New York, NY: Feminist Press at CUNY.

Ross, Loretta, and Rickie Solinger. 2017. *Reproductive Justice: An Introduction.* Vol. 1. Oakland, CA: University of California Press.

Rothman, Barbara Katz. 2007. "Laboring Then: The Political History of Maternity Care in the United States." In *Laboring on: Birth in transition in the United States*, W. Simonds, B. K. Rothman, and B. M. Norman (eds.), pp. 3–28. New York, NY: Routledge.

Sadler, Michelle, Mário J. D. S. Santos, Dolores Ruiz-Berdún, Gonzalo Leiva Rojas, Elena Skoko, Patricia Gillen, and Jette A. Clausen. 2016. "Moving Beyond Disrespect and Abuse: Addressing the Structural Dimensions of Obstetric Violence." *Reproductive Health Matters* 24(47): 47–55. https://doi.org/10.1016/j.rhm.2016.04.002.

Say, Lale, João Paulo Souza, Robert C. Pattinson, and World Health Organization (WHO) Working Group on Maternal Mortality and Morbidity Classifications. 2009. "Maternal Near Miss–Towards a Standard Tool for Monitoring Quality of Maternal Health Care." *Best Practice & Research Clinical Obstetrics & Gynaecology* 23(3): 287–296. https://doi.org/10.1016/j.bpobgyn.2009.01.007.

Schiller, Rebecca. 2016. "Dignity in Childbirth Is a Human Right." *J Fam Health* Mar-Apr;26(2): 14–16.

Schneider, Eric C., M. Susan Ridgely, Denise D. Quigley, Lauren E. Hunter, Kristin J. Leuschner, RAND Health, Saul N. Weingart, Joel S. Weissman, Karen P. Zimmer, and Robert C. Giannini. 2016. "Developing and Testing the Health Care Safety Hotline: A Prototype Consumer Reporting System for Patient Safety Events." Accessed August 22, 2024. https://www.ahrq.gov/patient-safety/reports/hotline.html.

Scott, Karen A. 2018. "A SACRED Birth Model of Care for Obstetric Quality Improvement." Black Maternal Health Week Black Mammas Matter Alliance. Online Presentation.

Scott, Karen A. 2019a. "Redesigning Perinatal Quality Improvement: Community Driven Measures, Meanings, and Methods." Brooklyn Grows Blog. November 3, 2019. Accessed July 28, 2024. https://brooklyngrows.squarespace.com/blog/2019

/11/3/redesigning-perinatal-quality-improvement-community-driven-measures-meanings-and-methodsnbsp.

Scott, Karen. 2019b. "Advancing Racial Equity: A Hospital-Based Birth Equity Quality Improvement Initiative." Invited Podium Presentation at Pennsylvania Convention Center, American Public Health Association Annal Meeting and Expor, Philadelphia, November 5, 2019.

Scott, Karen A. 2021. "The Rise of Black Feminist Intellectual Thought and Political Activism in Perinatal Quality Improvement: A Righteous Rage About Racism, Resistance, Resilience, and Rigor." *Feminist Anthropology* 2(1): 155–160. https://doi.org/10.1002/fea2.12045.

Scott, Karen A. 2023. "Advancing Community-led Accountability and Transformation in Research and Data Sovereignty." Black Maternal Health Data + Innovation Black Maternal Health Week Virtual "Popcorn" Presentation. Black Mamas Matter Alliance.

Scott, Karen A., Brittany D. Chambers, Rebecca J. Baer, Kelli R. Ryckman, Monica R. McLemore, and Laura L. Jelliff-Pawlowski. 2020. "Preterm Birth and Nativity Among Black Women with Gestational Diabetes in California, 2013–2017: A Population-Based Retrospective Cohort Study." *BMC Pregnancy and Childbirth* 20, no. 593. https://doi.org/10.1186/s12884-020-03290-3.

Scott, Karen A., Brittany D. Chambers, S. McKenzie-Sampson, TaNefer L. Camara, Emily W. VanGompel, Dána-Ain Davis, and Audrey Lyndon. 2021. "The Virtual Perinatal Quality Improvement Prioritization by Affected Communities (V-QPAC) Protocol." *Health Services Research* 56: 56–57.

Scott, Karen A., and Dána-Ain Davis. 2021. "Obstetric Racism: Naming and Identifying a Way Out of Black Women's Adverse Medical Experiences." *American Anthropologist* 123(3): 681–684. https://doi.org/10.1111/aman.13559.

Scott, Karen A., and Dána-Ain Davis. 2022. "Destigmatizing and Democratizing Postpartum Care: A 'Black Woman-Person First' Approach." *Clinical Obstetrics and Gynecology* 65(3): 663–675.

Scott, Karen A., and Indra Lusero. 2023. "The First Tool to Name Obstetric Racism Might Finally Push Policymakers Into Action." Ms. Magazine. October 14, 2023. Accessed August 11, 2024. https://msmagazine.com/2023/10/04/obstetric-racism-black-women-childbirth-maternal-health-discrimination/.

Scott, Karen A., Laura Britton, and Monica R. McLemore. 2019. "The Ethics of Perinatal Care for Black Women: Dismantling the Structural Racism in 'Mother Blame' Narratives." *The Journal of Perinatal & Neonatal Nursing* 33(2): 108–115.

Scott, Karen A., Stephanie Bray, and Monica R. McLemore. 2020. "First, Do No Harm: Why Philanthropy Needs to Re-examine Its Role in Reproductive Equity and Racial Justice." *Health Equity* 4(1): 17–22.

Shachar, Carmel, Tess Wise, Gali Katznelson, and Andrea Louise Campbell. 2020. "Criminal Justice or Public Health: A Comparison of the Representation of the Crack Cocaine and Opioid Epidemics in the Media." *Journal of Health Politics, Policy and Law* 45(2): 211–239.

Shaikh, Ulfat. 2020. "Improving Patient Safety and Team Communication through Daily Huddles." Patient Safety Network (PSNet). Rockville, MD: Agency for Healthcare Research and Quality (AHRQ), US Department of Health and Human Services. January 20, 2020. Accessed May 2, 2024. https://psnet.ahrq.gov/primer/improving-patient-safety-and-team-communication-through-daily-huddles.

Sharp, Lesley A. 2000. "The Commodification of the Body and Its Parts." *Annual Review of Anthropology* 29(1): 287–328.

Shoemaker, Nancy. 2015. "A Typology of Colonialism." *Perspectives on History* 53(7): 29–30. Accessed May 8, 2024. https://www.historians.org/perspectives-article/a-typology-of-colonialism-october-2015/.

Shorter-Gooden, Kumea, and Leslie C. Jackson. 2000. *The Interweaving of Cultural and Intrapsychic Issues in the Therapeutic Relationship*. New York, NY: The Guilford Press.

Simms, Rupe. 2001. "Controlling Images and the Gender Construction of Enslaved African Women." *Gender & Society* 15(6): 879–897.

Singh, S., G. K. Shakti, S. Arya, D. K. Sharma, and V. Aggarwal. 2015. "Adverse Drug Reaction Policy in a Tertiary Care Hospital." *International Journal of Research Foundation of Hospital And Healthcare Administration* 3: 41–47.

SisterSong. n.d. "SisterSong: About Us." Accessed August 16, 2024. https://www.sistersong.net/about-x2.

Smith, Richard. 2003. "Limits to Medicine. Medical Nemesis: The Expropriation of Health." *Journal of Epidemiology & Community Health* 57(12): 928–928.

Snipe, Margo. 2022. "Clinicians Dismiss Black Women's Pain. The Consequences Are Dire." Capital B News. Accessed April 5, 2024. https://capitalbnews.org/black-women-pain/.

Snively, Elizabeth. 2022. "Six Domains of Health Care Quality – New Considerations." Relias blog. November 15, 2022. Accessed April 2, 2024. https://www.relias.com/blog/six-domains-of-health-care-quality-new-considerations.

Sokol, Daniel. 2007. "Aequanimitas." *The British Medical Journal* 335(7628): 1049. https://doi.org/10.1136/bmj.39385.642315.FA.

Somer, Sarah J. Holdt, Rachel G. Sinkey, and Allison S. Bryant. 2017. "Epidemiology of Racial/Ethnic Disparities in Severe Maternal Morbidity and Mortality." *Seminars in Perinatology* 41(5): 258–265.

Starfield, Barbara. 20111. "Is Patient-Centered Care the Same as Person-Focused Care?" The *Permanente Journal* 15: 63–69.

Stephen Ekpenyong, Mandu, Mathew Nyashanu, Chioma Ossey-Nweze, and Laura Serrant. 2021. "Exploring the Perceptions of Dignity Among Patients and Nurses in Hospital and Community Settings: An Integrative Review." *Journal of Research in Nursing* 26(3): 517–537.

Suarez, Alicia. 2020. "Black Midwifery in the United States: Past, present, and Future." *Sociology Compass* 14(11): 1–12.

Sue, Derald Wing, and Lisa Spanierman. 2020. *Microaggressions in Everyday Life*. Hoboken, NJ: John Wiley & Sons.

Thomas, Anita Jones, Karen McCurtis Witherspoon, and Suzette L. Speight. 2004. "Toward the Development of the Stereotypic Roles for Black Women Scale." *Journal of Black Psychology* 30(3): 426–442.

Thomasson, Melissa A., and Jaret Treber. 2008. "From Home to Hospital: The Evolution of Childbirth in the United States, 1928–1940." *Explorations in Economic History* 45(1): 76–99.

Tillis, Tiffany Vanese. 2017. "When and Where I Enter: A Phenomenological Study of Black Women at a Selective Predominantly White Institution." PhD diss., University of Chicago. ProQuest (13865986).

Todd, Knox H., Christi Deaton, Anne P. D'Adamo, and Leon Goe. 2000. "Ethnicity and Analgesic Practice." *Annals of Emergency Medicine* 35(1): 11–16. https://doi.org/10.1016/s0196-0644(00)70099-0-.

Toufeeq, M., M. V. R. M. Kodali, S. Gunturu, K. Kumar, and K. Surapaneni. 2019. "Bilateral Dislocation of Mandibular Condyles Following General Anesthesia–An Overlooked Problem: A Case Report." *European Journal of Dentistry* 13(2): 291–293.

Trost, S. L., J. Beauregard, F. Njie, et al. 2022. "Pregnancy-Related Deaths: Data From Maternal Mortality Review Committees in 36 US States, 2017–2019." Centers for Disease Control and Prevention (CDC), US Department of Health and Human Services. Accessed May 8, 2024. https://www.cdc.gov/maternal-mortality/php/data-research/mmrc-2017-2019.html#cdc_research_or_data_summary_suggested_citation-suggested-citation.

Trust Black Women. n.d. "Trust Black Women: Our Roots." Accessed August 16, 2024. https://trustblackwomen.org/our-roots.

United States Census Bureau. 2020. "2019 Population Estimates by Age, Sex, Race and Hispanic Origin." Accessed May 8, 2024. https://www.census.gov/newsroom/press-kits/2020/population-estimates-detailed.html.

University of California-San Francisco (UCSF). n.d. "SACRED Birth During COVID-19." Accessed August 20, 2024. https://sacredbirth.ucsf.edu/.

University of California San Francisco (UCSF) Benioff Children's Hospitals (BCH). n.d. "Anti-Racism." Accessed August 5, 2024. https://diversitybch.ucsf.edu/bch-anti-racism.

Unknown Author. 2024. "Black Maternal Health Week 2024: U.S. News Recognizes U.S. Hospitals with Excellent Black Patient Outcomes." *US News and World* Report, April 11, 2024. Accessed May 7, 2024. https://www.usnews.com/info/blogs/press-room/articles/2024-04-11/black-maternal-health-week-2024-u-s-news-recognizes-u-s-hospitals-with-excellent-black-patient-outcomes.

U.S. Government Accountability Office. 2023. "Midwives: Information on Births, Workforce, and Midwifery Education." GAO-23-105861. Published April 26, 2023. Released May 8, 2023. Accessed August 21, 2024. https://www.gao.gov/products/gao-23-105861#:~:text=Midwives%20provide%20care%20during%20pregnancy,can%20provide%20varies%20by%20state.

Valencia, Zehra, Aditi Sen, and Katie Martin. 2023. "NICU Admissions and Spending Increased Slightly from 2017–2021." Health Care Costs Institute. July 25,

2023. Accessed May 7, 2024. https://healthcostinstitute.org/hcci-originals-dropdown/all-hcci-reports/nicu-use-and-spending-1.

Van der Waal, Rodante, Veronica Mitchell, Inge van Nistelrooij, and Vivienne Bozalek. 2021. "Obstetric Violence within Students' Rite of Passage: The Reproduction of the Obstetric Subject and Its Racialised (M)other." *Agenda (Durban)* 35(3): 36–53.

Vedam, Saraswathi, Kathrin Stoll, Tanya Khemet Taiwo, Nicholas Rubashkin, Melissa Cheyney, Nan Strauss, Monica McLemore, Micaela Cadena, Elizabeth Nethery, Eleanor Rushton, et al. 2019. "The Giving Voice to Mothers Study: Inequity and Mistreatment During Pregnancy and Childbirth in the United States." *Reproductive Health* 16: 1–18.

Vollers, Anna Claire. 2023. "The Hidden History of What Happened to Thousands of Black Midwives in the South." Reckon, February 24, 2023. Accessed May 8, 2024. https://www.reckon.news/family/2023/02/the-hidden-history-of-what-happened-to-thousands-of-black-midwvies-in-the-south.html.

Washington, Harriet A. 2006. *Medical Apartheid: The Dark History of Medical Experimentation on Black Americans from Colonial Times to the Present.* New York: Books.

Weinbaum, Alys Eve. 2019. *The Afterlife of Reproductive Slavery: Biocapitalism and Black Feminism's Philosophy of History.* Durham: Duke University Press.

Wertz, Richard W., and Dorothy C. Wertz. 1989. *Lying-in: A History of Childbirth in America.* New Haven, CT: Yale University Press.

West, C. 2012. "Mammy, Jezebel, Sapphire, and Their Homegirls: Developing an 'Oppositional Gaze' Toward the Images of Black Women." In *Lectures on the Psychology of Women,* J. C. Chrisler, C. Golden, and P. D. Rozee (eds.), 4th ed., pp. 286–299. Long Grove, IL: Waveland Press, Inc. (Original work published 2008).

Whitehead, Margaret. 1992. "The -Concepts and Principles of Equity and Health." *International Journal of Health Services* 22(3): 429–445.

White VanGompel, Emily, Jin-Shei Lai, Dána-Ain Davis, Francesca Carlock, Tamentanefer L. Camara, Brianne Taylor, Chakiya Clary, Ashlee M. McCorkle-Jamieson, Safyer McKenzie-Sampson, et al. 2022. "Psychometric Validation of a Patient-Reported Experience Measure of Obstetric Racism© (The PREM-OB Scale™ suite)." *Birth (Berkeley, Calif.)* 49(3): 514–525. https://doi.org/10.1111/birt.12622.

WHO. 1969. International Drug, Monitoring: The Role of the Hospital. Technical Report Series No. 425. Geneva: WHO. Accessed May, 2004. https://iris.who.int/bitstream/handle/10665/40747/WHO%20TRS%20425.pdf?sequence=1.

WHO. 1972. "Technical Report No. 498: International Drug Monitoring: The Role of National Centres." Geneva: WHO. Accessed May 4, 2024. https://who-umc.org/media/2680/who-technical-report-498.pdf.

WHO. 2009. Patient Safety. The Conceptual Framework for the International Classification for Patient Safety Version 1.1 Final Technical Report. Accessed May 2, 2024. https://iris.who.int/bitstream/handle/10665/70882/WHO_IER_PSP_2010.2_eng.pdf?sequence=1.

WHO. 2011. Working Group on Maternal Mortality and Morbidity Classifications and the WHO Multicountry Survey on Maternal and Newborn Health Research Group. "The WHO Near-Miss Approach for Maternal Health." Accessed August 3, 2024. https://iris.who.int/bitstream/handle/10665/44692/9789241502221_eng.pdf.

Wiegman, Robyn. 1995. *American Ānatomies: Theorizing Race and Gender*. Durham: Duke University Press.

Wilkie, L. A. 2003. *The Archaeology of Mothering: An African-American Midwife's Tale*. New York, NY: Routledge.

Wyatt, Gail Elizabeth. 1997. *Stolen Women: Reclaiming Our Sexuality, Taking Back Our Lives*. New York, NY: John Wiley.

Yancy, George. 2016a. *Black Bodies, White Gazes: The Continuing Significance of Race in America*. Lanham and Plymouth: Rowman & Littlefield, 2016.

Yancy, George. 2016b. "White Embodied Gazing, the Black Body as Disgust, and the Aesthetics of Un-Suturing." In *Body Aesthetics*, Sherri Irvin (ed.). Oxford, 2016; online edn, Oxford Academic. Accessed August 8, 2024. https://doi.org/10.1093/acprof:oso/9780198716778.003.0014.

Zinn Education Project. n.d. "Dec. 17, 1951: "We Charge Genocide" Petition Submitted to United Nations." Accessed May 8, 2024. https://www.zinnedproject.org/news/tdih/we_charge_genocide_petition.

Zorn, Theodore E., Juliet Roper, Kirsten Broadfoot, and C. Kay Weaver. 2006. "Focus groups as Sites of Influential Interaction: Building Communicative Self-Efficacy and Effecting Attitudinal Change in Discussing Controversial Topics." *Journal of Applied Communication Research* 34(2): 115–140.

Index

About the Author

Karen Antoinette Scott, MD, MPH, FACOG, is an improvement and implementation scientist activist, community OBGYN, and applied epidemiologist currently serving as the Chief Black Feminist Physician Scientist, CEO, and Owner of Birthing Cultural Rigor, LLC. She is the author of a self-titled chapter in *Thinking About Quitting Medicine?* and a contributing author to "Accountability for Obstetric Violence and Obstetric Racism: New Pathways for Families Seeking Justice" in *The Routledge Companion to Gender and Reproduction.*